Biochemistry of Exercise

Medicine and Sport

Vol. 3

Editor: E. JOKL, Lexington, Ky.

Advisory Board: P. O. ÅSTRAND, Sweden; ROGER BANNISTER, England; P. BECKMANN, Germany; H. N. BLEASDALE, England; D. BRUNNER, Israel; A. CARLSTEN, Sweden; G. LA CAVA, Italy; R. DIETRICH, German Democratic Republic; A. DIRIX, Belgium; F. N. DUKES-DOBOS, Switzerland; B. EISEMAN, United States; J. FERRER-HOMBRAVELLA, Spain; S. FIRSOV, Soviet Union; E. GADERMANN, Germany; A. GALLEGO, Spain; E. GEBHARDT, Germany; L. GEDDA, Italy; A. M. GEISSA, United Arab Republic; L. GUTTMANN, England; M. HALHUBER, Germany; K. HÄNTZSCHEL, German Democratic Republic; E. HAY, Mexico; W. HOLLMANN, Germany; M. IKAI, Japan; S. ISRAEL, German Democratic Republic; F. JANDA, Czechoslovakia; E. JOKL, United States; P. JOKL, United States; M. KARVONEN, Finland; E. J. KLAUS, Germany; A. V. KOROBKOV, Soviet Union; J. KRAL, Czechoslovakia; H. KRAUS, United States; F. KREUZER, Holland; K. LANGE ANDERSEN, Norway; S. P. LETUNOV, Soviet Union; R. MARGARIA, Italy; H. MELLEROWICZ, Germany; A. METZNER, Germany; N. NEMESSURI, Hungary; J. PARIZKOVA, Czechoslovakia; F. PLAS, France; L. PROKOP, Austria; L. G. C. E. PUGH, England; W. RAAB, United States; H. REINDELL, Germany; H. ROSKAMM, Germany; BENGT SALTIN, Sweden; G. SCHOENHOLZER, Switzerland; E. SIMON, Israel; M. STEINBACH, Germany; E. STRAUSZENBERG, German Democratic Republic; K. TITTEL, German Democratic Republic; F. ULMEANO, Rumania; A. VENERANDO, Italy; N. K. ZIMKIN, Soviet Union.

Published for and on behalf of Research Committee
International Council of Sport and Physical Education
UNESCO

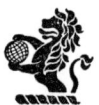

University Park Press, Baltimore, Maryland and Manchester, England

Biochemistry of Exercise

Proceedings of the first International Symposium on Exercise Biochemistry, Brussels 1968

Edited by J. R. POORTMANS
Chef de Travaux at the Laboratoire de l'Effort,
Université Libre de Bruxelles, Brussels (Belgium)

Organization Committee: M. SEGERS, J. R. POORTMANS, L. LEWILLIE, V. CONARD, H. DENOLIN, J. FRANCKSON, M. HEBBELINCK, J. S'JONGERS from the Laboratoire de l'Effort and the Faculty of Medicine of the Université Libre de Bruxelles, Brussels (Belgium)

With 127 figures and 83 tables

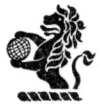

University Park Press, Baltimore, Maryland and Manchester, England

Originally published by S. Karger AG, Basel, Switzerland
Distributed exclusively in the United States of America and Canada by
University Park Press, Baltimore, Maryland and Manchester, England

Library of Congress Catalog Card Number 71–92729
Standard Book Number (SBN) 8391–0027–2

S. Karger AG, Arnold-Böcklin-Strasse 25, 4000 Basel 11 (Switzerland)

All rights, including that of translation into foreign languages, reserved. Photomechanic reproduction (photocopy, microcopy) of this book or part of it without special permission of the publishers is prohibited.

© Copyright 1968 by S. Karger AG, Basel
Printed in Switzerland by Buchdruckerei National-Zeitung AG, Basel
Blocks by Aberegg-Steiner & Cie. AG, Bern

Table of Contents

Preface IX

Acknowledgements X

I. Blood Gases and Metabolites in Acid-Base Chemistry

SCHERRER, M. (Berne): Acid-Base Imbalance and Gas Exchange During Heavy Work 2

COSTER, A. DE; DENOLIN, H.; MESSIN, R.; DEGRE, S. and VANDERMOTEN, P. (Brussels): Role of the Metabolites in the Acid-Base Balance During Exercise 15

DOLL, E. and KEUL, J. (Freiburg i. Br.): pO_2, pH, and pCO_2 in the Coronarvenous and Femoralvenous Blood During Exercise and Hypoxia 35

KEUL, J. and DOLL, E. (Freiburg i. Br.): The Influence of Exercise and Hypoxia on the Substrate Uptake of Human Heart and Human Skeletal Muscles 41

SHEPHARD, R. J. (Toronto): Oscillations of Acid-Base Equilibrium During Maximum Exercise 47

BANISTER, E. W. (Burnaby): The Potentiating Effect of Low Oxygen Tension Exposure on Acid-Base Balance During Exhaustive Work in Humans 52

AGNEVIK, G.; KARLSSON, J.; DIAMANT, B. and SALTIN, B. (Stockholm): Oxygen Dept, Lactate in Blood and Muscle Tissue During Maximal Exercise in Man 62

HARTLEY, L. H. and SALTIN, B. (Stockholm): Blood Gas Tensions and pH in Brachial Artery, Femoral Vein, and Brachial Vein During Maximal Exercise 66

CURETON, T. K. (Illinois): The Relative Value of Stress Indicators, Related to Prediction of Strenuous Athletic (Treadmill) Performance 73

HOLLMANN, W. and KASTNER, K. (Köln): The Behaviour of Arterial Blood Gases, Arterial Substrates, pH and Haematocrit in Different Ergometric Work 81

VANROUX, R. (Charleroi): L'acidose métabolique au cours de l'effort musculaire 89

TOPI, G. C.; GANDOLFO D'ALESSANDRO, L. et PIOVANO, G. (Roma): Quelques modifications hématochimiques causées par le travail musculaire chez des sujets d'âge moyen 96

II. Carbohydrate and Lipid Metabolisms

FRÖBERG, S. O. (Stockholm): Metabolism of Lipids in Blood and Tissues during Exercise 100

CONARD, V.; BRUNNENGRABER, H.; VANROUX, R.; DESCHAEPDRIJVER, A.; MOERMANS, E. and FRANCKSON, J. R. M. (Brussels): Influence of Muscular Exercise on Glucose Regulation 114
MORGAN, T. E.; SHORT, F. A. and COBB, L. A. (Seattle, Wash.): Alterations in Human Skeletal Muscle Lipid Composition and Metabolism Induced by Physical Conditioning 116
SHORT, F. A.; COBB, L. A. and MORGAN, T. E. (Seattle, Wash.): Influence of Exercise Training on *In Vitro* Metabolism of Glucose and Fatty Acid by Human Skeletal Muscle 122
SPITZER, J. J. (Philadelphia, Pa.): Oxidation of Free Fatty Acids by Skeletal Muscle During Rest, Electrical Stimulation and Administration of 2,4-dinitrophenol. 128
KEPPLER, D.; KEUL, J. and DOLL, E. (Freiburg i. Br.): The Influence of the Form of Exercise on the Arterial Concentrations of Glucose, Lactate, Pyruvate, and Free Fatty Acids 132
PAŘÍZKOVÁ, J. (Prague): The Effect of Age and Various Motor Activity on Fat Content, Lipoproteinase Activity and Experimental Necrosis in the Rat Heart. 137
KOSIEK, J.-P.; KERSTING, U.; KÜSTERS, F. and KLAUS, E. J. (Münster): Comparative Investigations on the Daily Rhythm of Blood Glucose after Rest, after Exhaustive Interval Exercise, and after Exhaustive Continuous Exercise. 144
DOLEŽEL, J. (Olomouc): The Effect of Two Types of Physical Strain During Summer and Winter on Cholesterolemia in Young People 148
JIRKA, Z. and DOLEŽEL, J. (Olomouc): Changes in Cholesterol Serum Levels after Spiroergometric Examinations in Children 152
MOSKWA, J. (Warsaw): Repeated Determination of Glucose Concentration in the Synovial Fluid in Haemorrhages into the Knee Joint 156
OLSSON, K. E. and SALTIN, B. (Stockholm): Variation in Total Body Water with Muscle Glycogen Changes in Man. 159
MARMO, E. and MATERA, A. (Naples): Inhibition of the Depletion of Diaphragmatic and Cardiac Glycogen by one β-adrenolytic Drugs in Mus Musculus Subjected to Swimming Stress 163

III. Hormones

EULER, U. S. VON (Stockholm): Sympatho-Adrenal Activity and Physical Exercise. 170
NAYER, PH. DE; OSTYN, M. and VISSCHER, M. DE (Louvain): Influence of Exercise on Serum Free Thyroxine and Binding Proteins 182
BECKER, E. J. and KREUZER, F. (Nijmegen): Sympathoadrenal Response to Hypoxia 188
TIPTON, C. M.; SANDAGE, D. S. and MERGNER, W. (Iowa City, Iowa): Influence of Anterior Pituitary Hormones and Physical Activity Levels on Intact and Repaired Knee Ligaments of Hypophysectomized Rats 192
WRIGHT, P. H. and MALAISSE, W. J. (Brussels): Inhibition of Insulin Secretion During Exercise 199
SCHAEPDRYVER, A. DE and HEBBELINCK, M. (Brussels): Ergometric Exercise and Urinary Excretion of Noradrenaline, Adrenaline, Dopamine, Homovanillic and Vanilmandelic Acid 202
NOWACKI, P.; SCHMID, E. and WEIST, F. (Lübeck): The Turnover of Sympathico-Adrenal Hormones of Sportsmen in Training, Anticipation

Table of Contents

and During Competition, Judged by Measurements of the Urinary Excretion of 3-methoxy-4-hydroxy-mandelic Acid 205
GEROLA, A.; DRINGOLI, R.; RAVAIOLI, P. and ORSUCCI, P. L. (Siena): Adrenosympathetic Activation and NEFA Metabolism 209

IV. Enzymes

SCHMIDT, E. and SCHMIDT, F. W. (Hannover): Enzyme Modifications During Activity 216
GOLLNICK, P. D. and KING, D. W. (Pullman, Wash.): The Immediate and Chronic Effect of Exercise on the Number and Structure of Skeletal Muscle Mitochondria 239
YAKOVLEV, N. N. (Leningrad): L'influence du travail musculaire systématique sur l'activité des ferments du métabolisme du glycogène et de G-6-P dans les muscles et dans le foie 245
BÖHMER, D. (Frankfurt/Main): Enzymatic Activity in Normal, Trained and Inactivated Muscle 249
NOVOSADOVÁ, J. (Olomouc): Lactic Dehydrogenase Isoenzymes in Serum and Tissues after Exercise in Rats 254
BLOCK, P.; RIJMENANT, M. VAN; BADJOU, R.; MELSEM, A. Y. VAN and VOGELEER, R. (Brussels): The Effects of Exhaustive Effort on Serum Enzymes in Man 259
ŁUKASIK, S. and BUŁA, B. (Wrocław): Studies on the Influence of the Diminished Atmospheric Pressure on some Enzymes. Part I. Serum activity of aldolase (ALD), phospho-hexose isomerase (PHI), glutamic-oxalacetic transaminase (GOT), glutamic-pyruvic transaminase (GPT) and alkaline phosphatase (alk. P) in athletes exercising in a low-pressure chamber 268
ŁUKASIK, S. and BUŁA, B. (Wracław): Studies on the Influence of the Diminished Atmospheric Pressure on some Enzymes. Part II. The activity of aldolase (ALD), phospho-hexose isomerase (PHI), glutamic-oxalacetic transaminase (GOT) and glutamic-pyruvic transaminase (GPT) in serum and tissues of rabbits kept intermittently in a low-pressure chamber . . . 271
DRINGOLI, R.; RAVAIOLI, P.; ORSUCCI, P. L. and CIAMPOLINI, E. (Siena): Amylasic Activity of the Blood During Physical Exercise 274
TOPI, G. C.; GANDOLFO D'ALESSANDRO, L. et PIOVANO, G. (Roma): Modification enzymoplasmatiques causées par le travail musculaire chez des sujets d'âge moyen 280

V. Electrolytes

ROUGIER, G. et BABIN, J. P. (Bordeaux): Modifications des électrolytes au cours des activités physiques 284
KRÁL, J. A.; KOPECKÁ, J. and ŽENÍŠEK, A. (Prague): Difference in the Quantity and Concentration of Sweat Produced on the Same Place of the Forearm 294
MITOLO, M. † and LEONE, D. (Bari): Potassium and Physical Exercise . . 297
METIVIER, G. (Ottawa): Enzymatic and Ionic Changes in Man Associated with Physical Work 301

VI. Proteins in Biological Fluids

POORTMANS, J. R. (Brussels): Influence of Physical Exercise on Proteins in Biological Fluids 312

HARALAMBIE, G. et JEFLEA, G. (Bucarest): Tableau biochimique sérique chez la femme sportive 328
LILJEFORS, I.; PISCATOR, M. and RISINGER, C. (Uppsala): Exercise Proteinuria in Monozygotic and Dizygotic Twins 333
SEGERS, M.; POORTMANS, J. R.; s'JONGERS, J. et SEGERS, A. (Bruxelles): Etude qualitative de la protéinurie intermittente au repos et après effort modéré 340
MALOMSOKI, J. (Budapest): The Significance of Polarographic Pattern Changes in the Protein Double Waves of Sportsmen 343
ULMEANU, F. C.; PARTHENIU, A. et HARALAMBIE, G. (Bucarest): Rapports entre la variation de la tyrosinémie et certaines modifications de l'excitabilité neuromusculaire, déterminées par un effort dosé chez les sportifs . . 347
DELFORGE, E.; DELFORGE, B. and POORTMANS, J. R. (Brussels): Influence of Increasing Activity on the Protein Level in Serum, Urine and Sweat . 353
VANFRAECHEM, J. (Brussels): The Proteins of Sweat 356
SEGERS, A. (Bruxelles): Répercussions des activités physiques modérées sur le taux de la protéinurie intermittente des adolescents 361
DOMINICI, G.; ROTTINI, E.; MILIA, U. et COZZOLINO, G. (Perugia): Protéinurie de fatigue: Détermination quantitative de certaines fractions protéiques 365
ROTARU, C. (Iassy): Etude expérimentale sur le comportement des mucoprotéines dans les conditions de l'effort physique 371

Subject Index 378
Author Index 383

Preface

This volume contains the proceedings of the first symposium which was organized to fulfill the wish of a number of scientists involved in the field of biochemistry of muscular activity to have an opportunity for a plain discussion of problems of mutual interest.

Biochemistry of exercise may include such a variety of different aspects that to hold a meeting on that general subject was nearly a utopia. Therefore, it was decided that the discussion within a limited area would be best, namely the humoral modifications occurring during physical activity. This subject was chosen since the body fluids are able to reflect the more basic perturbations which occur at the cellular level. To know the modifications relevant to physical activity is of major interest not only for fundamental research but also for the determination of physical fitness. Concerning their biochemical aspect, it may be said that both points are in a toddling phase. This volume will permit to clarify ideas where there is agreement, and stimulate discussions and investigations where still unsettled problems are obvious.

The topics covered by the proceedings include: blood gases and metabolites in acid-base chemistry, carbohydrate and lipid metabolisms, enzymes, hormones, electrolytes, proteins in biological fluids. The current researches were summarised as an introductory lecture to each of these sections by eminent specialists, namely: Professors M. SCHERRER (Bern), A. DECOSTER (Brussels), J. R. M. FRANCKSON (Brussels), S. FRÖBERG (Stockholm), F. W. SCHMIDT (Hannover), U. S. VON EULER (Stockholm), G. ROUGIER (Bordeaux) and Dr. J. R. POORTMANS (Brussels).

In addition, the collection of numerous communications closely follows the latest trends of research and reports on recent results.

It is hoped that the present volume, which encloses valuable sources of up-to-date information, will be a stimulating guide for future research in the field of biochemistry of exercise.

The organisation Committee, February 1969, Brussels

Acknowledgements

We, the Members of the Organization Committee, are glad to have the opportunity of expressing our thanks to the Université Libre de Bruxelles for giving the practical facilities in the general organization of the Symposium.

We are also endebted to those who served as chairmen of the various sessions and helped in developing the program: J. KRÁL (Prague), J. KEUL (Freiburg i.Br.), F. KREUZER (Nijmegen), Z. JIRKA (Olomouc), T. CURETON (Urbana), G. SCHÖNHOLZER (Macolin), D. GOLLNICK (Pullman), G. METIVIER (Ottawa), P. HALONEN (Helsinki), N. JAKOVLEV (Leningrad), B. SALTIN (Stockholm).

We wish to express our gratitude to the staff of the Laboratoire de l'Effort, and especially to the secretary, Mrs M. PLASCH, and technicians, Mrs.. O. RUBIN and Mr. R. ROBEAUX, who gave unstintingly of their time and effort to contribute to the success of this symposium.

It is also a pleasure to thank all those who made this meeting possible by their financial support, Université Libre de Bruxelles, Ministère de l'Education Nationale, Fonds National de la Recherche Scientifique, Analis, Bayer, Belgolabo, R. Bellon, Boehringer-Sohn, R. Coles, Labaz, Léo Pharmaceutical Products-Belgium, Merck, Sharp et Dohme, Organon, Pfizer, S.I.D. S.A. Pharbil, Roche, Sandoz, Simes International, U.C.B., Van der Heyden, A.L.R. Will et Co, Winthrop, Zyma Galen.

I. Blood Gases and Metabolites in Acid-Base Chemistry

Acid-Base Imbalance and Gas Exchange During Heavy Work[1]

M. SCHERRER

Division of Pneumology, Medical Clinic of the University, Berne

The O_2-transport way from the atmosphere to the muscles may be divided in 4 sections: (1) Pulmonary ventilation, (2) Pulmonary diffusion capactiy, (3) Circulation, (4) Muscular tissue diffusion capacity.

Ventilation and circulation are 2 convective systems requiring energy. The maintenance of a proper flux of O_2 over the diffusion systems, however, requires adequate O_2 pressure (p_{O_2})- gradients, which are maintained by the convective systems: the ventilation for the alveolar p_{O_2}, the circulation for the blood p_{O_2}. The O_2 transport capacity of the whole body depends on the capacities of each of the 4 departments [21]. The over-all O_2 transport system may be evaluated by the maximal O_2 uptake ($\dot{V}_{O_2max}$) found at maximal work load (aerobic work capacity [4]).

The present study will first show some relations between the aerobic work capacity and the acid-base imbalance. In a second part, some problems of exercise pulmonary diffusion capacity will be discussed.

Aerobic Work Capacity

In figure 1 is shown the non linear rise of minute ventilation ($\dot{V}_E$) and the linear rise of the O_2 consumption ($\dot{V}_{O_2}$) with increasing work load in a young man. The $\dot{V}_{O_2max}$ depends on a number of variables: body size and weight [24], age and sex [4, 39], physical fitness [11, 33], muscles involved [27, 35], inspired p_{O_2} [7, 14, 22, 30], total hemoglobin content [21] and others. The aerobic work capacity is strongly related to the submaximal work load at a given heart rate, f.i. 175 [5], and correlates also in a typical manner with different respiratory and acid-base parameters. During a submaximal work of f.i. 800 kg/min, the $\dot{V}_E$ of a woman with a $\dot{V}_{O_2max}$ = 1,8 l/min is found to be 70 l/min; the same work load performed by a trained man having a

---

[1] The investigations were carried out in Collaboration with T. ABELIN, A. BIRCHLER, J. HODLER, F. KUBICEK and K. KYD, and were supported by the Swiss National Foundation for Scientific Research.

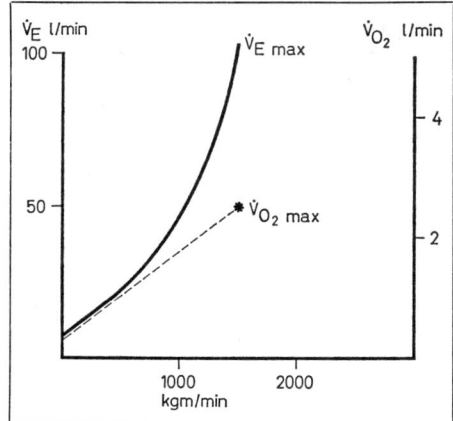

Figure 1. Minute ventilation ($\dot{V}_E$) and oxygen uptake ($\dot{V}_{O_2}$) in a young man during performance of increasing work on a bicycle ergometer.

$\dot{V}_{O_2max} = 3$ l/min requires only a $\dot{V}_E$ of 30 l/min. Furthermore, the increase of $\dot{V}_E$ with exercise seems to be linear for light work loads, but increases more rapidly when a threshold exercise is exceeded (figure 1). This threshold work load, which induces hyperventilation, depends on the $\dot{V}_{O_2max}$ and corresponds with the level of work at which the respiratory exchange ratio R begins to rise above its resting level and at which arterial lactate increases and, finally, at which also plasma bicarbonate falls (figure 2) [28, 37].

From these facts 3 work steps may be derived (figure 3):

1. A nearly alactacidemic step, performed in a perfect respiratory and humoral steady state.

2. A more severe step with considerable lactacidemia, still even performed apparently in a respiratory steady state. However, R increases approaching 1.0. Compensatory alveolar hyperventilation occurs and decreases the arterial p_{CO_2} below 40 mm Hg.

3. A slightly higher work-step, in which lactacidosis and hyperventilation increase rapidly in an irresistible manner. The work must be interrupted in a state of extreme acidosis and exhaustion. R exceeds 1.0, arterial p_{CO_2} falls below 30 mm Hg, the pH below 7,25 [1].

The threshold-work inducing acid-base imbalance of such degrees seems to depend on all 4 components determining the aerobic work capacity, i.e. ventilatory, circulatory and diffusing capacities. Inversely, the extreme alveolar hyperventilation and the metabolic acidosis at severe exercise have

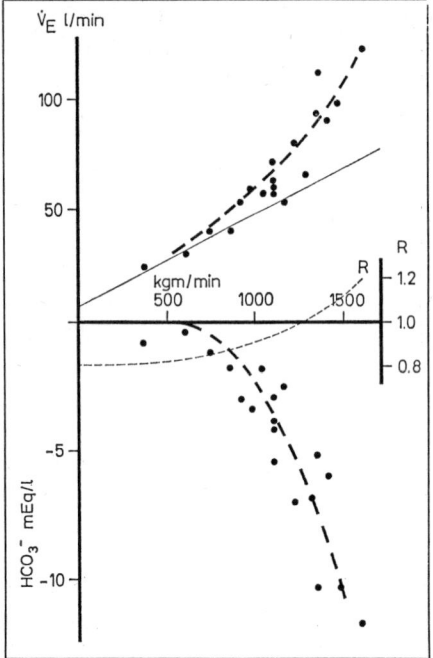

Figure 2. Minute ventilation ($\dot{V}_E$), exchange ratio (R) and fall of arterial plasma bicarbonate (HCO_3^-) 5 min after beginning of different bicycle work load (400–1,600 kgm/min) in 8 healthy, 20 years old students. From ABELIN and SCHERRER [1].

also typical influences on the gas exchange, increasing f.i. the alveolar p_{O_2} and shifting the Hb-O_2-dissociation curve on the right side.

Pulmonary Diffusion Capacity

Alveolar hyperventilation, hypocapnia and increasing R favour the pulmonary O_2 diffusion. At heavy work, indeed, the alveolar p_{O_2} tends to increase [2, 6, 8, 15, 16, 26]. A similar rise in the arterial p_{O_2} (p_{aO_2}) was not observed by all the cited authors; thus, one may be in presence of a rising alveolar-arterial p_{O_2}-difference (AaD_{O_2}) at strenuous work. There are, however, great discordances in the recent literature, not only about a possible plateau of the exercise diffusing capacity of the lung for CO [20, 23, 31], but also about the p_{aO_2} at heavy work (table I). Correcting p_{aO_2} on body

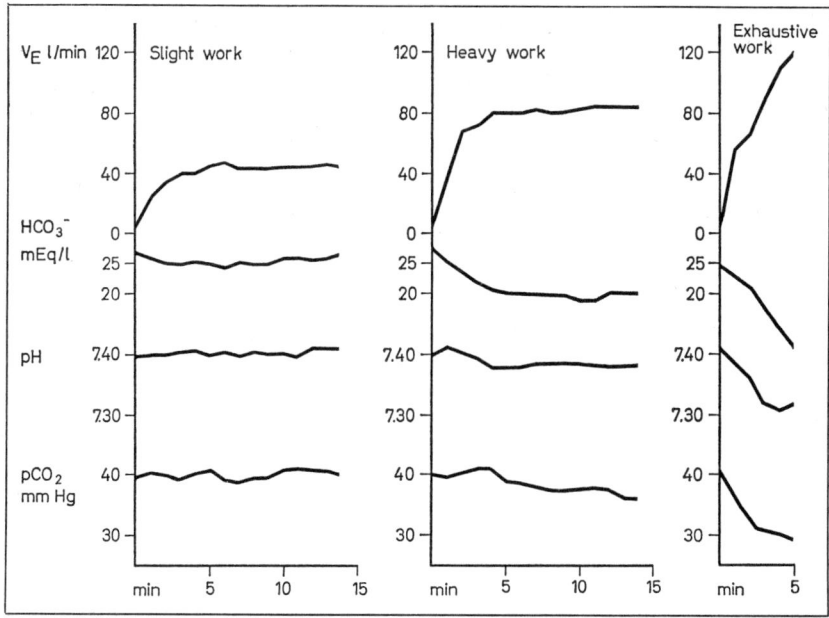

Figure 3. Continuous measurements of minute ventilation, bicarbonate ions in the arterial plasma, arterial pH and p$_{CO_2}$ during slight work (860 kgm/min) at left, heavy work (1,400 kgm/min) in the middle and exhaustive work (1,600 kgm/min) at right. 20 years old, healthy student. From ABELIN and SCHERRER [1].

temperature at heavy work, ASMUSSEN and NIELSEN [3], HOLMGREN and MCILROY [19], HESSER and MATELL [18] and HANSEN et al. [17] observed a considerable increase of p$_{aO_2}$. Other authors, renouncing on the temperature correction, found the same values at heavy work as at rest, or even a very important fall of p$_{aO_2}$ at severe exercise; these last data originate from athletes during brief, strenuous work [9, 32]. In order to keep more informations about an eventual diffusion limited work capacity, p$_{aO_2}$ should be known not only in normoxic conditions, at sea level, but also in hypoxic conditions, at altitude (table II): DOLL et al. [10] found a considerable fall of the p$_{aO_2}$ of olympic athletes exercising in Mexico City (2300 m), PUGH et al. observed the same phenomenon in 2 working european men, 32 and 51 years old, but not in a young native sherpa, 28 years old, at 5800 m of altitude (British Himalaya Expedition). ASMUSSEN and NIELSEN [3] and HANSEN et al. [17] reported unchanged p$_{aO_2}$ for young students during heavy work, compared to rest, in deep hypoxia resp. at 4300 m of altitude.

Table I. Arterial oxygen pressure (mm Hg) at rest and during exercise found by different authors

Authors	Individuals	Age years	Rest	Moderate to heavy exercise	Exhaustive exercise	Body-temp. correction
Asmussen and Nielsen, 1960 [3]	Students	young	88	85	88	+
Ulmer and Reichel, 1963 [36]	Miners	< 30	91	89		−
	Miners	> 50	80	82		−
Worth et al., 1963 [40]	Miners	< 30	90	91		−
	Miners	> 40	88	87		−
Holmgren and McIlroy, 1964 [19]	Students	< 40	90	97	97	+
Rowell et al., 1964 [32][1]	Untrained men	< 24	(95.8[1])		after 3': (93.4[1])	
	Trained men	< 24	(95.4[1])		(91.4[1])	
Hesser and Matell, 1965 [18]	Students	< 26	93	98		+
Ekelund and Holmgren, 1965 [12]	Students	< 30	92		10': 30': 60': 88 90 92	+
Doll et al., 1966 [9]	Students	< 30	98	98	96	−
	Athletes	< 30	102	90	88	−
Wasserman et al., 1967 [37]	Students	< 30	94	93	94	−
Hansen et al., 1967 [17]	Students	< 24	94	98	106	+

[1] % O_2-saturation

Table II. Arterial oxygen pressure (mm Hg) at rest and during exercise at hypoxia or at altitude found by different authors

Authors	Individuals	Age years	Rest	Moderate to heavy exercise	Exhaustive exercise	Body-temp. correction
ASMUSSEN and NIELSEN, 1960 [3] (Hypoxia, F_{IO_2} = 0.12)	Students	young	36	36	38	+
PUGH et al., 1964 [29] (Himalaya, 5800 m)	J. B. West	32	35	29	20	−
	L. G. Pugh	51	33	24	29	−
	Sherpa	28	32	32	29	−
DOLL et al., 1967 [10] (Mexico City, 2300 m)	Athletes		66	55	53	
HANSEN et al., 1967 [17] (Pikes Peak, 4300 m)	Students (newcomers)	< 24	44	43	45	+
	Students (acclimatized)	< 24	53	51	54	+

Table III. Alveolar (A) and arterial (a) oxygen pressure, alveolar-arterial difference (mm Hg) and standard deviations, at rest and at heavy work during room air breathing (F_{IO_2} = 0.21), hypoxia-breathing (F_{IO_2} = 0.16) and oxygen breathing (F_{IO_2} = 0.95). From SCHERRER and BIRCHLER [34]

	F_{IO_2}:	At rest 0.21	At heavy work 0.21	0.16	0.95	
12 male athletes	18–26 years old	100 ± 10	96 ± 3	70 ± 2	576 ± 8	A
	$\dot{V}_{O_2}$ = 2.7 l/min	96 ± 8	86 ± 5	65 ± 4	537 ± 33	a
		4 ± 4	10 ± 5	5 ± 3	39 ± 31	AaD_{O_2}
9 female athletes	17–21 years old	98 ± 6	98 ± 3	72 ± 4	585 ± 14	A
	$\dot{V}_{O_2}$ = 1.8 l/min	94 ± 6	91 ± 6	66 ± 5	558 ± 33	a
		4 ± 6	7 ± 8	6 ± 5	27 ± 24	AaD_{O_2}
9 well trained men	45–60 years old	103 ± 9	100 ± 3	74 ± 5	576 ± 7	A
	$\dot{V}_{O_2}$ = 1.8 l/min	80 ± 10	84 ± 9	56 ± 9	547 ± 24	a
		23 ± 13	16 ± 8	18 ± 8	29 ± 26	AaD_{O_2}

Our own experience concerns 3 groups of subjects [34]: 2 groups of young, 20 years old athletes, 12 male and 9 female, and a group of 9 well trained sportive men, 50 years old. The alveolar and arterial pO2 were measured during a steady state at lactacidemic work load ($\dot{V}_{O_2}$ = 2.6, resp. 1.8 l/min) on a bicycle ergometer in normoxia (F_{IO_2} = 0.21), hypoxia (F_{IO_2} = 0.16) and hyperoxia (F_{IO_2} = 0.95) (table III). The lactacidemia

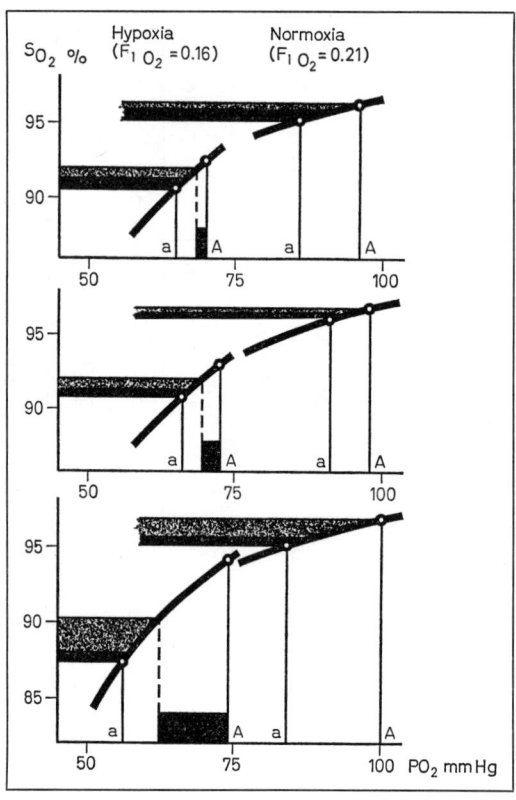

Figure 4. Alveolar (A) and arterial (a) oxygen pressures during room air and hypoxia breathing on the abscissa. The values are projected versus the *in vivo* measured Hb-O2-dissociation curves (saturation for O2 on the ordinate). Above: Means of 12 young male athletes. Middle: Means of 9 young female athletes. Below: Means of 9 well trained 50 years old men. All during heavy, lactacidemic bicycle work.
Black band: True shunt saturation deficit.
Grey band: Distribution related physiological shunt saturation deficit.
Black pO2 zone: Part of the hypoxia AaDO2 due to diffusion-limitation.
From SCHERRER and BIRCHLER [34].

was found to increase during hypoxia-breathing and to vanish during hyperoxia-breathing. The p_{aO_2} were corrected on body temperature using HOLMGREN and MCILROY's [19] correction procedure.

The AaD_{O_2} increased at heavy work in our young athletes, but decreased in the elderly men. Therefore, our results confirm those of DOLL et al. [9] concerning the decrease of p_{aO_2} in young athletes, but they do not confirm DOLL's findings for the elderly men. During hypoxia, according to ASMUSSEN and NIELSEN [3], HANSEN et al. [17] and PUGH et al. [29], we found relatively high p_{aO_2} in the young athletes and relatively low p_{aO_2} in the elderly men.

Knowing the AaD_{O_2} during hyperoxia (F_{IO_2} = 0.95), we calculated the arterial saturation deficit due to shunting, assuming that the shunts remain constant during all levels of inspired O_2 (figure 4). This shunt (black horizontal band in figure 4) lies in the order of less than 1 % of the cardiac output. Nevertheless, ¾ of the large normoxia AaD_{O_2} of athletes seem to be due to this 1 % shunt, the shunting venous blood being very deeply desaturated in trained athletes [11]. A quarter of the exercise AaD_{O_2} found in normoxia remains to be explained (grey horizontal band in figure 4). Probably, this part of the normoxia AaD_{O_2} has to be ascribed to a physiological shunt coming from distribution effects. Doubling this distribution-related deficit of the arterial saturation for the hypoxia condition [13], one

Table IV. Alveolar (A) and arterial (a) oxygen pressure and alveolar-arterial difference (mm Hg) at heavy exercise during room air breathing, hypoxia- and oxygen breathing, before and after abounding, volume compensated phlebotomy. From KUBICEK and SCHERRER [25].

33 years old man $\dot{V}_{O_2}$ = 2.5 l/min	F_{IO_2}:	17.0 g Hb/100 ml 0.21	0.16	0.75	
		100	75	434	A
		92	64	385	a
		8	11	49	AaD_{O_2}
	F_{IO_2}:	14.4. g Hb/100 ml 0.21	0.16	0.75	
		103	80	460	A
		91	57	420	a
		12	23	40	AaD_{O_2}

may estimate the hypoxia alveolar-endcapillary O_2-gradient due to diffusion: According to ASMUSSEN [2], this part of the hypoxia AaD_{O_2} is less than 2 mm Hg in young athletes (black zone of p_{O_2} in figure 4); the result leads to super-diffusion-capacities lying between 100 and 200 ml/min mm Hg. But in elderly men, despite their good training, the hypoxia endgradient amounts to 12 mm Hg, a surprisingly high and well measurable value. The corresponding O_2 diffusion capacity, 60 ml/min mm Hg, lies in the same range as the values found by earlier authors [8, 26].

We think that in *young* athletes O_2 diffusion capacity of the lung is never limiting the aerobic work capacity, not even at altitude; however, in *elderly* well trained men, the pulmonary O_2 diffusion clearly becomes a limiting factor for heavy work at altitude, or at hypoxia, causing a measurable arterial O_2 deficit. It is possible, speculating, that the same aging processus as in the lungs plays important parts also for an age dependent decrease of the muscular O_2 diffusion capacity.

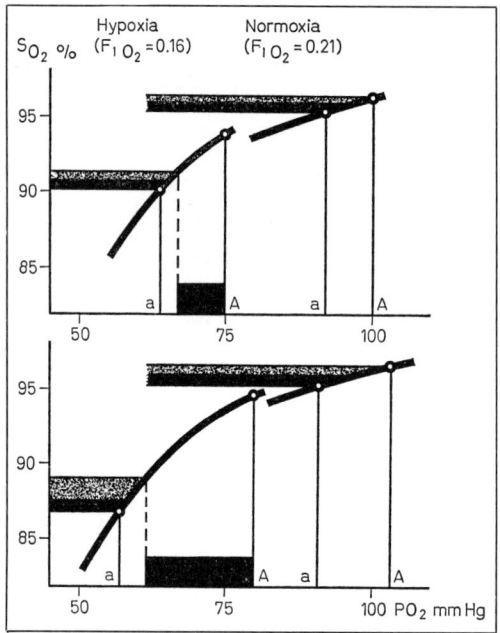

Figure 5. Same representation as figure 4; concerns a 33 years old, healthy student, at heavy, lactacidemic work on a bicycle ergometer. Before and after abounding volume compensated phlebotomy. From KUBICEK and SCHERRER [25].

Concerning the rôle of anemia for O_2 diffusion, a similar experience was realized in a 33 years old, healthy, well trained man, working on a bicycle ergometer with a $\dot{V}_{O_2}$ of 2.5 l/min (table IV). His AaD_{O_2} was found to be slightly higher than in young athletes. After the first step of investigations, a phlebotomy and a simultaneous volume-compensating plasma reinfusion were realized in order to decrease the arterial hemoglobin content from 17.0 to 14.4 g per 100 ml of blood. This procedure was well supported by the volunteer, a medical student, without any complaints about immediate or late troubles, exc. a much more pronounced dyspnoea on strong exertion. After one hour to take rest, the same work with $\dot{V}_{O_2}$ = 2.5 l/min was performed and all measurements repeated [25]. We found an important rise of lactates at all three O_2-levels compared to the state before phlebotomy, a considerable decrease of the hypoxia p_{aO_2} and an increase of the hypoxia AaD_{O_2}. The hypoxia endgradient was found to rise from 8 before, to 18 mm Hg after the phlebotomy (figure 5), the diffusion capacity of the lung to fall from 84 to 66 ml/min mm Hg.

This example illustrates the fact, that the hemoglobin content determines the pulmonary (and perhaps also the muscular) O_2 diffusion capacity; anemia may deteriorate the aerobic work capacity and favour the lactacidemia not only in the way of creating directly a tissue hypoxia, but also by impairing the O_2 diffusion capacities, inducing arterial hypoxemia, predominantly at altitude or at other hypoxia conditions.

Summary

The interdependence between lactacidemia at heavy work and maximal oxygen uptake (aerobic work capacity) is discussed. Three exercise levels are studied: 1. an alactacidemic one, performed in a perfect humoral and respiratory steady state. 2. a higher level with important lactacidemia, elevated R and compensatory alveolar hyperventilation. 3. an exhaustive work load with rapidly progressive acidosis and hyperventilation.

During severe work, alveolar hyperventilation leads to an increase of alveolar p_{O_2}. It is unknown, however, if the arterial p_{O_2} does also increase or decrease during severe exercise. In our findings, during heavy work p_{aO_2} decreases in young athletes (the decrease being due to shunting of deeply desaturated venous blood), but increases in elderly men. Despite these results, the exercise diffusion capacity of the lungs for oxygen is found to be extremely high in young athletes (super-O_2-diffusion capacities lying between 100 and 200 ml/min mm Hg), but critically deep in elderly men (60 ml/min mm Hg).

References

1. ABELIN, T. und SCHERRER, M.: Ventilation und Säurebasenhaushalt des Gesunden bei schwerer Arbeit. Schweiz. med. Wschr. *90:* 369–375 (1960).

2. ASMUSSEN, E.: Muscular exercise; in FENN and RAHN's Handbook of Physiol. Section 3: Respiration 2: 939–978 (Amer. Physiol. soc., Washington, D.C. 1965).
3. ASMUSSEN, E. and NIELSEN, M.: Alveolo-arterial gas exchange at rest and during work at different O_2-tensions. Acta physiol. scand. 50: 153–166 (1960).
4. ASTRAND, I.: Aerobic capacity in men and women with special reference to age. Acta physiol. scand. 149: Suppl. 169 (1960).
5. ASTRAND, P. O. and RYHMING, I.: A nomogram for calculation of aerobic capacity from pulse rate during submaximal work. J. appl. Physiol. 7: 218–221 (1954).
6. BARTELS, H.; BEER, R.; FLEISCHER, E.; HOFFHEINZ, H. J.; KRALL, J.; RODEWALD, G.; WENNER, J. und WILT, I.: Bestimmung von Kurzschluss-Durchblutung und Diffusionskapazität der Lunge bei Gesunden und Lungenkranken. Pflügers Arch. ges. Physiol. 261: 99–132 (1955).
7. BUSKIRK, E. R.; KOLLIAS, J.; AKERS, R. F.; PROKOP, E. K. and REATEGUI, E. P.: Maximal performance at altitude and on return from altitude in conditioned runners. J. appl. Physiol. 23: 259–266 (1967).
8. COHN, J. E.; CARROL, D.; ARMSTRONG, B. W.; SHEPARD, R. H. and RILEY, R. L.: Maximal diffusing capacity of lung in normal male subjects of different ages. J. appl. Physiol. 6: 588–597 (1954).
9. DOLL, E.; KEUL, J.; MAIWALD, C. und REINDELL, H.: Das Verhalten von Sauerstoffdruck, Kohlensäuredruck, pH, Standardbicarbonat, und base excess im arteriellen Blut bei verschiedenen Belastungsformen. Int. Z. angew. Physiol. 22: 327–355 (1966).
10. DOLL, E.; KEUL, J.; BRECHTEL, A.; LIMON-LASON, R. und REINDELL, H.: Der Einfluss körperlicher Arbeit auf die arteriellen Blutgase in Freiburg und in Mexico City. Sportarzt und Sportmedizin 8: 317–325 (1967).
11. EKBLOM, B.; ASTRAND, P. O.; SALTIN, B.; STENBERG, J. and WALLSTRÖM, B.: Effect of training on circulatory response to exercise. J. appl. Physiol. 24: 518–528 (1968).
12. EKELUND, L. G. and HOLMGREN, A.: Diffusion capacity for CO during prolonged non steady state sitting exercise in ordinarily trained young men. Acta physiol. scand. 65: 143–152 (1965).
13. FAHRI, L. E. and RAHN, H.: A theoretical analysis of the alveolar-arterial oxygen difference with special reference to the distribution effects. J. appl. Physiol. 7: 699–705 (1955).
14. FAULKNER, J. A.; DANIELS, J. T. and BALKE, B.: Effects of training at moderate altitude on physical performance capacity. J. appl. Physiol. 23: 85–89 (1967).
15. FILLEY, G. F.; GREGOIRE, F. and WRIGHT, C. W.: Alveolar and arterial oxygen tension and the significance of the alveolar-arterial oxygen tension difference in normal men. J. clin. Invest. 33: 517–529 (1954).
16. FRIEHOFF, F.: Gasaustausch bei gesunden Männern unter Ruhebedingungen und während körperlicher Arbeit. Pflügers Arch. ges. Physiol. 270: 431–441 (1960).
17. HANSEN, J. E.; STELTER, G. P. and VOGEL, J. A.: Arterial pyruvate, lactate, pH, and p_{CO_2} during work, at sea level and at altitude. J. appl. Physiol 23: 523–530 (1967).
18. HESSER, C. M. and MATELL, G.: Effect of light and moderate exercise on the AaD$_{O_2}$ in man. Acta physiol. scand. 63: 247–259 (1965).
19. HOLMGREN, A. and McILROY, M. B.: Effect of temperature on arterial blood gas tensions and pH during exercise. J. appl. Physiol. 19: 243–245 (1964).
20. HOLMGREN, A.: On the variation of the diffusion capacity of the lung for CO

with increasing oxygen uptake during exercise in healthy trained young men and women. Acta physiol. scand. *65:* 207–220 (1965).
21. HOLMGREN, A. and ASTRAND, P. O.: D_L and the dimensions and functional capacities of the oxygen transport system in humans. J. appl. Physiol. *21:* 1463–1470 (1966).
22. HUGHES, R. L.; CLODE, M.; EDWARDS, R. H. T.; GOODWIN, T. J. and JONES, N. L.: Effect of inspired O_2 on cardiopulmonary and metabolic responses to exercise in man. J. appl. Physiol. *24:* 336–347 (1968).
23. JOHNSON, R. L.; TAYLOR, H. S. and LAWSON, W. H.: Maximal diffusing capacity of the lung for CO. J. clin. Invest. *44:* 349–355 (1965).
24. KNUTTGEN, H. G.: Aerobic capacity of adolescents. J. appl. Physiol. *22:* 655–658 (1967).
25. KUBICEK, F. und SCHERRER, M.: Einfluss des Hämoglobingehaltes auf Säure-Basen-Haushalt, Ventilation und O_2-Diffusion beim Gesunden während schwerer Arbeit. Schweiz. med. Wschr. *92:* 415–419 (1962).
26. LILIENTHAL, J. R.; RILEY, R. L.; PROEMMEL, D. D. and FRANKE, R. E.: An experimental analysis in men of the oxygen pressure gradient from alveolar air to arterial blood during rest and exercise at sea level and at altitude. Amer. J. Physiol. *167:* 199–216 (1946).
27. MAGEL, J. R. and FAULKNER, J. A.: Maximum oxygen uptakes of college swimmers. J. appl. Physiol. *22:* 929–938 (1967).
28. NAIMARK, A.; WASSERMANN, K. and MCILROY, M. B.: Continuous measurement of ventilatory exchange ratio during exercise. J. appl. Physiol *19:* 644–652 (1964).
29. PUGH, Z. J. C. E.; GILL, M. B.; ZAHIRI, S.; MILLEDGE, J. S.; WARD, M. P. and WEST, J. B.: Muscular exercise at great altitudes. J. appl. Physiol. *19:* 431–440 (1964).
30. REEVES, J. T.; GROVER, R. F. and COHN, J. E.: Regulation of ventilation during exercise at 10,200 feet in athletes born at low altitude. J. appl. Physiol. *22:* 546–554 (1967).
31. REUSCHLEIN, P. S.; REDDAN, W. G.; BURPEE, J.; GEE, J. B. L. and RANKIN J.: Effect of physical training on the pulmonary diffusing capacity during submaximal work. J. appl. Physiol. *24:* 152–158 (1968).
32. ROWELL, Z. B.; TAYLOR, H. Z.; WANG, J. and CARLSON, W. S.: Saturation of arterial blood with oxygen during maximal exercise. J. appl. Physiol. *19:* 284–286 (1964).
33. SALTIN, B. and ASTRAND, P. O.: Maximal oxygen uptake in athletes. J. appl. Physiol. *23:* 353–358 (1967).
34. SCHERRER, M. und BIRCHLER, A.: Altersabhängigkeit des alveoloarteriellen O_2-Partialdruckgradienten bei Schwerarbeit in Normoxie, Hypoxie und Hyperoxie. Med. Thorac. *24:* 99–117 (1967).
35. STENBERG, J.; ASTRAND, P. O.; EKBLOM, B.; ROYCE, J. and SALTIN, B.: Hemodynamic response to work with different muscle groups, sitting and supine. J. appl. Physiol. *22:* 61–70 (1967).
36. ULMER, W. T. und REICHEL, G.: Untersuchung über die Altersabhängigkeit der alveolären und arteriellen O_2- und CO_2-Partialdrücke. Klin. Wschr. *41:* 1–19 (1963).
37. WASSERMAN, K.; BURTON, G. G. and VAN KESSEL, A. L.: Excess lactate concept and oxygen debt of exercise. J. appl. Physiol. *20:* 1299–1306 (1965).
38. WASSERMAN, K.; VAN KESSEL, A. L. and BURTON, G. G.: Interaction of physiological mechanisms during exercise. J. appl. Physiol. *22:* 71–85 (1967).

39. WILMORE, J. H. and SIGERSETH, P. O.: Physical work capacity of young girls, 7–13 years of age. J. appl. Physiol. *22:* 923–928 (1967).
40. WORTH, G.; MUYSERS, H. und SIEHOFF, F.: Zur Problematik der arteriellen O_2- und CO_2-Partialdrücke sowie der alveolo-arteriellen O_2- und CO_2-Druckgradienten im Rahmen arbeitsmedizinischer Fragen. Med. Thorac. *20:* 223–243 (1963).

Author's address: Prof. MAX SCHERRER, Division of Pneumology, Medical Clinic of the University, *Berne* (Switzerland).

Role of the Metabolites in the Acid-Base Balance During Exercise[1]

A. DE COSTER, H. DENOLIN, R. MESSIN, S. DEGRE and
P. VANDERMOTEN

Institute for Cardiological Research (Prof. J. LEQUIME), Department of Cardiology (Prof. H. DENOLIN) and Department of Respiratory Diseases (Dr. A. DE COSTER); Hôpital Saint-Pierre, Brussels

The increase of lactic acid during physical exercise is well known, since the classical works of HILL *et al.* [25, 26] and MARGARIA *et al.* [34].

Lactic and pyruvic acids are the two parameters which are most often studied during exercise and it may be of interest to mention here the methods employed and their accuracy.

Techniques

For *lactic acid* we use the enzymatic technique. Measurements are made on plasma. Arterial blood is taken from the humeral artery; a small amount of sodium fluoride is added. Under these conditions, there is no glycolysis and the results remain constant for 4 h.

The precision of the enzymatic method was estimated from 296 duplicate plasma samples and the values obtained were divided into three groups: lower than 25, from 25 to 50 and more than 50 mg/100 ml.

Table I shows the mean values of the two duplicate sets, the mean difference between duplicates, the standard deviation of differences and the standard error of one measurement. The precision of the method increases for the highest lactic acid level. The method seems to be rather satisfactory.

When applied to plasma, the enzymatic technique is as precise as the Barker-Summerson technique for values below 50 mg/100 ml. For higher concentrations, the lactic dehydrogenase (LDH) technique is definitely more accurate. When applied to total blood on the contrary, the LDH technique shows a lower precision [11].

The dosage of *pyruvic acid* is still more delicate. We also applied it to plasma. It should be stressed that the pyruvic acid concentration decreases when fluoride or iodoacetate is added. The best technique consists in centrifugating the blood sample immediately in ice and in precipitating the proteins as soon as centrifugation is completed.

250 samples were divided into three groups: lower than 1 mg, from 1 to 2 mg and more than 2 mg/100 ml.

The mean values of the two samples, the mean difference between duplicates with standard deviation of differences and standard error of one measurement are reported in table II. It appears from these results that the standard error is about the same whatever

---

[1] This study was made possible by a grant from the High Authority of the European Community for Coal and Steel in Luxemburg.

Table I. Accuracy of the enzymatic technique for lactic acid (LA)

LA Plasma mg/100 ml	Number duplicates	X_1	X_2	Differences between duplicates $\bar{d} \pm S_{\bar{d}}$	S_d	Standard error one determination mg/100 ml	% of $\overline{X}$
<25	100	13.75	13.67	0.08 ± 0.15	1.53	1.08	7.9
25–50	100	37.41	37.56	0.15 ± 0.13	1.32	0.93	2.5
>50	96	77.26	77.36	0.10 ± 0.27	2.64	1.86	2.4

Table II. Accuracy of the enzymatic technique for pyruvic acid (PA)

PA Plasma mg/100 ml	Number Duplicates	X_1	X_2	Differences between duplicates $\bar{d} \pm S_{\bar{d}}$	S_d	Standard error one determination mg/100 ml	% of $\overline{X}$
<1	50	0.697	0.706	0.0088 ± 0.0080	0.057	0.040	5.7
1–2	100	1.468	1.455	0.0134 ± 0.0080	0.080	0.057	4
>2	100	2.642	2.645	0.0025 ± 0.0065	0.065	0.046	1.8

the pyruvic acid level can be and that, just as for lactic acid, the precision of the method increases with the pyruvic acid level.

This technique is quite satisfactory.

We checked – and this is most important – the validity of our measurements by adding increasing amounts of pyruvic acid to plasma samples. In these experiments known as 'recovery experiments', we recovered from 95 to 105% of the added pyruvic acid. This indirectly proves the validity of the method.

Relationship Between Lactic and Pyruvic Acids and Total CO_2

In 23 patients the increase in lactic and pyruvic acids during exercise on one hand and the simultaneous decrease in total CO_2 on the other were compared. The increase in lactic and pyruvic acids is by far more important than the decrease in CO_3H^-, the regression equation being $Y = 1.58\ X$ (figure 1). This means that the increase in lactic and pyruvic acids is by 60% higher than the decrease in total CO_2. In the cases we studied these changes are of metabolic origin only, as we only chose patients in whom, during the

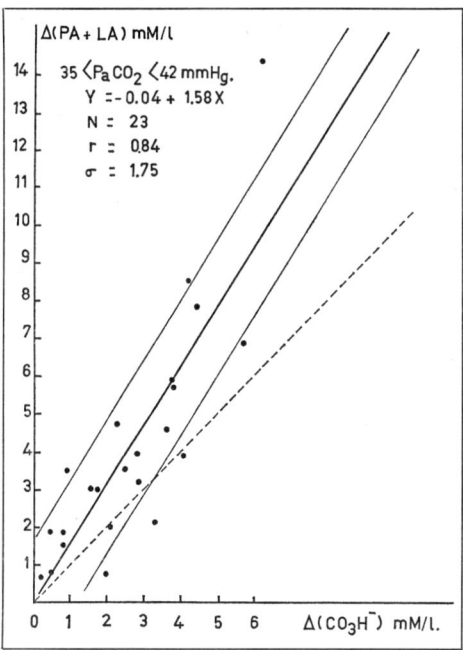

Figure 1. Relation between the increase in LA + PA and the decrease in total CO_2 (Pa CO_2 between 35 and 42 mm Hg).

blood sampling, the $PaCO_2$ was between 35 and 42 mm Hg, which excludes the possible role of any ventilatory factor. In all cases, we simultaneously observed a sometimes very important decrease in pH due to a metabolic acidosis and the impossibility for the subject to counterbalance efficiently and quickly the huge amount of H^+ ions poured into the blood stream (figure 2).

Such observations do not fit with some data of the literature according to which there would most often be a relationship between the decreasing total CO_2 and the increasing lactic acid [20]; this relationship is not always satisfactory. In 1930, DILL *et al.* [16] already stressed that the increase in lactic acid is often less marked than the decrease in total CO_2.

More recently, HARRIS [24] observed a larger increase in lactic acid than the decrease in standard bicarbonates. Anyway, the regression equation we calculated is very different from VISSER'S [40] who found a close volume correlation between changes in lactic acid and in CO_3H^- ions.

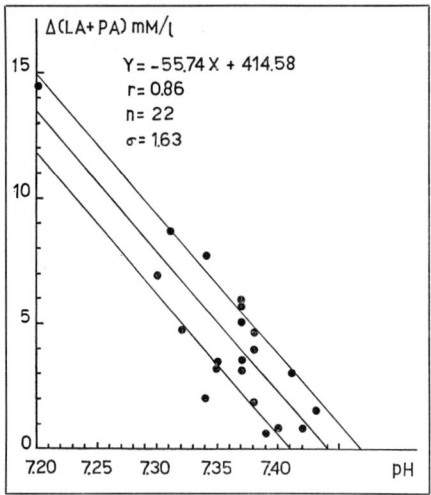

Figure 2. Relation between the increase in LA + PA and the decrease in pH ($PaCO_2$ between 35 and 42 mm Hg).

Factors Influencing the Amount of Acid Metabolites During Exercise

1. Lactic acid can be measured in total blood or in plasma and the results are quite different. The lactic acid concentration was measured by the technique of Barker-Summerson on the red cells fraction and on plasma. The sum of the so obtained values was compared with a dosage on total blood. It appeared from these investigations that the percentage of plasmatic lactic acid was systematically higher that the red cells percentage (figure 3). The regression line showed that the concentration was at least 30% higher in plasma.

These findings are in agreement with those of HILL et al. [25], GESELL et al. [18], HALDI [21], DEVADATA [15], HUCKABEE [27] and many others. The plasma-red cell gradient cannot be considered to be due to differences in proteins or free water concentrations in the two media. Indeed these differences are taken into account in our calculations: moreover, these are too high and differ from one subject to another; in addition, they change with time [11].

One explanation thereof could be that lactates pass more slowly through cell membranes than other anions such as chlorides and bicarbonates, an hypothesis which was proposed by JOHNSON in 1945 [30].

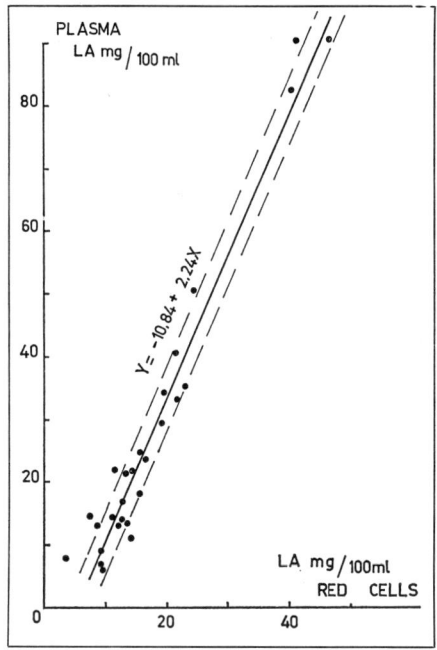

Figure 3. Relation between LA in red cells and in plasma.

The same studies were made for pyruvic acid by measuring it in total blood and in plasma, using the enzymatic method and by calculating the amount of pyruvic acid in red cells from hematocrit.

The difference in pyruvic acid concentration between plasma and red cells is still more marked than for lactic acid, being at least 50% higher in plasma than in red cells (figure 4).

Practical implications are obvious and we prefer to measure lactic and pyruvic acids in plasma because this allows us to detect much smaller and earlier changes in lactic and pyruvic acid concentrations and these changes can be more easily compared with those of other ions such as potassium.

2. Arterial or venous sampling. In a subject exercising on a bicycle, the difference in lactic acid concentration in the brachial artery and in the cubital vein may be important. This arterio-venous difference changes according to the arterial lactic acid level. If it is low, the arterio-venous difference will decrease, even to zero at the 10th min of exercise. If the lactic

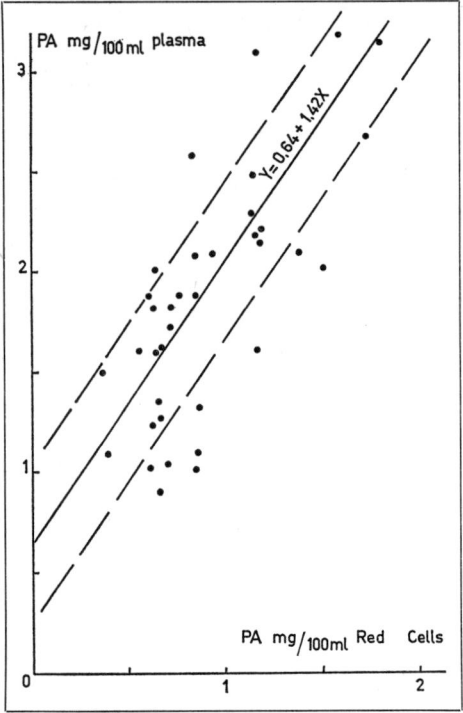

Figure 4. Relation between PA in red cells and in plasma.

acid level is very high, the arterio-venous difference in lactates entirely remains even during the recovery period (figure 5). If the lactic acid level is moderately raised, arterial and venous lactate levels may become equal during recovery but not during exercise (figure 6).

It is thus necessary that all studies on acidosis during physical exercise should be based on arterial blood, as mentioned a long time ago by MARGARIA et al. [34], HUCKABEE [27], CARLSON et al. [5], DE COSTER et al. [14] and many others. Studies on venous blood unquestionably entail errors; arterialized blood can be possibly used. Rather satisfactory comparisons have been made between arterialized capillary blood and arterial blood by HARRIS et al. [24] among others. The method is reliable, except perhaps in very particular clinical conditions such as shock or circulatory insufficiency.

The fact that the arterio-venous difference in lactates persists also proves that it can be hazardous to extrapolate the arterial lactic acid level

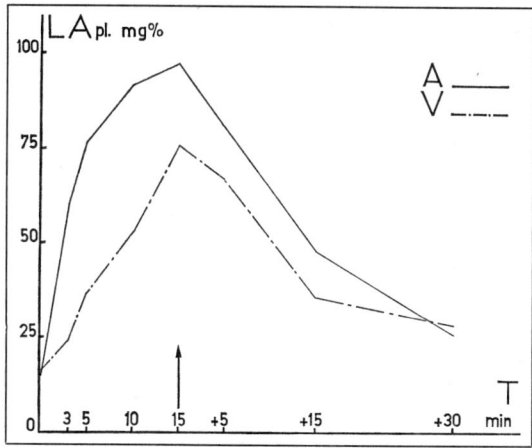

Figure 5. LA level in the humeral artery (A) and the cubital vein (V) in a subject exercising on a bicycle. The arterio-venous difference exists during work and recovery.

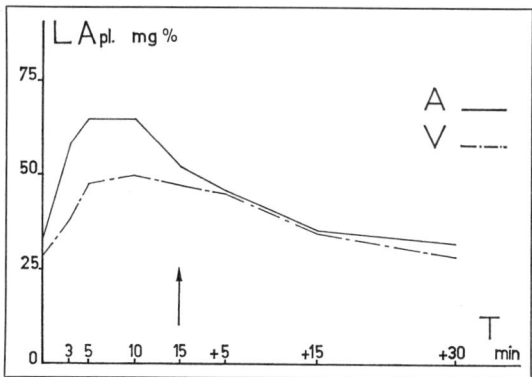

Figure 6. LA level in the humeral artery (A) and the cubital vein (V) in a subject exercising on a bicycle. The arterio-venous difference remains during physical work and disappears during the recovery period.

to total body water. Indeed, if an arterio-venous difference remains at the 15th min of exercise in a resting limb, it really proves that the saturation of tissues in lactic acid is not complete. However, the calculation of total lactic acid in order to evaluate the oxygen debt for instance supposes a perfect distribution in the different parts of the body.

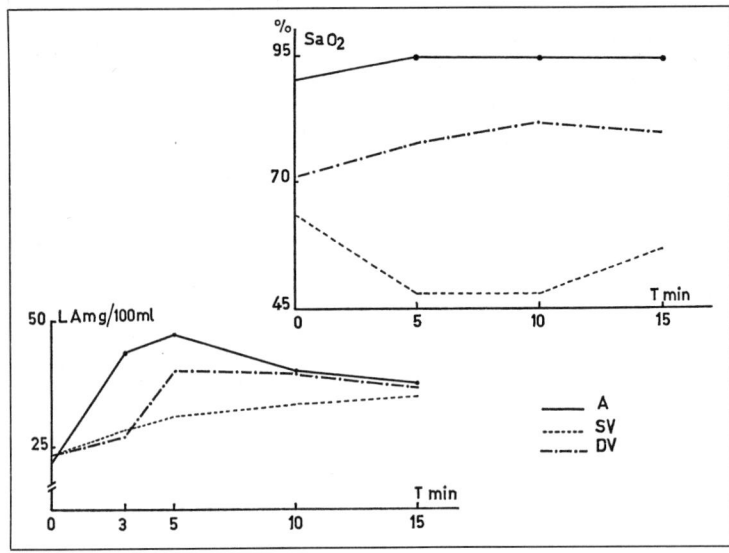

Figure 7. Evolution of Sa O$_2$ and LA in the brachial artery (A), a superficial vein (SV) and the humeral vein (DV) of a subject exercising on a bicycle.

Moreover, lactic acid concentration has a different evolution during exercise on the bicycle ergometer when blood is taken from a superficial or from a deep vein. In a superficial vein of the arm we can observe a decrease in oxygen saturation during the first part of exercise, and a slowly progressive increase in lactic acid that has not yet reached the arterial lactic acid level at the 15th min.

In a deep vein, on the contrary, arterial saturation increases and the arterio-venous difference in lactates is less marked (figure 7). These various changes are due to a difference in the local circulation: in a superficial vein, circulation is rather slow and this probably causes a decrease in oxygen saturation and a slow increase in lactates, while in the deep veins where circulation is more active, a partial arterialization of the venous blood occours. These differences in local circulation have been already stressed and investigated by BISHOP et al. [3], CARLSON et al. [7] and DONALD et al. [17].

3. *The moment when blood sampling is done* should always be mentioned. In fact, the lactic and pyruvic acids levels are never constant during exercise. Either a progressive increase, or an initial increase followed by a plateau, or even an initial increase followed by a progressive decrease can be observed [13]. The result thereof is that any correlation between a circula-

Table III. Evolution of V_E, V_{O_2}, f, V_T, f_h, LA, PA, Q and Q_S in progressive load and in constant load. Measurements are made at the 5th min of the same load.

	n	Constant $\overline{X}_1 \pm S\overline{X}_1$	Progressive $\overline{X}_2 \pm S\overline{X}_2$	$\overline{d} \pm S\overline{d}$	P
$\dot{V}_E$ l/min	10	37.1 ± 4.7	38.1 ± 6.5	1.0 ± 2.5	—
V_{O_2} cc/min	13	1,461 ± 143	1,413 ± 125	48 ± 52	—
f	10	27 ± 5	32 ± 6	5 ± 2	+
V_T cc	10	1,402 ± 151	1,202 ± 126	200 ± 62	+ +
f_h	10	135 ± 11	139 ± 14	4 ± 6	—
LA mg/100 ml	20	51.6 ± 10.9	35.3 ± 13.4	16.3 ± 1.2	+ + +
PA mg/100 ml	6	2.3 ± 0.4	1.8 ± 0.4	0.5 ± 0 2	P = 0.05
LA/PA	6	19.8 ± 3.6	17.0 ± 1.8	2.8 ± 1.7	—
$\dot{Q}$ l/min	9	13.6 ± 2.2	13.8 ± 1.8	0.2 ± 1.0	—
Q_S ml	9	102 ± 18	101 ± 20	1 ± 9	—

— non significant; + 0.05 > P > 0.01; + + 0.01 > P > 0.001; + + + P < 0.001

tory or ventilatory parameter and the concentration of acid metabolites must be done between simultaneous measurements.

4. *The type of effort* should be mentioned as the metabolic effect is not the same when a subject performs a constant exercise, for example 600 kg-m/min during 15 min, or a progressive exercise, for example 250 kg-m/min during 5 min, followed by 400 kg-m/min during 5 min and 600 kg-m/min during 5 min.

Under these conditions, the comparison between the lactic and pyruvic acids levels measured at the 5th min of a constant or progressive exercise gives for the same load statistically different results, the lactic and pyruvic acids levels being definitely lower during a progressive work (table III).

On the contrary, there is no significant difference for ventilation, oxygen consumption, heart rate, cardiac output and stroke volume.

The comparison of lactates production during exercise on the bicycle ergometer and on a treadmill shows a lower level in lactic acid in the latter, probably owing to the use of more important muscle groups (figure 8). This is at least the explanation most often given by authors who sometimes report important differences in lactates for similar oxygen consumptions.

All these factors we have mentioned tend thus to influence the lactic acid as well as the pyruvic acid level. That is the reason why it is so important that the experimental conditions under which measurements have been made should by made very precise.

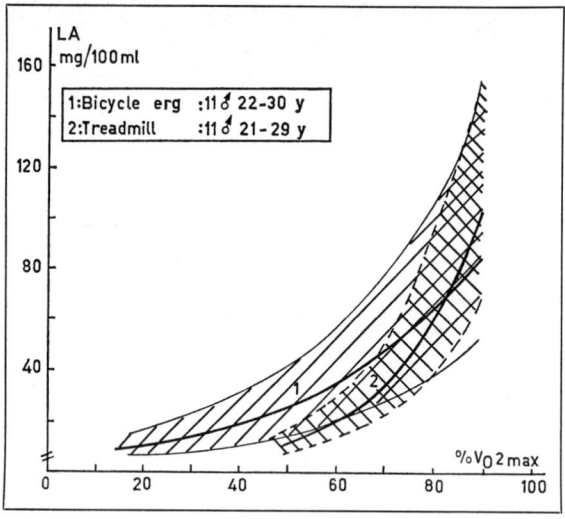

Figure 8. Relationship between LA and $\dot{V}_{O_2}$ for the same subjects exercising on a bicycle or on a treadmill.

Evolution of Lactic and Pyruvic Acids During Exercise on the Bicycle

1. Lactic Acid

At the beginning of exercise, the lactic acid level increases very quickly. For a load of 600 kg-m/min lactic acid is not detectable during the first 30 sec.

At the end of the first minute the lactic acid level is significantly higher in all cases and it steadily increases in a more or less linear way until the 3rd or 5th min (figure 9).

During exercise, this increase may go on beyond the 5th min especially during exhaustive work.

The evolution of lactic acid in 53 normal subjects or patients with light anthracosilicosis who performed a load of 600 kg-m/min on the bicycle is reported on figure 10. The following criteria of good tolerance were considered: the exercise can be sustained for 15 min; difference in ventilation is lower than 15% from the 5th to the 15th min; difference in oxygen consumption is lower than 10% from the 5th to the 15th min; the respiratory equivalent for oxygen is lower than or equal to 30 and the respiratory rate is lower than 35. In this group, we observe:

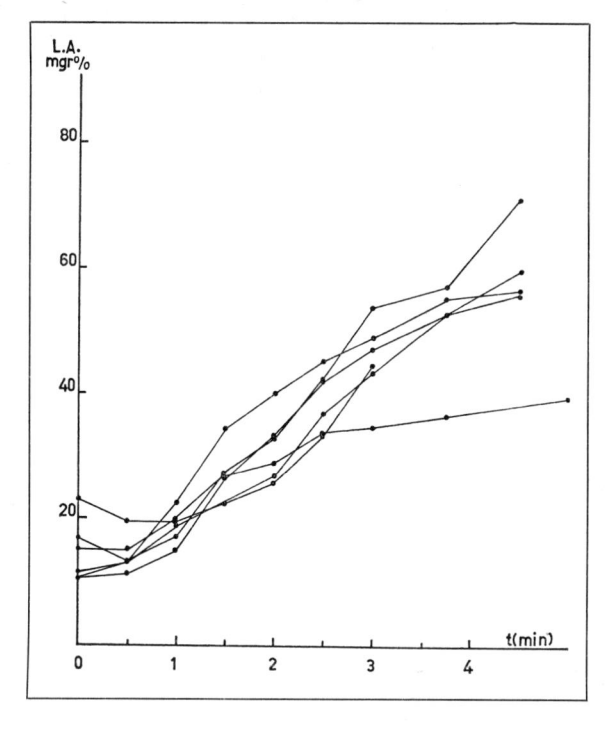

Figure 9. Increase of LA at the beginning of exercise (sample from the brachial artery; exercise of 600 kg-m/min on a bicycle).

– an important scattering of lactates values for rather identical respiratory conditions;
– a scattering that increases with the length of exercise;
– a tendency to a decrease in lactic acid during exercise. This is much more evident during prolonged work when subjects performed 400 kg-m/min during 45 to 60 min (figure 11).

This particular evolution of lactate during prolonged exercise has already been emphasized by LUNDIN et al. [33], ÅSTRAND et al. [2], HARRIS et al. [22] and SALTIN et al. [38].

Four factors can theoretically explain that decrease or even the normalization of lactates during exercise:

– A diffusion of lactates into inactive tissues. We have seen for instance that when the level in lactic acid is low the arterio-venous difference soon disappears probably owing to a progressive saturation in lactates of the

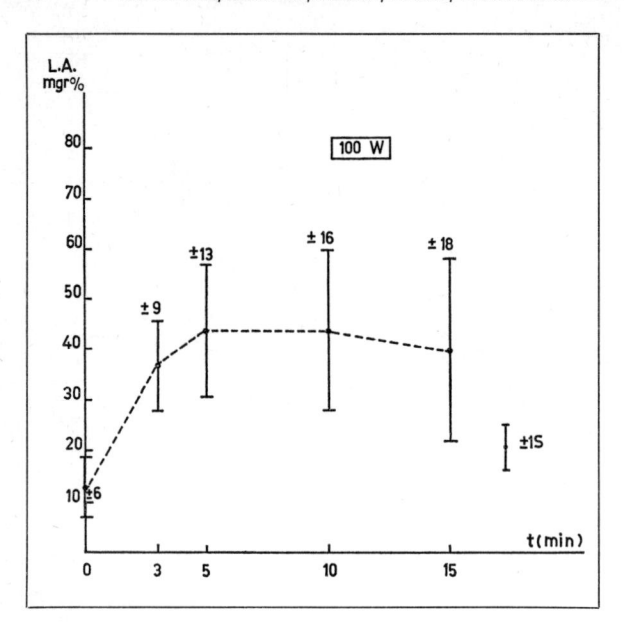

Figure 10. Evolution of LA in 53 patients with light anthracosilicosis who tolerated 600 kg-m/min for 15 min.

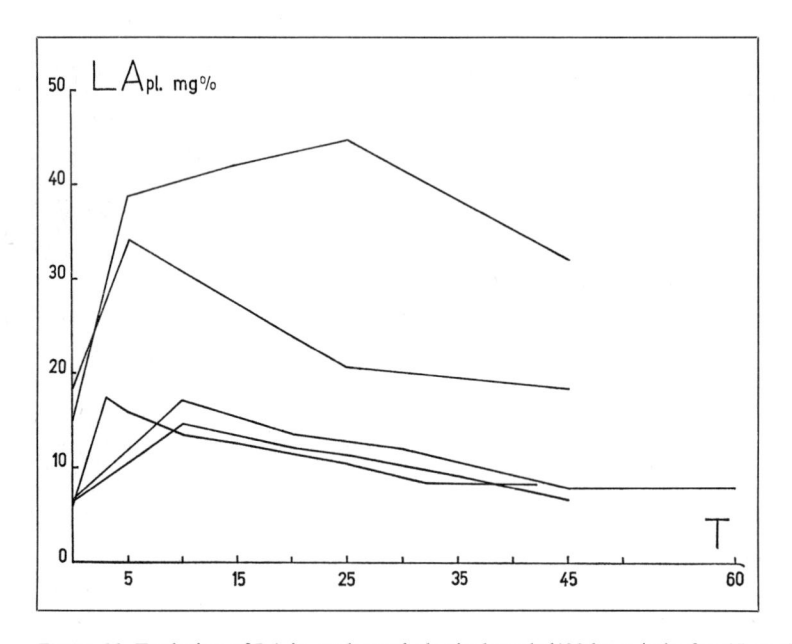

Figure 11. Evolution of LA in prolonged physical work (400 kg-m/min for 45 to 60 min).

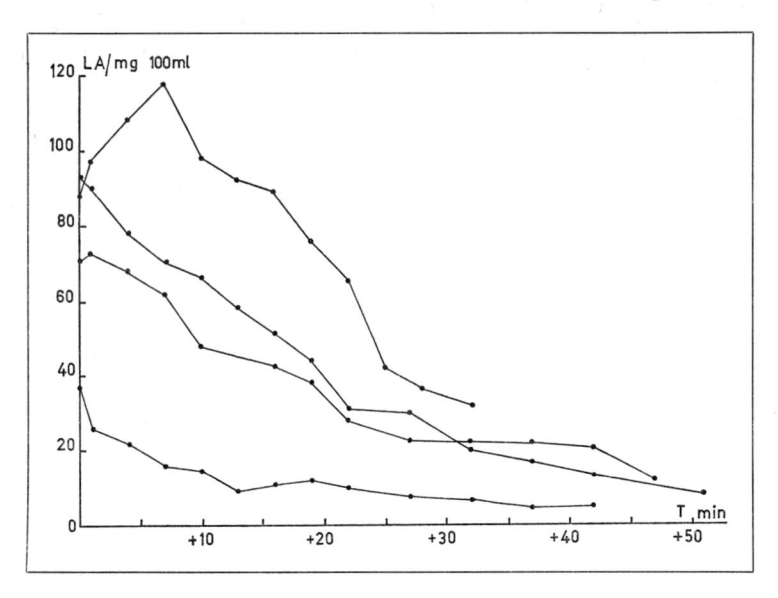

Figure 12. Different types of evolution of LA after work.

perfused tissues. Such are probably our cases where the lactic acid level is rather moderate;

— A progressive diffusion of lactic acid into the cells cannot explain its progressive decrease with time since, as we have seen it, its gradient between intra- and extracellular water is still more important during exercise than at rest [11];

— An increase of the extracellular compartment cannot explain the progressive decrease in lactates. Indeed, we measured in several cases the evolution of the extracellular compartment during exercise by the thiocyanate technique: this compartment does not change at all during work [12];

— One should admit some active metabolism of lactic acid at the hepatic or muscular level to explain its normalization during prolonged exercise.

After exercise, different evolutions can be observed (figure 12). When exercise is very heavy, lactates still increase after work and then progressively decrease, four or five min after the muscular work is completed.

When effort is not exhaustive, the decrease in lactic acid is very clear within the 30 first seconds after the test and the time required for normalization depends on the lactic acid level which was reached at the end of exercise. When lactates are very high, it can sometimes take as much as 40 to 50 min before normalization is obtained.

The recovery curves are not simple or double exponential curves as it was stated by MARGARIA [34, 35]. This is not surprising since the decrease in lactic acid after exercise is due to several mechanisms:

A. There are Two Sources of Lactic Acid Output: (a) the lactic acid contained in the working muscles diffuses into the circulation after work. Its level in the working muscles is in fact higher than in venous blood [37]; that is probably why lactates sometimes increase after work is completed; (b) the level of lactic acid in the cells progressively decreases as it diffuses back into the extracellular compartment.

B. Three mechanisms for lactate decrease can be considered: (a) patients often show profuse transpiration immediately after work in connection with a peripheral vasodilatation; (b) lactic acid is changed into glycogen; (c) lactic acid is oxydated into CO_2 and water.

It is obvious that the relative importance of these different mechanisms cannot lead to a simple curve. That is probably why its mathematical interpretation proves to be very difficult.

2. Pyruvic Acid

During exercise on the bicycle ergometer the pyruvic acid evolution is by far less systematic.

Sometimes its level is only moderate in comparison with the lactic acid level (figure 13) and sometimes it shows two peak values.

In other cases pyruvic and lactic acid levels are parallel, the lactates being however always definitely higher (figure 14).

Sometimes pyruvic acid increases with the intensity of exercise when lactic acid decreases. There is sometimes an increase in pyruvates during recovery (figure 15) which could be due to the transformation of lactic acid and to the reintroduction of the latter into the aerobic metabolism. This evolution, which has been observed by GOLDSMITH *et al.* [19], ASMUSSEN [1], DAVIS *et al.* [10] and HARRIS *et al.* [22, 23], is however far from being constant.

So, during muscular exercise pyruvic acid evolves in very different ways and this evolution seems to be independent of the degree of training, the kind of patient, the lactic acid level, and the ventilatory or circulatory parameters.

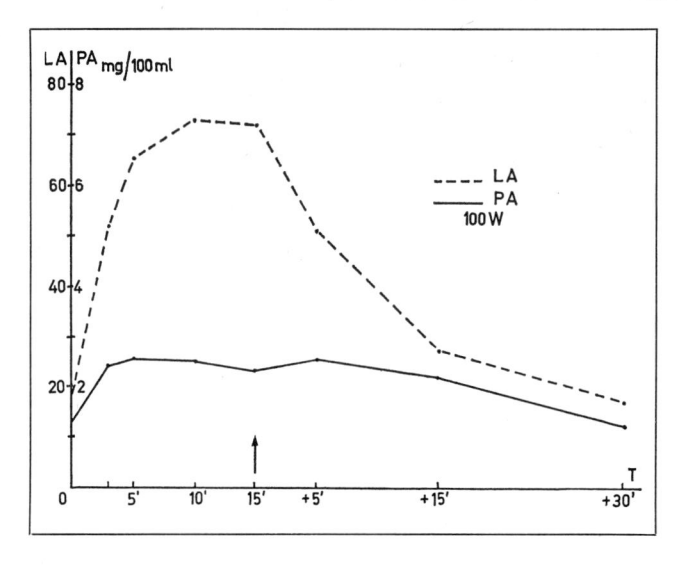

Figure 13. Evolution of LA and PA during and after work on a bicycle (samples from the brachial artery).

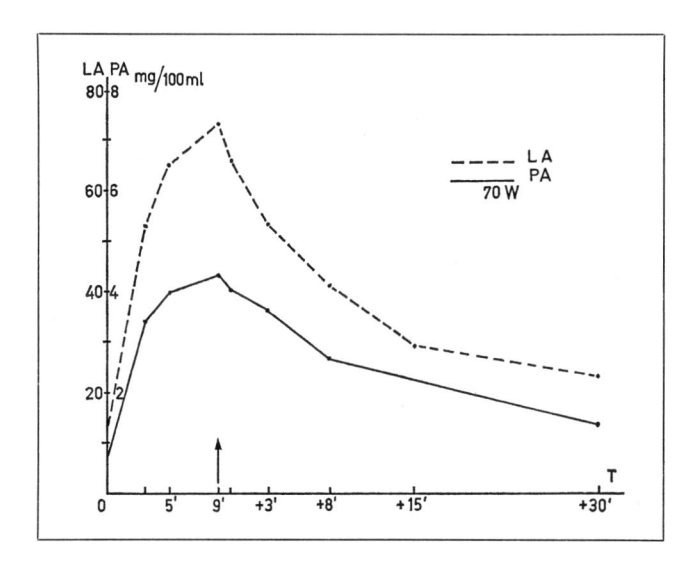

Figure 14. Evolution of LA and PA during and after work on a bicycle (samples from the brachial artery).

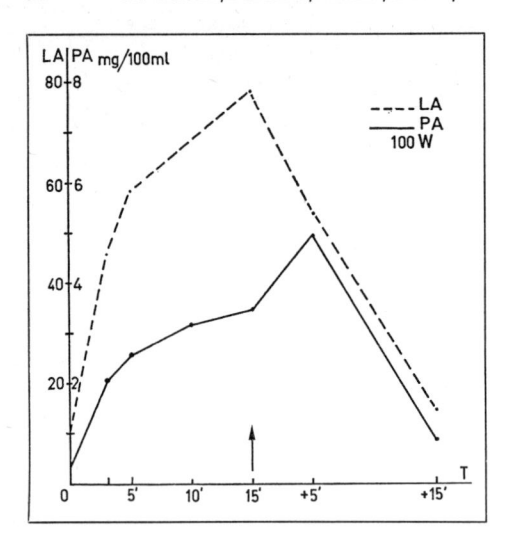

Figure 15. Evolution of LA and PA during and after work on a bicycle (samples from the brachial artery).

Lactic-Pyruvic Acid Ratio

Like all authors [1, 28, 29, 23, 24, 31, 39], we observed a very significant increase in the lactic-pyruvic acid ratio which at the beginning of exercise is always higher than at rest. It seems however difficult to provide quantitative values for this ratio, because pyruvic and lactic acid levels continuously change with time and have no parallel evolution. We studied the lactic-pyruvic acid ratio in 10 normal subjects, in 10 patients suffering from mitral stenosis and in 8 cases of lung disease. Table IV shows that the ratio varies in different ways even in the same group of patients. It sometimes increases continuously with time and sometimes at the beginning of exercise with a final plateau; sometimes, after an initial increase, it decreases during exercise. The reasons why this lactic-pyruvic acid ratio changes and its biochemical significance are not clear. No correlation could be made with the respiratory or circulatory parameters which were recorded and measured simultaneously in these cases.

The Excess Lactate Concept

In 1958, HUCKABEE showed that an isolated increase in lactic acid could be subsequent to metabolic or respiratory changes without any cellular hypoxia [28]. He proposed a formula for the calculation of what he

Table IV. Evolution of LA, PA, LA/PA ratio and XL in 10 normal subjects, 10 patients with mitral stenosis and 8 patients with respiratory insufficiency

		Normal subjects 10 cases	Mitral stenosis 10 cases	Pulm. disease 8 cases
AL	↗	4	6	4
	↗ →	1		2
	↗ ↘	5	4	2
AP	↗	2	4	4
	↗ →	4	3	4
	↗ ↘	4	3	
AL/AP	↗	1	2	2
	↗ →	5		2
	↗ ↘	4	8	4
XL	↗	4	4	3
	↗ →	3	1	4
	↗ ↘	3	5	1

called 'excess lactate', *i.e.* the fraction of lactic acid connected with cellular hypoxia only. In his work, the author showed a remarkable parallelism between the oxygen debt and the amount of oxygen necessary for oxidizing the excess lactate. This correlation would not exist between the oxygen debt and the amount of oxygen necessary to oxidize the lactic acid really measured.

This concept of 'excess lactate' was applied by many authors [4, 6, 8, 9, 32, 36] to various pathological conditions and it is obvious that the excess lactate is always important in cases of intensive exercise or in cases of badly tolerated exercise where lactic acid progressively increases. But when exercise is well tolerated, there can be a decrease in lactic acid as well as in the excess lactate even during exercise as shown in table IV. During recovery, we sometimes obtained negative values for excess lactate as it has been reported by WASSERMAN *et al.* [41], THOMAS *et al.* [39] and HARRIS *et al.* [24]. On the other hand, we did not find the excellent correlation reported by HUCKABEE [29] between oxygen debt and excess lactate. Nor did we find the high lactic acid levels obtained by this author when respiratory or metabolic alcalosis is only present. Indeed we never found important lactates values in patients with respiratory insufficiency who were well oxygenated and submitted to artificial ventilation with respiratory alcalosis and pH sometimes reaching 7.50 or 7.55. In our opinion, the excess lactate concept has no precise significance and the results obtained by HUCKABEE need further confirmation [13].

Conclusion

We think we have pointed out the various factors which, independently of the load, can influence the arterial level of lactic acid. The interpretation of some of our observations seems to be rather difficult, particularly the decrease of the lactic acid level during prolonged exercise and even sometimes during effort of rather short duration. Finally, the relationship between the oxygen debt and the lactates level is probably much more complex than it was stated before.

Summary

The precision of the enzymatic technique for lactic and pyruvic acids dosage in plasma is calculated from duplicates and proves to augment with larger acid concentrations.

The increase in lactic and pyruvic acids blood level during exercise is by 60% higher than the decrease in total CO_2.

Several factors influence the amount of acid metabolites during exercise: analysis of total blood or plasma, arterial or venous sampling, moment of sampling and type of exercise.

In normal subjects exercising on the bicycle ergometer, lactic acid increases after 30 sec until the 3rd or 5th min. When exercise is prolonged and not too heavy the lactic acid level decreases yet during effort. Recovery curves are complex and hard to analyse mathematically.

The evolution of pyruvic acid as well as of lactic-pyruvic acid ratio is much less systematic.

The 'excess lactate' concept is criticized on the basis of personal observations.

References

1. ASMUSSEN, F.: Pyruvate and lactate content of the blood during and after muscular work. Acta physiol. scand. *20:* 125 (1950).
2. ÅSTRAND, P. O.; HALLBÄCK, I.; HEDMAN, R. and SALTIN, B.: Blood lactates after prolonged severe exercise. J. appl. Physiol. *18:* 619 (1963).
3. BISHOP, J. M.; DONALD, K. W.; TAYLOR, S. M. and WORMALD, P. W.: The blood flow in the human arm during supine leg exercise. J. Physiol. *137:* 294 (1957).

4. BRUCE, R. A.; JONES, J. W. and GAIL, B.: Anaerobic metabolic responses to acute maximal exercise in male athletes. Circulation 26: 692 (1962).
5. CARLSON, L. A. and PERNOW, B.: Oxygen utilization and lactic acid formation in the legs at rest and during exercise in normal subjects and in patients with arteriosclerosis obliterans. Acta med. scand. 164: 39 (1959).
6. CARLSON, L. A. and PERNOW, B.: Studies on the peripheral circulation and metabolism in man. I. O_2 utilization and lactate pyruvate formation in the legs at rest and during exercise in healthy subjects. Acta physiol. scand. 52: 328 (1961).
7. CARLSON, L. A.; PERNOW, B. and ZETTERQUIST, S.: Studies on the peripheral circulation and metabolism in man. III. O_2 utilization and lactate pyruvate formation in the legs at rest and during exercise in subjects with hyperkinetic circulation and low physical capacity (vasoregulatory asthenia) and in healthy females. Acta med. scand. 172: 389 (1962).
8. COBB, L. A.; JOHNSON, W. P.; STRAIT, G. and BRUCE, R. A.: Circulatory and metabolic responses to strenuous exercise in trained and untrained normal men. Clin. Res. 10: 100 (1962).
9. COBB, L. A. and JOHNSON, W. P.: Hemodynamic relationship of anerobic metabolism and plasma free fatty acids during prolonged strenuous exercise in trained and untrained subjects. J. clin. Invest. 42: 800 (1963).
10. DAVIS, H. and GAZETOPOULOS, N.: Dyspnea in cyanotic congenital heart disease. Brit. Heart J. 27: 28 (1965).
11. DE COSTER, A.; MESSIN, R. et FRANCKSON, J. R. M.: Répartition de l'acide lactique entre plasma et globules rouges chez l'homme. Comparaison des résultats fournis par différentes méthodes de dosage. Arch. Int. Physiol. Bioch. 74: 251 (1966).
12. DE COSTER, A.: Les espaces extracellulaires au cours de l'effort physique. Fonds de la Recherche Scientifique Médicale; p. 136 (1966).
13. DE COSTER, A.; MESSIN, R. et DEGRE, S.: Etude critique de la notion d'excess lactate. Fonds de la Recherche Scientifique Médicale; p. 129 (1966).
14. DE COSTER, A. et MESSIN, R.: Evolution des acides lactiques artériel et veineux au cours des épreuves d'effort. Arch. Int. Phys. Bioch. 72: 567 (1964).
15. DEVADATA, S. C.: Distribution of lactate between the corpuscles and the plasma in blood. Quart. J. exp. Physiol. 24: 294 (1935).
16. DILL, D. B.; TALBOT, J. H. and EDWARDS, H. T.: Studies in muscular activity. VI. Response of several individuals to a fixed task. J. Physiol. 69: 267 (1930).
17. DONALD, K. W.; WORMALD, P. N.; TAYLOR, S. H. and BISHOP, J. M.: Changes in the O_2 content of femoral venous blood and leg blood flow during leg exercise in relation to cardiac output response. Clin. Sci. 16: 567 (1957).
18. GESELL, R.; KRUEGER, H.; NICHOLSON, H.; BRASSFIELD, C. and BELECOVICH, M.: A comparison of the response of the anesthetized dog to i. v. administration of CNNa during uniform artificial ventilation and during normally controlled ventilation with additional observations on the effects of methylene blue. Amer. J. Physiol. 100: 227 (1932).
19. GOLDSMITH, G. A. and FONTNOTE, A.: The blood lactate-pyruvate relationship in various physiologic and pathologic states. Amer. J. med. Sci. 215: 182 (1948).
20. GROAG, B. und SCHWARZ, H.: Der Einfluss der Muskelarbeit auf die Blutmilchsäure, Alkalireserve, Azidität des Harns usw. bei Kreislaufkrankən. Arch. exp. Path. Pharmakol. 121: 23 (1927).
21. HALDI, J.: Lactic acid in blood and tissues following intravenous injection of sodium bicarbonate. Amer. J. Physiol. 106: 134 (1933).
22. HARRIS, P.; BATEMAN, M. and GLOSTER, J.: Relations between the cardio-

respiratory effects of exercise and the arterial concentration of lactate and pyruvate in patients with rheumatic heart disease. Clin. Sci. *23:* 531 (1962).
23. HARRIS, P.; BATEMAN, M. and GLOSTER, J.: The regional metabolism of lactate and pyruvate during exercise in patients with rheumatic heart disease. Clin. Sci. *23:* 545 (1962).
24. HARRIS, P.; BATEMAN, M.; BAYLEY, T. J.; GLOSTER, J. and WHITEHEAD, T.: Observation on the course of the metabolic events accompanying mild exercise. Quart. J. exp. Physiol. *53:* 43 (1968).
25. HILL, A. V.; LONG, C. N. H. and LUPTON, H.: Muscular exercise, lactic acid and supply and utilization of oxygen. V. The recovery process after exercise in man. Proc. Roy. Soc. B. *97:* 96 (1924).
26. HILL, A. V.; LONG, C. N. H. and LUPTON, H.: Muscular exercise, lactic acid and supply and utilization of oxygen. Proc. Roy. Soc. B. *97:* 84 (1924).
27. HUCKABEE, W. E.: Control of concentration gradients of pyruvate and lactate across cell membranes in blood. J. appl. Physiol. *9:* 163 (1956).
28. HUCKABEE, W. E.: Relationships of pyruvate and lactate during anaerobic metabolism. I. Effects of infusion of pyruvate or glucose and of hyperventilation. J. clin. Invest. *37:* 244 (1958).
29. HUCKABEE, W. E.: Relationships of pyruvate and lactate during anaerobic metabolism. II. Exercise and formation of O_2 debt. J. clin. Invest. *37:* 255 (1958).
30. JOHNSON, R. E.; EDWARDS, H. T.; DILL, D. B. and WILSON, J. W.: Blood as a physiochemical system. XIII. The distribution of lactate. J. biol. Chem. *157:* 461 (1945).
31. JONES, W. B.; THOMAS, H. D. and REEVES, T. S.: Circulatory and ventilatory responses to postprandial exercise. Amer. Heart J. *69:* 668 (1965).
32. KNUTTGEN, H. G.: Oxygen debt, lactate, pyruvate and excess lactate after muscular work. J. appl. Physiol. *17:* 639 (1962).
33. LUNDIN, G. and STRÖM, G.: The concentration of blood lactic acid in man during muscular work in relation to the partial pressure of oxygen of the inspired air. Acta physiol. scand. *13:* 253 (1947).
34. MARGARIA, R.; EDWARDS, H. T. and DILL, D. B.: The possible mechanism of contracting and paying the oxygen debt and the role of lactic acid in muscular contraction. Amer. J. Physiol. *106:* 689 (1933).
35. MARGARIA, R.: Biochemistry of muscular contraction and recovery. J. Sport. Med. *3:* 145 (1963).
36. MUYSERS, K.; WORTH, G. and SIEHOF, F.: L'équilibre acidobasique chez les silicotiques. Ent. Phys. Resp., Nancy, octobre 1964.
37. SACHS, J. and SACHS, W.: Blood and muscle lactic acid in the steady state. Amer. J. Physiol. *118:* 697 (1937).
38. SALTIN, B. and STENBERG, J.: Circulatory response to prolonged severe exercise. J. appl. Physiol. *19:* 833 (1964).
39. THOMAS, H. P.; BOSHELL, B.; GAOS, C. and REEVES, T. J.: Cardiac output during exercise and anaerobic metabolism in man. J. appl. Physiol. *19:* 839 (1964).
40. VISSER, B. F.; KREUKNIET, J. and MASS, A. H. V.: Increase of whole blood lactic acid concentration during exercise as predicted from pH and PCO_2 determination. Pflügers Arch. ges. Physiol. *281:* 300 (1964).
41. WASSERMAN, K.; BURTON, G. G. and VAN KESSEL, A. L.: Excess lactate concept and O_2 debt of exercise. J. appl. Physiol. *20:* 1299 (1965).

Author's address: Dr. A. DE COSTER, Department of Respiratory Diseases, Hôpital Saint-Pierre, *Brussels* (Belgium).

pO_2, pH, and pCO_2 in the Coronarvenous and Femoralvenous Blood During Exercise and Hypoxia

E. Doll and J. Keul

Department of Internal Medicine, University of Freiburg i. Br.

In 26 healthy persons aged 20–30, we measured the oxygen pressure of the coronarvenous blood and of the venous blood of the working muscles, further the arterial-coronarvenous and the arterial-femoralvenous oxygen content difference. The measurements were made at rest, under submaximal and maximal steady state stress, and during recovery. Simultaneously, the subjects were made to breath air of 20.9%, 15.9%, and 12.7% oxygen content, corresponding to an altitude of 260 m, 2500 m, and 4250 m above sea level. The coronarvenous blood was drawn by a catheter in the sinus coronarius, the venous blood from the working muscles was drawn by a catheter in a deep femoral vein.

The arterial oxygen pressure does not sink significantly during respiration of normal air, even during extreme physical exertion. At 15.9% hypoxia, it already falls during rest to 69 Torr. At 12.7% hypoxia it falls at rest to 47 Torr. At both 15.9% and 12.7% hypoxia, in contrast to normal atmospheric conditions, the arterial oxygen pressure continues to fall, since the diffusion capacity of the lungs is diminished under these conditions.

The coronarvenous oxygen pressure (figure 1) under normal atmospheric conditions amounts to 24 Torr at rest. During strenuous exercise it decreases an average 3 Torr. A further decrease of 2–3 Torr is avoided by the fact that during exertion the pH of the coronarvenous blood sinks to an average of 7.266, causing the oxygen dissociation curve to be moved to the right.

In the third minute of recovery, the coronarvenous oxygen pressure shows a rapid decrease. This rise results partly from a further adjustment of the oxygen dissociation curve towards the right, partly from the increase (relative to heart activity) in blood supply to the heart muscle.

Although the coronarvenous oxygen pressure under hypoxia was lower at rest than during normal atmospheric conditions – particularly at 12.7% – the subsequent decrease is seen to be only slight, and not significant, even during maximal exertion. The critical coronarvenous oxygen pressure,

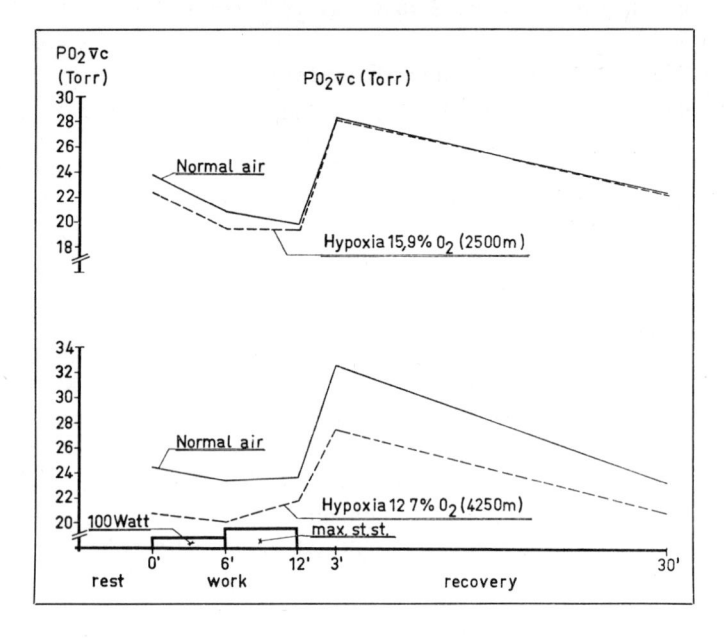

Figure 1. Coronarvenous oxygen pressure at rest, during exercise and recovery.
────── normal atmospheric conditions
------ hypoxia
max. st. st. = maximal steady state

which BRETSCHNEIDER has identified as 7 Torr, was not approached at any time.

The arterial-coronarvenous oxygen content difference (figure 2) under 15.9% hypoxia is not different at rest and in normal atmosphere. At 100 watts and during maximal steady state stress, the arterial-coronarvenous oxygen content difference is reduced 9% compared to normal atmosphere.

Under 12.7% hypoxia, the arterial-coronarvenous oxygen content difference decreases at rest 17.7% compared to normal. During submaximal *and* maximal steady state stress, the decrease amounts to 30%.

The relatively slight decrease in coronarvenous oxygen pressure even during intensive work under hypoxic conditions corresponding to 4250 m above sea level shows that even in this situation the oxygen supply to the heart is guaranteed. It is important to note that under severe hypoxic conditions – as compared to normal atmosphere or moderately hypoxic conditions – no rise in the arterial-coronarvenous oxygen difference is ob-

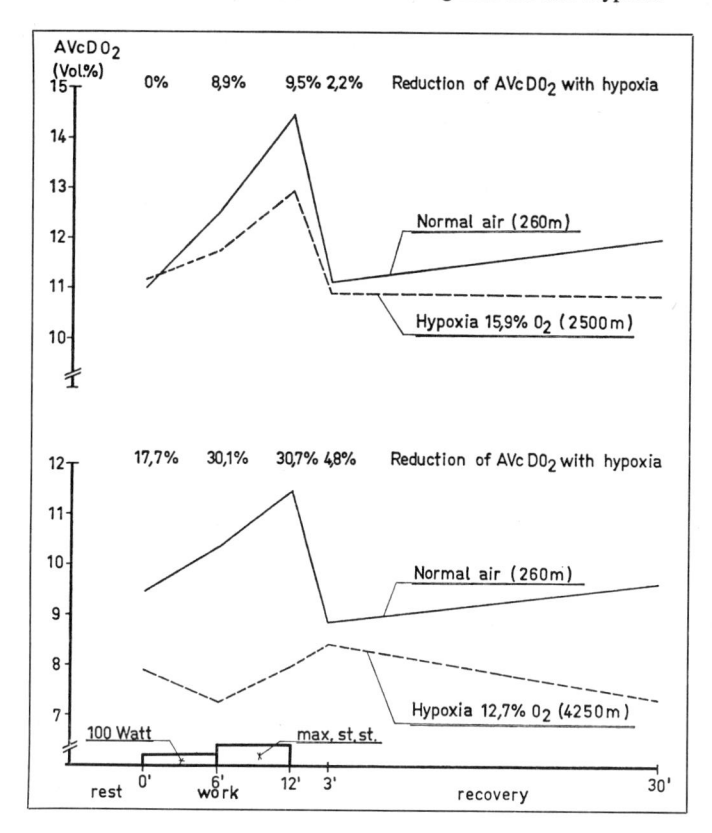

Figure 2. Arterial-coronarvenous oxygen content difference in normal atmosphere (———) and under hypoxic conditions (------), at rest, during exercise and recovery.

served under increased stress. This difference, which at 12.7% hypoxia is already reduced during rest, shows no further alteration under increased stress. This demonstrates that in healthy persons the oxygen supply to the heart muscle is assured even in situations of maximal stress, thanks mainly to the extraordinary adaptability of coronary circulation, and *not* primarily to intensified oxygen uptake from the venous blood.

The oxygen supply to the working muscles does not react in the same way as that to the heart muscle. During rest the oxygen pressure at 15.9% and 12.7% hypoxia already lies about 10 Torr below the value for normal atmospheric conditions (figure 3). Whereas the oxygen pressure of the coronarvenous blood did not sink significantly during exertion, that of the venous blood leaving the working muscles shows a considerable further

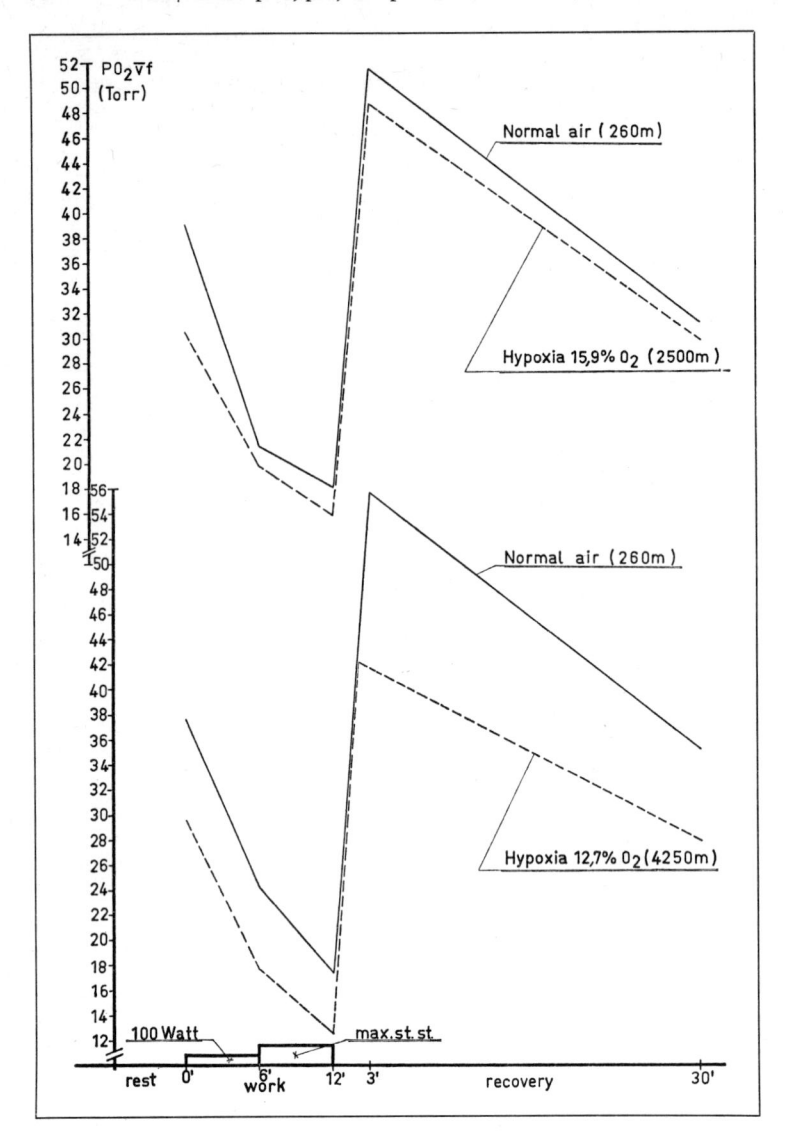

Figure 3. Femoralvenous oxygen pressure at rest, during exercise and recovery.
─────── normal atmospheric conditions
------ hypoxia

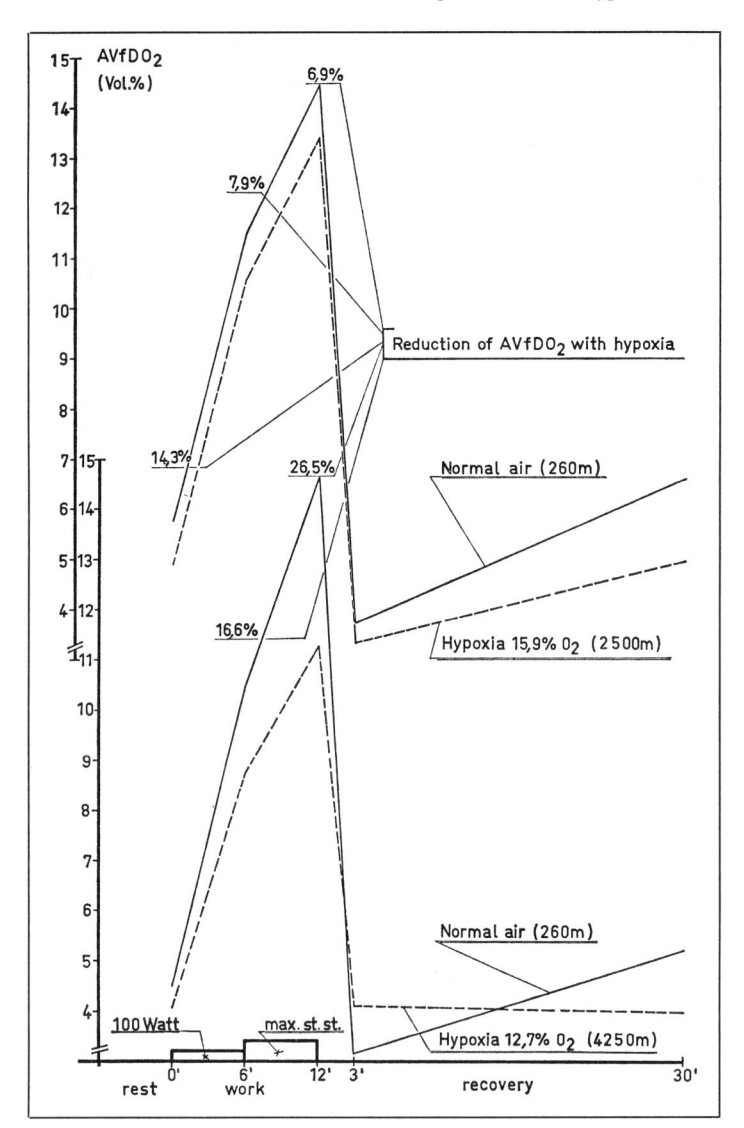

Figure 4. Arterial-venous oxygen content difference of skeletal muscles at rest, during exercise and recovery.
——— normal atmospheric conditions
------ hypoxia

decrease under stress, both under normal atmospheric conditions and hypoxia. At 12.7% hypoxia, corresponding to an altitude of 4250 m above sea level, the average of 12.6 Torr nearly reaches the critical venous oxygen pressure for skeletal muscles; in a few cases STAINSBY's critical value of 10 Torr was passed, so that metabolism could no longer be carried on aerobically and the oxygen supply to the working muscles became a limiting factor for performance. Dr. KEUL will show in his paper that in these cases changes in metabolism are observed indicating an increased role of anaerobic energy output.

The arterial-venous oxygen content difference of the skeletal muscles (figure 4) at rest and during stress is less under hypoxic conditions than during respiration of normal air, although this effect is less pronounced than in the heart muscle. Under stress, however, the increase in the arterial-venous oxygen content difference of the skeletal muscles in normal air is three to four times as high as that of the heart muscle. At 15.9% hypoxia corresponding to 4250 m above sea level, the oxygen content difference under stress climbs still higher, from 4.1 to 11.3 vol%, whereas in the heart muscle it remains unchanged under the same circumstances.

Under the conditions described, a decisive difference is observed between the oxygen supply to the heart and that to the skeletal muscles. Under the same stress conditions, the heart muscle is capable of filling its oxygen requirements through increased circulation for a longer period. In performing the same physical work, the skeletal muscle, which exhausts its possibilities of increasing circulation more rapidly, must turn earlier to an extensive oxygen extraction from the venous blood. The result is that the critical venous oxygen pressure of the working muscles is finally reached and that – in contrast to the heart muscle – a point is reached by which physical performance is limited.

Authors' address: Dr. E. DOLL and Dr. J. KEUL, Medizinische Universitätsklinik, Hugstetterstrasse 55, *78 Freiburg i.Br.* (Germany).

The Influence of Exercise and Hypoxia on the Substrate Uptake of Human Heart and Human Skeletal Muscles

J. Keul and E. Doll

Department of Medicine, University Hospital, Freiburg i. Br.

29 healthy male persons were examined during heavy work on a bicycle ergometer under normal barometric conditions and hypoxia [3]. Arterial, coronary venous and femoralvenous blood were drawn off for analysis of glucose, lactate, pyruvate, free fatty acids, β-hydroxybutyrate, acetacetate, amino acids and ammonia and also oxygen content [3].

Under hypoxia with 15.9% oxygen, the arterial substrate levels show no important changes during the steady-state. Under conditions of 12.7% oxygen, the arterial levels of glucose, lactate and free fatty acids, as well as ammonia, are significantly higher than in normal air [14].

The reason for the rise in the lactate level during physical work under hypoxic conditions is an increased anoxidative energy production by the skeletal muscle (figure 1). The arteriovenous differences of the various substrates such as glucose, lactate, pyruvate and free fatty acids do not alone provide sufficient evidence for a quantitative evaluation of the substrate metabolism under hypoxic conditions. The decrease in the arteriovenous oxygen differences [3, 4, 5], and unknown changes in blood flow in the muscles must be taken into account for such a quantitative evaluation. The arteriovenous substrate differences must be correlated with the arteriovenous oxygen difference. For this reason the chief energy-producing substrates were computed first as oxygen equivalents, and then compared.

In normal air, the arteriovenous difference for glucose decreases during exercise, but much more in relation to the oxygen uptake. The free fatty acids show an absolute increase as well as a relative increase compared to oxygen uptake (figure 2). Glycogen is not involved in energy production at rest, but contributes considerably during physical stress. The quantity involved can be established on the basis of the known arteriovenous oxygen and substrate differences, or of the local respiratory quotient and the lactate and pyruvate output of the muscle. With hypoxia of 15.9% oxygen, no important difference is found. However, in relation to the smaller arteriovenous oxygen differences at 12.6% oxygen, the oxygen equivalents of glucose and glycogen are significantly higher and those of free fatty acids

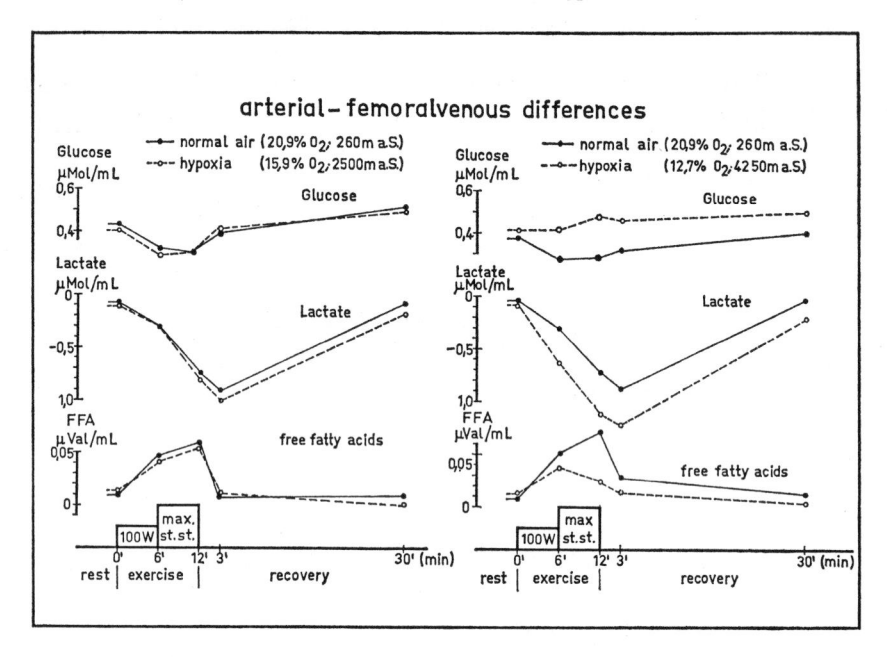

Figure 1. The arterial-femoralvenous differences for glucose, lactate and free fatty acids under normal air and hypoxia in rest, during submaximal work (100 W) and maximal steady state (normal air: 200 W, 15.9% hypoxia: 190 W, 12.7% hypoxia: 165 W).

are lower. Under these circumstances, despite the diminished arteriovenous oxygen difference, the highest lactate output is observed.

On the basis of the oxygen and substrate uptake by the muscle, the amount of ATP produced per unit of blood flowing through the muscle can be calculated (table I). The results show that under normal atmospheric conditions the amount of ATP metabolized per unit of blood increases from rest to maximal steady-state. The energy produced anoxidatively during maximal steady-state under normal air amounts to 7.8%. Under conditions of 15.9% hypoxia the amount of energy produced oxidatively per unit of blood is slightly decreased, the amount produced anaerobically slightly increased. A distinct change is observed at 12.7% hypoxia during submaximal and maximal work, there is an unmistakable decrease of ATP-production relative to the amount of blood flow in the muscles. The amount of *additional* energy produced anaerobically under 12.7% oxygen is about 5% during maximal steady-state [9, 14].

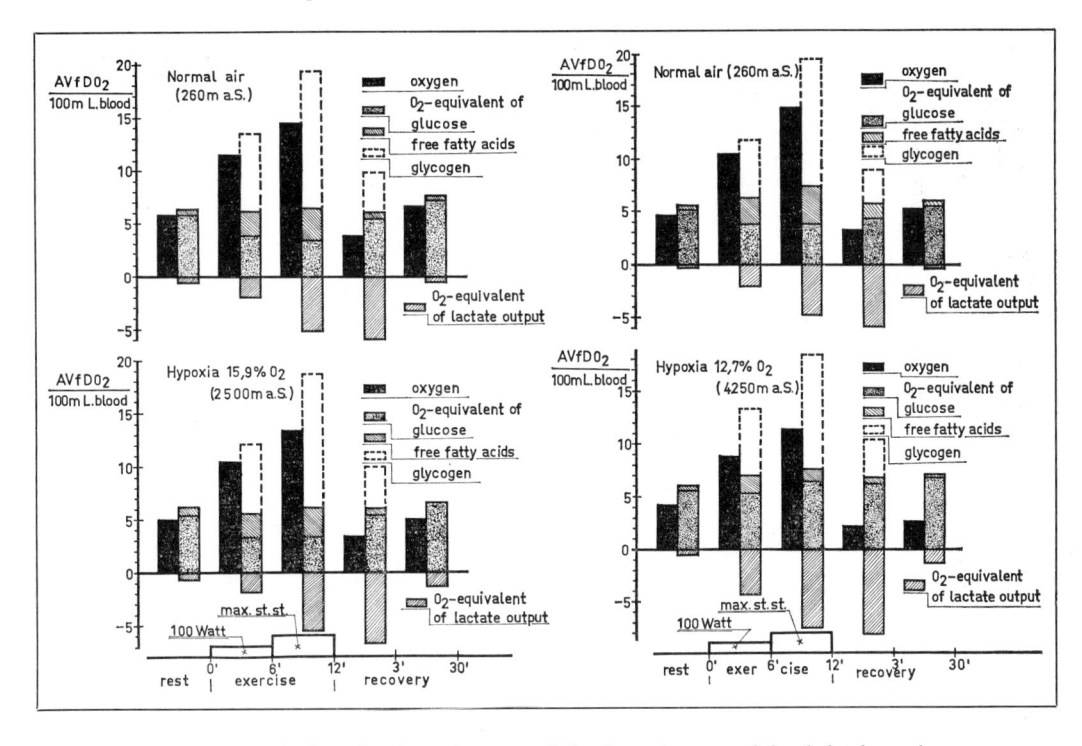

Figure 2. The oxygen equivalents for the main energy delivering substrates of the skeletal muscle.

Table I. The theoretical energy production in skeletal muscle counted from arterial femoralvenous oxygen and substrate differences

| | \multicolumn{6}{c}{Energy production (mM ATP/L blood)} |||||||
| | normal air (260 m a.S.) || | Hypoxia 15.9% O_2 (2500 m a.S.) || | Hypoxia 12.7% O_2 (4250 m a.S.) || |
	rest		exercise	rest		exercise	rest		exercise
		100 W	max.st.st.		100 W	max.st.st.		100 W	max.st.st.
oxidative	15.4	31.3	39.2	14.2	27.2	35.9	12.8	24.0	28.8
unoxidative	0.9	1.6	3.1	0.8	1.6	3.1	0.8	2.0	3.6
unoxidative in % of oxidative	5.8	5.1	7.8	5.6	5.9	8.6	6.3	8.4	12.5

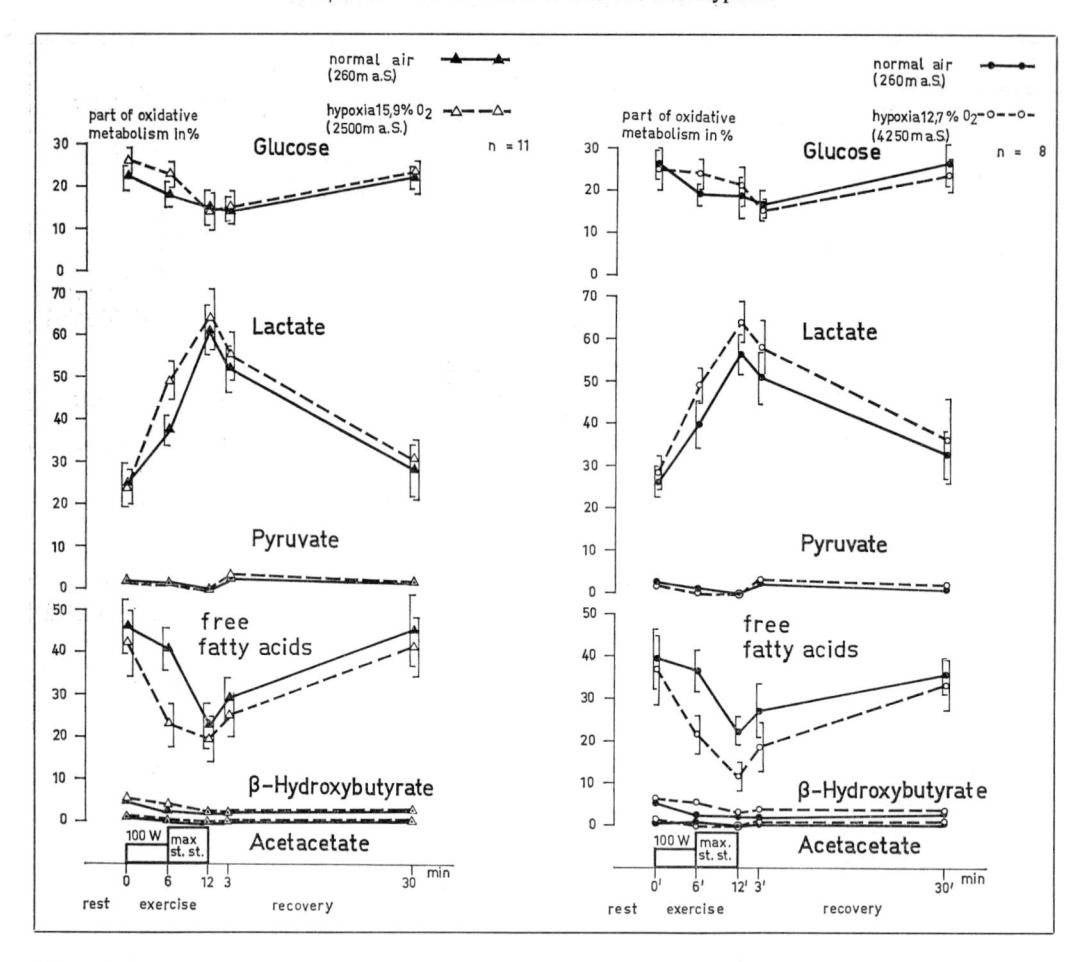

Figure 3. The per cent of oxidative metabolism of the human heart in normal air and hypoxia in rest and during exercise. (Coronary-venous blood was drawn off by a catheter).

Considering the human heart, the situation is fundamentally different [4, 5, 10, 11, 12, 13]. At altitudes up to 4250 m, there is no lack of oxygen for the heart muscle. This fact is proven not only by the behavior of the coronary-venous oxygen pressure, but also by the lactate/pyruvate ratio and the lactate uptake [6].

There is no difficulty in discovering the role of the various substrates in the oxidative metabolism of the heart muscle, since, (1) no lactate is discharged, (2) the extracted substrates are all completely metabolized, – there is no storage worth mentioning.

During work and under the conditions of hypoxia (15.9% O_2) there was no important difference in substrate uptake in the human heart as compared to the values under normal barometric conditions (figure 3).

During inhalation of an oxygen mixture of 12.7%, the per cent of free fatty acids employed in energy production during and immediatly following physical exercise is reduced. This is compensated for by an increased utilisation of lactate and glucose for energy production. The carbohydrate metabolites play an increased role in energy production under hypoxic conditions.

What causes lie behind these changes in the role of the various substrates in energy production of the heart when there is no oxygen deficit? (1) Changes in the arterial substrate levels, particularly of lactate, free fatty acids, and β-hydroxybutyrate [14]. Increased levels of lactate and β-hydroxybutyrate in the arterial blood reduce the uptake of free fatty acids [7, 8, 10, 11, 12, 13]. (2) The increased velocity of blood flow through the myocardium. The diffusion of lactate in the myocardium could be unaffected by the increased velocity of coronary blood flow; whereas the active transport of free fatty acids or glucose through the heart muscle cells might be insufficient at such high velocity. – According to these results, the substrate and oxygen supply of the heart is not endangered for healthy persons at an altitude up to 4250 m [1, 2, 9, 14].

The reason for the diminished performance in man under hypoxia is the oxygen deficit in skeletal muscle, which cannot be totally compensated by anoxidative processes.

Supported by Deutsche Forschungsgemeinschaft and Kuratorium für Sportmedizin.

References

1. DOLL, E.; KEUL, J.; BRECHTEL, A. und REINDELL, H.: Die arteriellen Blutgase bei Verminderung der Sauerstoffkonzentration in der Inspirationsluft während körperlicher Arbeit. Int. Z. angew. Physiol. 25: 46 (1968).
2. DOLL, E.; KEUL, J.; BRECHTEL, A.; LIMÓN-LASON, R. und REINDELL, H.: I. Der Einfluss körperlicher Arbeit auf die arteriellen Blutgase in Freiburg und Mexico City. Sportarzt u. Sportmed. 8: 317 (1967).
3. DOLL, E. and KEUL, J.: Oxygen pressure and oxygen saturation in the coronarvenous' and femoralvenous' blood during exercise and hypoxia. (This Journal in press.)
4. DOLL, E.; KEUL, J.; STEIM, H.; MAIWALD, Ch. und REINDELL, H.: Über den Stoffwechsel des menschlichen Herzens. II. Das Verhalten von PO_2, PCO_2, pH, Standardbikarbonat und base excess im coronarvenösen Blut in Ruhe,

während und nach körperlicher Arbeit. Pflügers Arch. ges. Physiol. *282:* 28 (1965).

5. DOLL, E.; KEUL, J.; STEIM, H.; MAIWALD, CH. und REINDELL, H.: Über den Stoffwechsel des Herzens bei Hochleistungssportlern. II. Mitt., Z. Kreisl-Forsch. *3:* 248 (1966).
6. HERMAN, M.V.; ELLIOTT, W.C. and GORLIN, R.: An electrocardiographic, anatomic, and metabolic study of zonal myocardial ischemia in coronary heart disease. Circulation *35:* 834 (1967).
7. HIRCHE, HJ. und RÖHNER, G.: Änderungen der Substrataufnahme des Herzmuskels bei induzierten Änderungen der arteriellen Substratkonzentration. Pflügers Arch. ges. Physiol. *278:* 408 (1963).
8. HIRCHE, HJ. und LOCHNER, W.: Über den Stoffwechsel des Herzens bei vermehrtem Milchsäureangebot. Verh. dtsch. Ges. Kreisl-Forsch. *27:* 207–212 (Steinkopff Verlag, Darmstadt 1961).
9. KEUL, J.; DOLL, E.; LIMÓN-LASON, R.; MERZ, P. und REINDELL, H.: II. Der Einfluss körperlicher Arbeit auf die arteriellen Glucose-, Lactat- und Pyruvatspiegel in Freiburg und in Mexico City. Sportarzt u. Sportmed. *8:* 327 (1967).
10. KEUL, J.; DOLL, E. and KEPPLER, D.: The substrate supply of the human skeletal muscle at rest, during and after work. Experientia *23:* 974 (1967).
11. KEUL, J.; KEPPLER, D. and DOLL, E.: Lactate-pyruvate ratio and its relation to oxygen pressure in arterial, coronarvenous and femoralvenous blood. Arch. int. Physiol. Bioch. *75:* 573 (1967).
12. KEUL, J.; DOLL, E.; STEIM, H.; HOMBURGER, H.; KERN, H.; SINGER, U. und REINDELL, H.: Über den Stoffwechsel des menschlichen Herzens. I. Die Substratversorgung des menschlichen Herzens in Ruhe, während und nach körperlicher Arbeit. Pflügers Arch. ges. Physiol. *282:* 1 (1965).
13. KEUL, J.; DOLL, E.; STEIM, H.; FLEER, U. und REINDELL, H.: Über den Stoffwechsel des menschlichen Herzens. III. Der oxidative Stoffwechsel des Herzens unter verschiedenen Arbeitsbedingungen. Pflügers Arch. ges. Physiol. *282:* 43 (1965).
14. KEUL, J.; DOLL, E.; ERICHSEN, H. und REINDELL, H.: Die arteriellen Substratspiegel bei Verminderung der Sauerstoffkonzentration in der Inspirationsluft während körperlicher Arbeit. Int. Z. angew. Physiol. *25:* 89 (1968).

Authors' address: Dr. J. KEUL and Dr. E. DOLL, Department of Medicine, University Hospital, *78 Freiburg i.Br.* (Germany).

Oscillations of Acid-Base Equilibrium During Maximum Exercise

R. J. Shephard

Department of Physiological Hygiene, School of Hygiene, University of Toronto

Respiratory oscillations of alveolar carbon dioxide tension are of practical importance when estimating the mean gradient of CO_2 tension between alveolar gas and arterial blood. If transmitted to the arterial blood stream, they could also have important implications for the respiratory control mechanism. Previous studies [Dubois et al., 1951; Lamb et al., 1965 and Lacoste, 1958] have been confined to rest and moderate exercise. The present communication describes a theoretical and experimental study of maximum exercise now in progress in my laboratory.

The computer programme used to calculate the oscillation is outlined in fig. 1. The breathing cycle is divided into equal segments of 10 ms length, and a number of simple calculations are carried out for each segment. The method of calculation is modified, Dubois et al. [1951], when the dead space is inhaled, and, Lamb et al. [1965], when the tidal volume is inhaled. An estimate of the end-tidal CO_2 concentration is initially inserted in the programme, and iteration continues through successive breathing cycles until input and output coincide to 0.001%.

The figures used in the calculation are based for convenience on personal experience, but contain no unusual values. The distribution of alveolar volumes, ventilation and perfusion in a nine slice model of the lung is based on published work, particularly that of Dr. Anderson from this laboratory.

The extent of theoretical respiratory oscillations during maximum exercise is shown in fig. 2. Oscillations are of similar magnitude in all lung slices, and amount to about 5 mm Hg. The mean alveolar CO_2 tension in a given slice exceeds the mid-plateau value by about 0.7 mm Hg, but is about 0.7 mm Hg less than the end-tidal value; there is also a gradient of 3–4 mm Hg in the mean alveolar CO_2 tension from the first to the ninth slice. The lung as a whole mirrors the behaviour of the sixth slice.

If it is assumed that 55% of the pulmonary blood flow occurs during inspiration, this has the effect of damping the oscillations slightly.

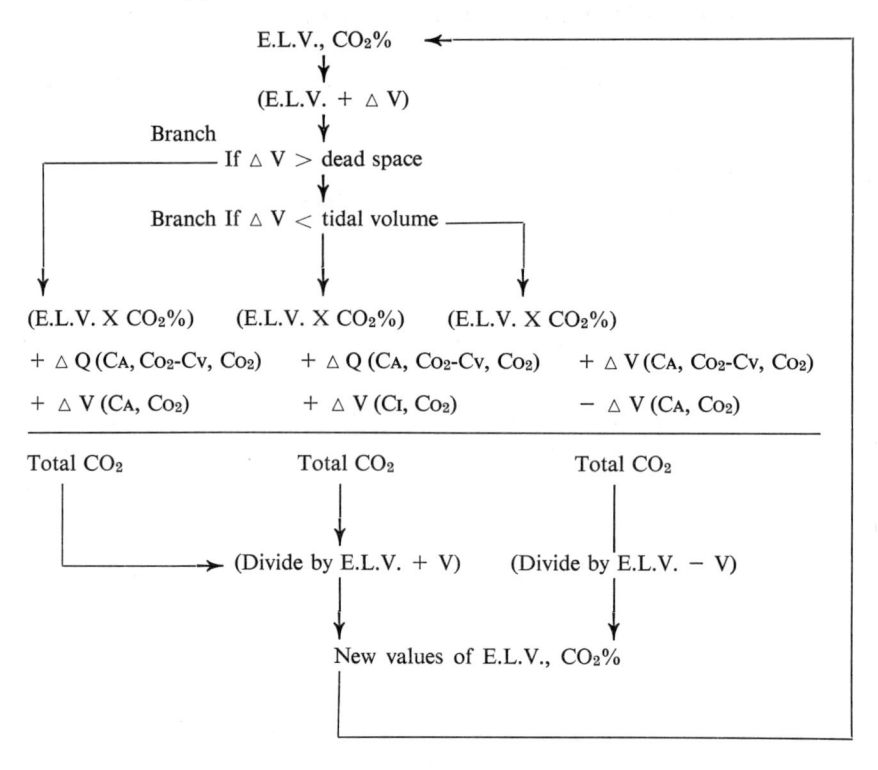

```
                        E.L.V., CO₂% ←─────────────┐
                             ↓                      │
                        (E.L.V. + Δ V)              │
            Branch            ↓                     │
        ┌──────────── If Δ V > dead space           │
        │                     ↓                     │
        │   Branch If Δ V < tidal volume ──────┐    │
        │            │            │            │    │
        ↓            ↓            ↓            ↓    │
  (E.L.V. × CO₂%)  (E.L.V. × CO₂%)  (E.L.V. × CO₂%) │
  + Δ Q(Cₐ,Co₂-Cv,Co₂)  + Δ Q(Cₐ,Co₂-Cv,Co₂)  + Δ V(Cₐ,Co₂-Cv,Co₂)
  + Δ V(Cₐ,Co₂)     + Δ V(Cᵢ,Co₂)          − Δ V(Cₐ,Co₂)
  ─────────────────────────────────────────────────
  Total CO₂        Total CO₂          Total CO₂
     │                 ↓                  │
     └──────────→ (Divide by E.L.V. + V)  (Divide by E.L.V. − V)
                       ↓                  ↓
                  New values of E.L.V., CO₂%
```

Figure 1. Method of calculating changes in alveolar carbon dioxide concentration during breathing cycle. The entire cycle shown is repeated every 10 ms throughout a respiratory cycle. Iteration continues until the CO_2 concentration at the beginning and end of the cycle are equal. (E.L.V. = effective lung volume, $CO_2\%$ = alveolar CO_2 percentage, Δ V and Δ Q = ventilation and blood flow in unit time)

However, the discrepancy between the true mean alveolar tension and the two estimates based on mid-plateau and end-tidal samples is unchanged.

Respiratory rate has a marked effect on the extent of oscillations (fig. 3). At low rates, the oscillations are exaggerated, and at high rates they are suppressed. At any given respiratory rate, an increase of tidal volume increases the oscillations; this is because in maximum exercise the increase tends to occur at the expense of the expiratory reserve, and the mean alveolar volume falls. An increase of physiological dead space increases both the mean alveolar CO_2 tension and the discrepancy between inspired and expired CO_2 tensions. However it has little influence upon the total extent of the oscillations. The damping of oscillations is increased with an increase in the

Oscillations of Acid-Base Equilibrium During Maximum Exercise

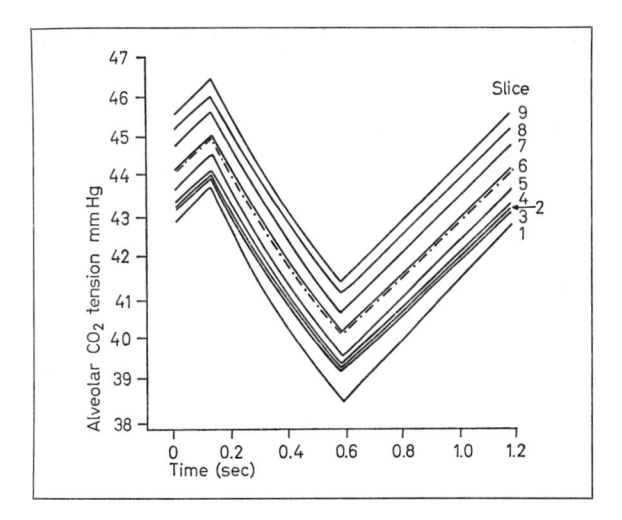

Figure 2. Oscillations of alveolar CO_2 tension during maximum exercise. Data for 9 slice model of the lung, with subjects exercising at maximum aerobic power. Average data for whole lung coincide closely with slice six.

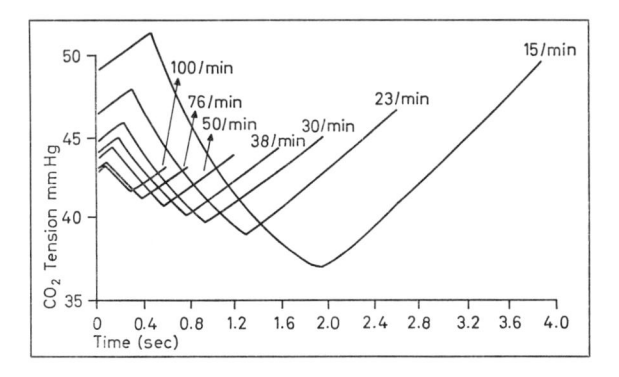

Figure 3. The influence of respiratory rate upon the fluctuations of alveolar CO_2 tension. Theoretical curves for subjects exercising at 80% of their aerobic power.

effective lung volume. However, the effect is not large over the likely range of values.

The extent of oscillations has been examined experimentally by means of a rapid-response infra-red CO_2 analyser sampling at the mouth. A typical expiratory record shows a phase of rapidly increasing CO_2 concentration, and then an upward sloping 'alveolar plateau'. There is a phase lag

Table I. Oscillations of expired CO_2 tension at selected respiratory rates. Experimental and theoretical data for 8 subjects exercising at 80% of aerobic power

Respiratory rate	Measured oscillation[1] mm Hg	Estimated total oscillation mm Hg[2]	mm Hg[3]	Theoretical oscillation (fig. 3) mm Hg
25	6.2	10.4	6.4	8.2
35	5.6	9.4	5.4	5.4
45	5.2	8.6	4.6	3.7
55	4.4	7.4	3.4	2.3

[1] Measured from the commencement of the alveolar plateau to the end-tidal point.

[2] Measured value increased by two-thirds to allow for transit through a dead space equal to 25% of tidal volume, and a further increase of alveolar CO_2 tension with inhalation of dead space gas.

[3] Previous column corrected by 4 mm Hg to allow for contribution of ventilation/perfusion effects to slope of alveolar plateau.

between alveolar gas and mouthpiece concentrations, due to transit time through the dead space, and the commencement of the alveolar plateau thus coincides in time with the minimum point of the oscillation. The end-tidal point falls short of the peak oscillation due to transit time through the dead space and the continuing increase of CO_2 tension during the early part of inspiration. The observed oscillation (table I) is thus only about 60% of the true oscillation. However, it is reinforced by the effect of ventilation/perfusion inequalities; these can amount to about 4 mm Hg. If correction is applied for these two sources of error, there is fair agreement between the observed oscillation and the theoretical prediction.

The alveolar-arterial gradient may be re-examined in the light of this work (table II). Traditionally, the end-tidal sample has been assumed representative of alveolar gas. This study suggests the true value in heavy exercise is mid-way between the mid-plateau and end-tidal values; further, a correction must be applied to the apparent end-tidal value to allow for the influence of ventilation/perfusion ratio on the slope of the alveolar plateau. If these factors are taken into account, the Aa gradient in heavy exercise amounts to 1–2 mm Hg. The contribution of spatial and temporal inequalities of ventilation to this gradient is about 0.1 mm Hg, shunts account for about 0.3 mm Hg, and the residual gradient of perhaps 1 mm Hg is due to the relatively slow rate of reaction of CO_2 that has entered the blood stream.

Table II. Effect of respiratory rate on CO_2 gradient between end-tidal sample and arterialized capillary blood. Experimental data for subjects exercising at 80% of aerobic power

Respiratory Rate	CO_2 Gradient (end-tidal)	Corrected alveolar-arterial gradient[1]
Group (a) (n = 8)		
25	−5.1 mm Hg	−1.5 mm Hg
35	−3.0	+0.4
45	−1.2	+2.1
55	−1.8	+1.3
Group (b) (n = 10)		
50	−0.7±2.9	
50 (HV)[2]	+4.1±7.0	
100 (HV)	+3.4±4.6	
50 (CO_2 HV)[3]	+4.1±4.7	
100 (CO_2 HV)	+0.8±6.5	

[1] The mean concentration of alveolar gas has been assumed to lie midway between the mean mid-plateau and end-tidal concentrations, and a correction of 2 mm Hg has been applied to the end-tidal reading to allow for VA/Q effects (see text).
[2] Voluntary hyperventilation
[3] CO_2 hyperventilation.

It is unlikely that the oscillations we have observed have practical significance for respiratory control mechanisms. In the blood stream, they are immediately damped to about a quarter of their alveolar size (1–2 mm Hg), and further damping undoubtedly occurs before they reach the chemosensitive tissues of the carotid body and fourth ventricle. Thus we may conclude that the oscillations are of vital importance to physiologists who use alveolar gas to calculate dead space, cardiac output and other parameters, but that the body in its wisdom is able to ignore them with impunity.

References

1. DUBOIS, A. B.; BRITT, A. G. and FENN, W. O.: Alveolar CO_2 during the respiratory cycle. U.S.A.F. Wright Field, Tech. Rept. *6528:* 419–432 (1951).
2. LACOSTE, J.: L'antagonisme ventilation – diffusion au cours du cycle respiratoires; Ph. D. Thesis, University of Nancy, France (1958).
3. LAMB, T. W.; ANTHONIESEN, N. R. and TENNEY, S. M.: Controlled frequency breathing during muscular exercise. J. appl. Physiol. *20:* 244–248 (1965).

Author's address: Dr. R. J. SHEPHARD, Department of Physiological Hygiene, School of Hygiene, University of Toronto, *Toronto* (Canada).

The Potentiating Effect of Low Oxygen Tension Exposure on Acid-Base Balance During Exhaustive Work in Humans

E. W. BANISTER

Human Performance Laboratory, Physical Development Centre, Simon Fraser University, Burnaby

Introduction

As a classical index of athletic performance, oxygen intake cannot differentiate between highly trained states. Indeed the recent papers of JONES [1967] and CAMPBELL [1967] have indicated that expired carbon dioxide and its blood gas concentrations may be more useful as indices of limited exercise tolerance. The term aerobic capacity itself may not adequately describe exergonic reactions which proceed by hydrogen transport and electron transfer and use atmospheric oxygen only in the terminal stage.

It is the purpose of this paper to show that increased performance ability with training is secondary to changes in physiological parameters other than oxygen uptake. These changes may even be potentiated by limited oxygen availability during the training process.

Materials and Methods

Schedule

A high calibre olympic athlete (182 cm, 84 kg) was trained under hypoxic conditions FIO_2 0.115–0.125 in a chamber previously described by BANISTER et al. [1967]. The training followed the procedure of PIWONKA and ROBINSON [1965] consisting of interval riding on a bicycle ergometer (Monark AB Cyclefabriken) for three minute intervals with 2 minute rest pauses. Six intervals were completed during each training session at work loads ranging from 1,500 kg-m/min to 1,800 kg-m/min. The training program was in effect for one month under the hypoxic conditions followed by similar training in normoxia for one month and a further month under hypoxic conditions. Test rides to exhaustion were made bi-weekly throughout the training in normoxia or hypoxia. Previous to the training the responses of the subject to work tasks of 1,080, 1,260, 1,620 and 2,100 kg-m/min respectively were measured. These evaluations were repeated over the same range of work rates at the end of the training.

Testing Procedure

The exercise measurements followed similar patterns with a variation depending upon whether all-out tests were being made during the training or whether the subject's responses to a standard work rate were being measured prior to, or after the completion of, training. In the all-out tests, after a 5 min warm-up period (60 rpm, no load, heart rate 87± 8 b/min), the subject overcame, at 1 min intervals, work rates of 960, 1,500, and 2,160 kg-m/min respectively until exhaustion (figure 1). In the standard work task after the same warm-up period the appropriate standard work rate was performed for several minutes. Expired gas was directed through a short length of Collins non-kinkable hose (1D 1 ½ in.) to a 5 l mixing chamber from which aliquot gas samples were removed during the middle 30 sec. of each of the last 4 min of exercise for micro-Scholander analysis. Ventilation was measured at the terminal end of the apparatus by a Parkinson-Cowan gas meter. Expired air temperature was measured by a thermometer inserted in the gas flow. Continuous electrocardiogram records were obtained throughout the experiment by radiotelemetry. Samples of arterialized capillary blood were drawn from an ear lobe, prewarmed for 5 min, in 50–75μl heparinized capillary tubes periodically before the commencement

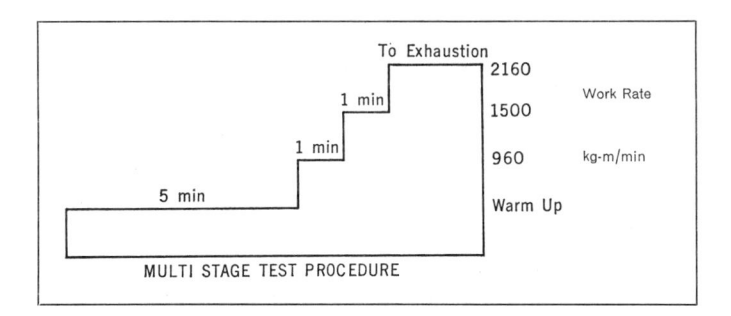

Figure 1. Showing the procedure in the all-out tests. The combinations of speed and load at the various working rates were: 80 rpm and 2 kg at 960 kg-m/min; 100 rpm and 2.5 kg at 1,500 kg-m/min; 120 rpm and 3 kg at 2,160 kg-m/min respectively.

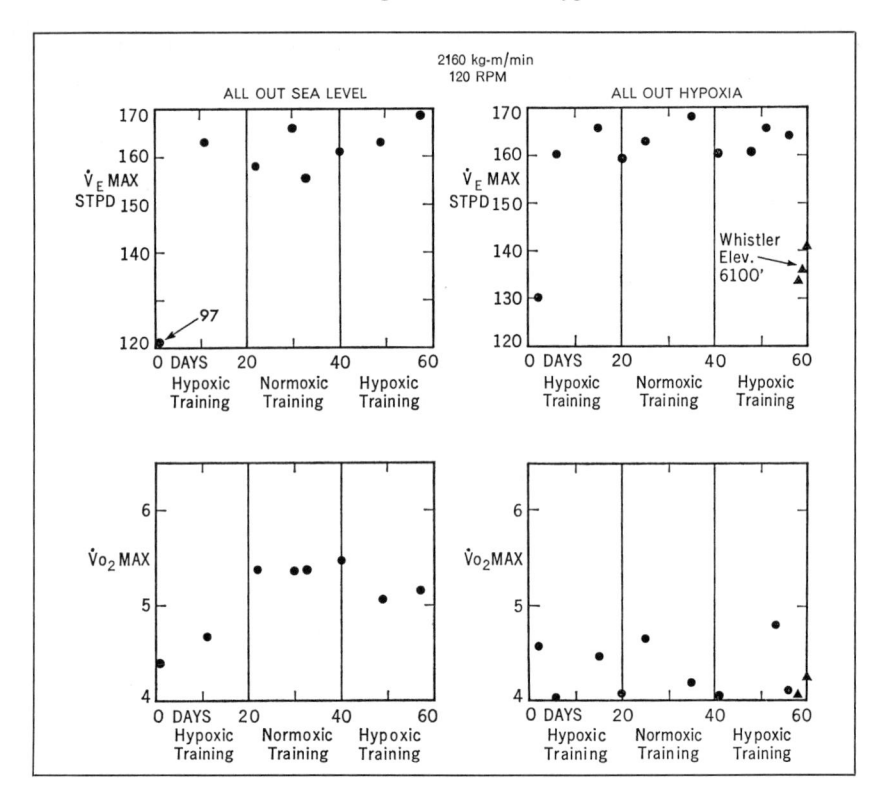

Figure 2. Respiratory gas exchange rates in tests to exhaustion in normoxia and hypoxia during the course of training. Triangles indicate actual altitude performance at 6,100 ft. elevation.

of exercise, and always 5 min after the cessation of exercise. The subject recovered from the hypoxic exhaustive rides in normoxia outside the chamber and the PaO$_2$ values reflected these conditions. Blood samples were analysed by the Radiometer Astrup blood gas analysis system. The pH electrode was standardized with Radiometer precision buffers to ±.002 and the oxygen electrode with deoxygenated water and water equilibrated with the atmosphere, both at 37°C. Arterial PaCO$_2$ mmHg, standard bicarbonate (HCO$_3^-$) mEq/l were calculated by the manner of Siggard-Andersen after equilibration of the blood sample at two known carbon dioxide tensions previously determined by micro-Scholander analysis. An approximate value for the equivalent lactic acid (LA) accumulation mEq/l was

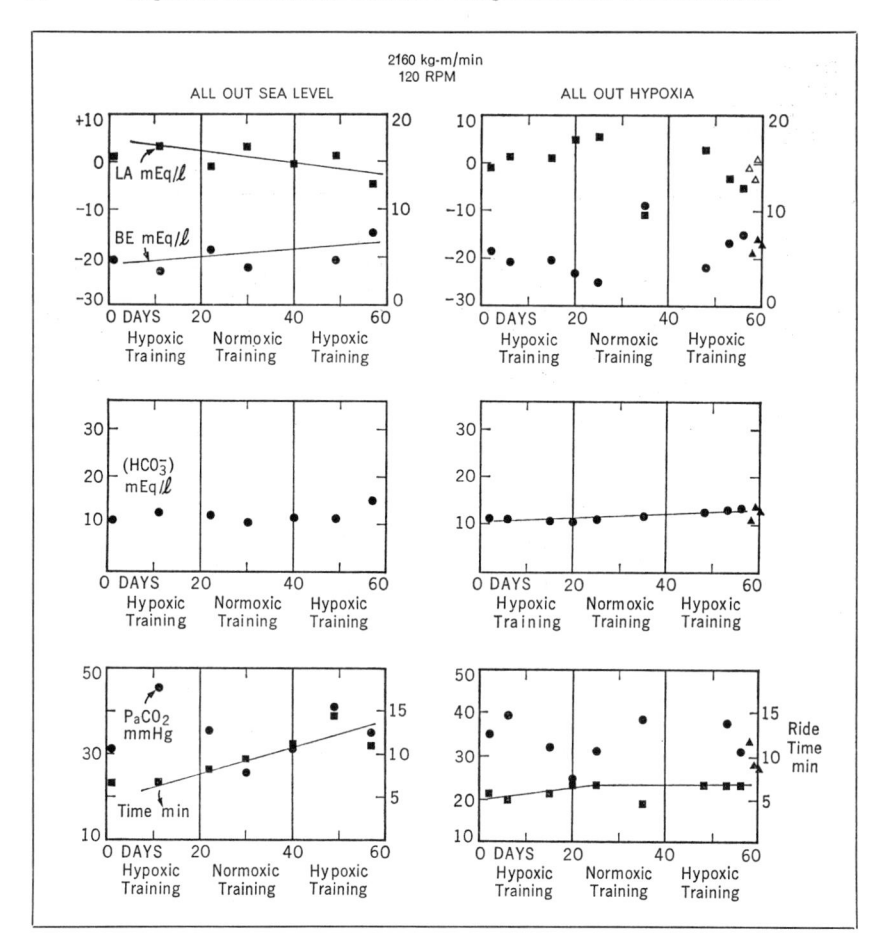

Figure 3. Changes in BE, calculated LA accumulation [BOUHUYS et al., 1966], standard bicarbonate, PaCO₂ and endurance time in all-out performance in normoxia and hypoxia during the course of hypoxic training. Actual altitude values at 6,100 ft. elevation are indicated by open triangles (rest) and closed triangles (all-out performance).

calculated from the regression of BE on LA determined by BOUHUYS et al. (1966).

After completing the final month of hypoxic training the subject lived for 3 days at 6,100 ft. altitude and performed one exhaustive ride on each day when the same physiological measurements as described above were made except for the electrocardiogram.

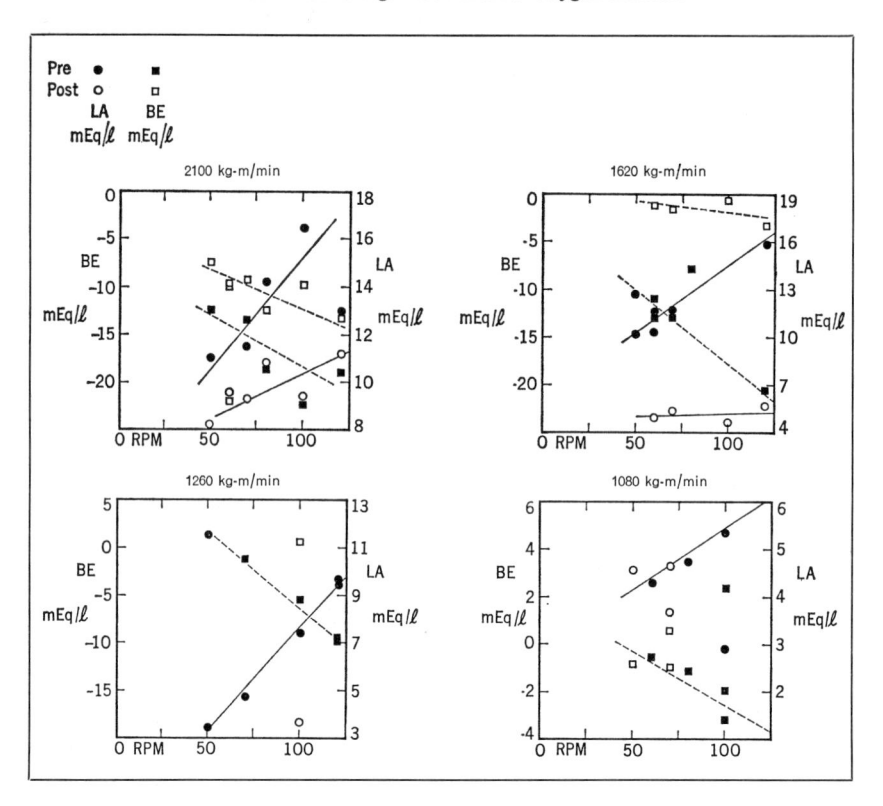

Figure 4.

Results

Figure 2 shows that during the course of the hypoxic training maximum oxygen uptake in normoxia increased. The subject's developing tolerance for exhaustive work in normoxia was shown also in the increased endurance time, a less negative base excess level and lactic acid accumulation and less depleted bicarbonate reserves (figure 3). After an initial improvement exhaustive performance in the hypoxic environment remained constant for oxygen uptake but showed a continued training trend in the blood acid-base variables.

The subject's acid-base balance at the submaximal standard work rates before and after the hypoxic training (figure 4) show the same improvement. The heart rate increase (figure 5) for identical submaximal work

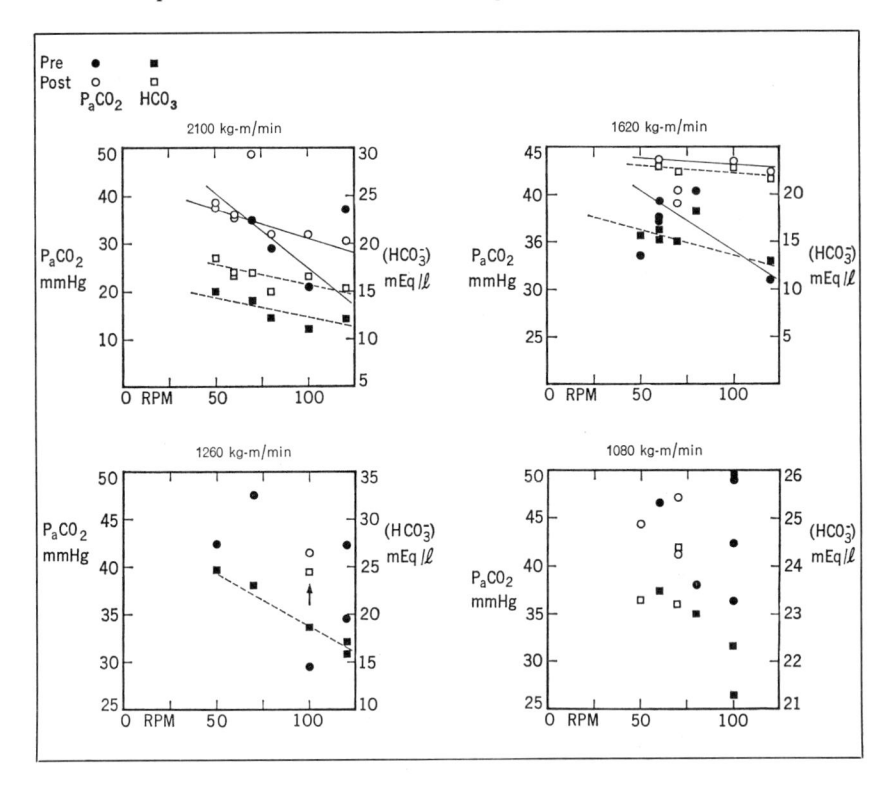

Figure 4. Showing pre and post hypoxic training responses of the subject in acid-base balance variables during standard submaximal work rates. The lactic acid accumulation is shown as a more conventional interpretation of the BE value. It is an aproximate value only, calculated after the manner of BOUHUYS et al. [1966].

rates was greatly reduced after the hypoxic training while previously reported $\dot{V}_{O_2}$ values, BANISTER and JACKSON [1967] in these tasks showed no consistent change. A clear separation between pre and post training values for BE, LA (calculated) and (HCO_3^-) levels was observable at the higher work rates, no consistent change was shown at the lower work rates which did not stress the subject sufficiently. Figure 6 shows that there was also an increased oxygen extraction at higher comparable ventilation rates, after the training, in submaximal work tasks. In tests to exhaustion, at an actual altitude of 6,100 ft., the developed acidemia according to BE and standard bicarbonate levels was less than that developed at sea level at the beginning of the training and the endurance time of the test considerably improved.

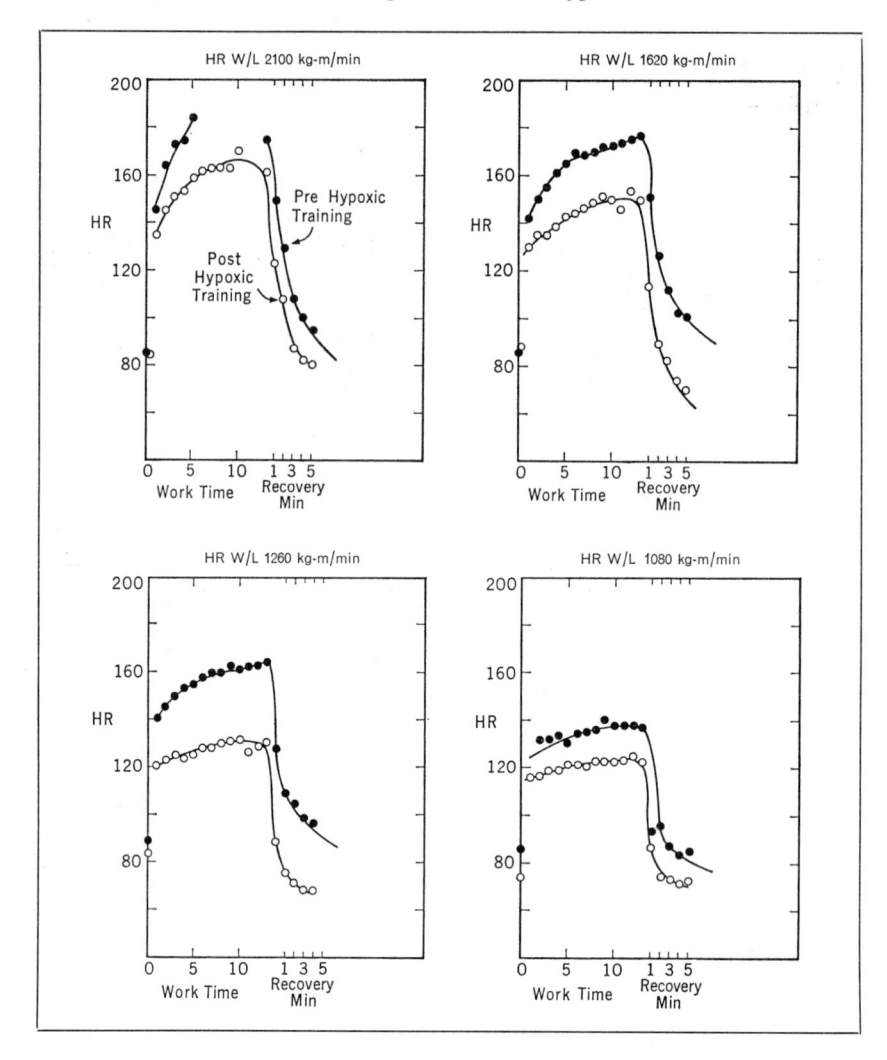

Figure 5. Heart rate increase response to standard work rates before (full circles) and after (open circles) hypoxic training.

Discussion

The initial development of high BE in exhaustive exercise in hypoxia tends to support the conclusion of HANSEN, STELTER, and VOGEL [1967a] that large amounts of non-volatile acid are to be found in arterial

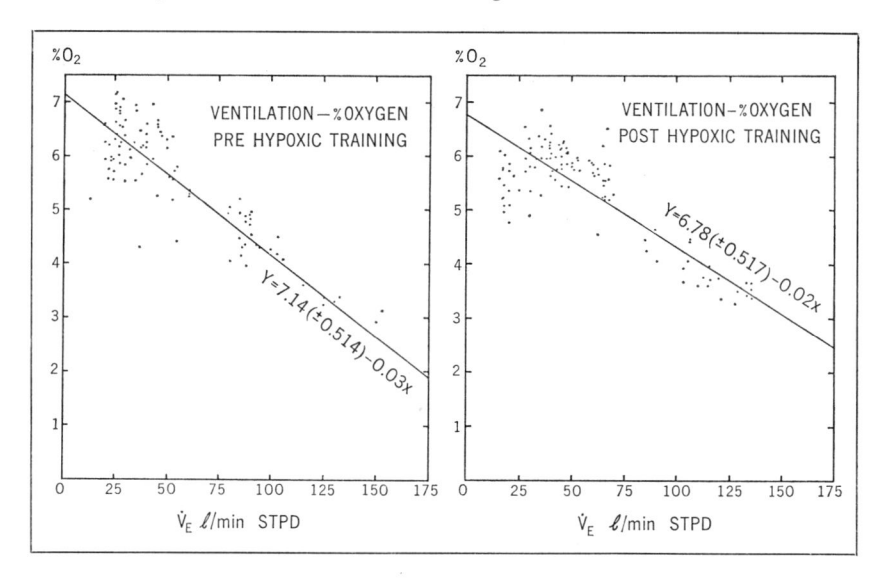

Figure 6. Regression of % oxygen extraction on ventilation (STPD) before and after hypoxic training. [Reproduced with permission Int. Z. angew. Physiol. (in Press)].

blood during heavy exercise at high altitude. Their finding of declining resting and exercise levels of non-volatile acid with adaptation is similar to the findings demonstrated during the course of training in this study, even though performance time and $\dot{V}_{O_2}$ max. in hypoxia had reached limiting values. In normoxia although $\dot{V}_{O_2}$ max. reached a plateau value, performance time continued to increase paralleling the continued decline in non-volatile acid accumulation.

An attractive hypothesis integrating the acid-base changes with known serum enzyme changes resulting from exercise and hypoxic exposure [ALTLAND, HIGHMAN and NELSON, 1968], involves the changed cellular membrane permeability with increased hydrogen ion concentration. Following the concept of MEERSON et al. [1964] 'That in the process of adaptation of the differentiated cell to a continuous increase of physiological load the mass of energy-producing structures is augmented prior to that of the structures immediately effectuating the specific physiological function of the cell', one may speculate that mitochondrial changes are effected first. As a reaction to increased cellular permeability, loss of enzymes, degeneration of the cristae SULKIN and SULKIN [1967] with consequent uncoupling of oxidative phosphorylation an intense proliferation of mitochondria could occur acting to contain the developed hypoxemia and consequent acidemia [KING and GOLLNICK, 1968]. With adaptation, control of hydrogen ion concentration, restoration of the integrity of the mitochondrial membrane and oxidative phosphorylation, an enhanced oxygen transport at the cellular level would result in a continuing reduction of non-volatile acid levels as seen in this study.

Another proposed mechanism of adaptation, both to training and exercise in a hypoxic environment, is better directed blood flow, specifically to the muscle mass involved in the movement [ANDREW et al., 1966]. The lowered cardiac output required for a given work rate which might result from such adaptation would be reflected in a reduced heart rate as shown in figure 5. Similarly at rest or in mild exercise the oxygen extraction for any given ventilatory rate would decrease as seen in the data of HANSEN et al. [1967b] and in this study. On the other hand in exhaustive exercise where local oxygen demand is high and the tissue oxygen transfer mechanisms are preserved by the cellular adaptations described above oxygen extraction may be expected to be higher than pre-training values where oxidative phosphorylation was disrupted. Figure 6 shows this type of adaptation and this data is contrary to that of HANSEN et al. [1967b] who found a lower oxygen extraction from respired air after acclimatization. However, these investigators made their comparison between pre- and post-training extraction values without reference to the ventilation rate so that although the percentage extraction of oxygen was slightly lower after acclimatization the ventilatory rate was considerably higher.

Further studies integrating changes in gross performance characteristics to morphological, enzymatic and acid-base parameters, in serial data, during adaptation to hypoxia will be necessary to reveal the mechanisms and kinetics involved.

References

1. ALTLAND, P. D.; HIGHMAN, B. and NELSON, B. D.: Serum enzyme and tissue changes in rats exercised repeatedly at altitude: effects of training. Amer. J. Physiol. *214:* 28–32 (1968).
2. ANDREW, G. M.; GUZMAN, C. A. and BECKLAKE, M. R.: The effect of exercise training on cardiac output. J. appl. Physiol. *21 (2):* 603–608 (1966).
3. BANISTER, E. W.; BROWN, S. R.; LOWEN, H. R. and NORDAN, H. C.: The royal Canadian 5BX program: a metabolic analysis. Med. services J. Canada. *23:* 1237–1244 (1967a).
4. BANISTER, E. W. and JACKSON, R. C.: The effect of speed and load changes

on oxygen intake for equivalent power outputs during bicycle ergometry. Int. Z. angew. Physiol. *24:* 284–290 (1967b).
5. BANISTER, E. W.; JACKSON, R. C. and CARTMEL, J.: The potentiating effect of low oxygen tension during training on subsequent cardiovascular performance. Int. Z. angew. Physiol. (in press, 1968).
6. BOUHUYS, J. P.; BINKHORST, R. A. and LEENWEN, P. VAN.: Metabolic acidosis of exercise in healthy males. J. appl. Physiol. *21:* 1040–1046 (1966).
7. CAMPBELL, E. J. M.: Exercise Tolerance. Lect. scient. Basis Med. Annual Review 128–144 (1967).
8. HANSEN, J. E.; STELTER, G. P. and VOGEL, J. A.: Arterial pyruvate, lactate, pH and PCO_2 during work at sea level and high altitude. J. appl. Physiol. *23:* 523–530 (1967a).
9. HANSEN, J. E.; VOGEL, J. A.; STELTER, G. P. and CONSOLAZIO, C. F.: Oxygen uptake in man during exhaustive work at sea level and high altitude. J. appl. Physiol. *23:* 511–522 (1967b).
10. JONES, N. J.: Exercise testing. Brit. J. dis. chest. *61:* 169–189 (1967).
11. KING, D. W. and GOLLNICK, P. D.: The immediate and chronic effect of exercise on the number and structure of skeletal muscle mitochondria. American College Sports Medicine 5th Annual Meeting, Pennsylvania, USA (1968).
12. MEERSON, F. Z.; ZALETAYEVA, T. A.; LAGUTCHEV, S. S. and PSCHENNIKOVA, M. G.: Structure and mass of mitochondria in the process of compensatory hyperfunction and hypertrophy in the heart. Exp. Cell Res. *36:* 568–578 (1964).
13. PIWONKA, R. W. and ROBINSON, S.: Pre-acclimatization of men to heat by training. J. appl. Physiol. *20:* 379 (1965).
14. SULKIN, D. F. and SULKIN, N. M.: The effects of age on the fine structure of autonomic ganglion and cardiac muscle cells in chronically hypoxic rats. The gerontologist *7:* 17 (1967).

Author's address: Dr. E. W. BANISTER, Human Performance Laboratory, Physical Development Centre, Simon Fraser University, *Burnaby 2, B. C.* (Canada).

Oxygen Debt, Lactate in Blood and Muscle Tissue During Maximal Exercise in Man[1]

G. Agnevik, J. Karlsson, B. Diamant and B. Saltin

Department of Physiology, Gymnastik- och idrottshögskolan, and Department of Pharmacology, Karolinska Institutet, Stockholm

Blood lactate determinations are routine in combination with exercise tests, and there are several reports on the relationship between blood lactate and oxygen debt [5]. From many standpoints the use of blood lactate determination in this connection can be critisized. Recently a method has been developed to determine lactate in muscle samples [4] obtained by a biopsy technique [2]. It was then though of interest to investigate whether the tissue concentration of lactate in exercising muscle at exhaustion of a maximal effort was related to the observed oxygen debt.

Four well-trained and well motivated physical education students with almost the same body weight (about 70 kg) and conditioning background performed maximal work on a bicycle ergometer, chosen so that the working time at exhaustion was about three minutes. Prior to the work the subject was resting on a bed for 30 min. Resting values were then determined for oxygen uptake using the Douglas bag technique with the gas samples analyzed according to a modified Haldane method, blood lactate using arterialized finger tip blood and an enzymatic method [7], and muscle tissue lactate [4] using a biopsy technique. The muscle tissue samples, 15–30 mg wet weight, were obtained from the lateral part of M. quadriceps femoris.

During the work period the total oxygen uptake was measured. Oxygen debt using the conventional concept was determined with the subjects resting on a bed for 60 min following the termination of the work (figure 1). Immediately after the work was terminated (within 5 sec) and 10, 30 and 60 min after the termination samples were taken for muscle tissue lactate and blood lactate determinations.

The oxygen deficit was calculated as the difference between the calculated oxygen requirement and the oxygen uptake during the work period.

[1] Supported from project No. K67-14X-740-02, Swedish Medical Research Council.

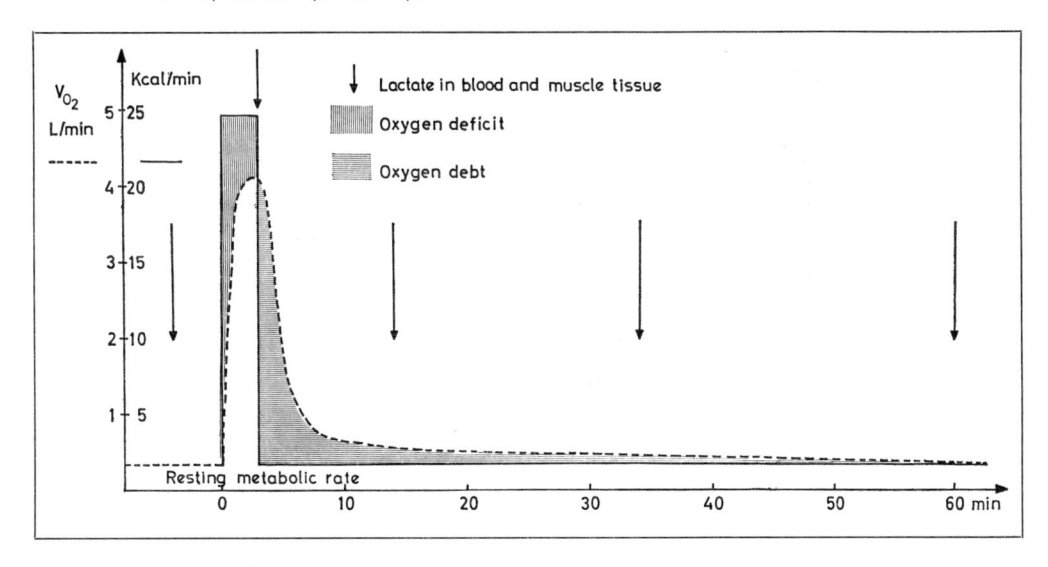

Figure 1. The procedure for the experiment. Oxygen uptake, oxygen debt and oxygen deficit in connection with 3 min of maximal work. At the arrows muscle tissue lactate and blood lactate were determined.

Table I. Results from maximal work on a bicycle ergometer where the oxygen deficit was calculated assuming a mechanical efficiency of 22.7%.

Subject	Total work KPM	Required oxygen L	Oxygen uptake L	Oxygen deficit L	Oxygen debt L	O_2 def. O_2 debt	Muscle tissue mM per kg	Blood lactate mM
O. S.	6,080	14.3	10.3	4.0	10.5	38%	11.2	7.3
B. J.	7,200	17.0	11.2	5.8	14.7	39%	19.0	11.2
H. L.	5,913	13.9	7.1	6.8	16.5	41%	24.6	14.5
J. S.	5,316	12.6	7.6	5.0	12.5	40%	21.6	12.4
Average	6,130	14.5	9.1	5.4	13.6	40%	19.1	11.4

Results and Discussion

The individual results are presented in table I.

ASMUSSEN reported 1946 that the anaerobic efficiency is only between 40 and 50% of the aerobic [1]. CHRISTENSEN – HÖGBERG found in 1950 that the corresponding figure was around 50% [3]. Both figures are in

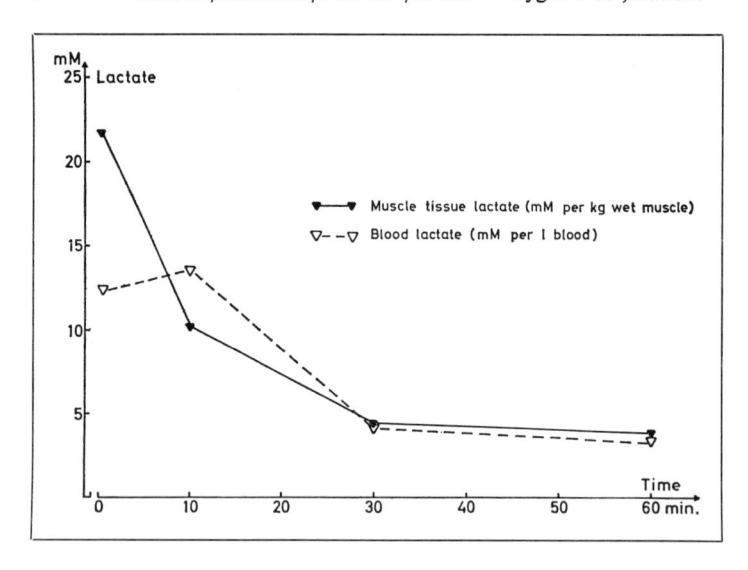

Figure 2. Muscle tissue lactate and blood lactate in one subject after 3 min of maximal work. [Diamant *et al.*, Acta physiol. scand. *72:* 383–384 (1968)].

good agreement with Meyerhof's results based on myothermal determinations [6]. Our results of 40% are somewhat low compared to the ones of the above mentioned authors. In our experiment we have assumed that the mechanical efficiency remained unchanged (about 22.7%) during the work period. There are reasons to believe that the mechanical efficiency decreases during the latter part of exhaustive work. This would then at least partly explain our rather low figures. It should be remembered that in our figure for oxygen debt is included the volume of oxygen needed for saturation of myoglobin, hemoglobin and resynthesizing of ATP and CP.

In one of the four subjects the muscle tissue lactate also was determined 10, 30 and 60 min after the work was terminated. Unfortunately the samples from the remaining three subjects were destroyed when a freezer broke down (figure 2).

There seems to be a correlation – although our material is too small to be the base for definite conclusions – both between oxygen deficit and muscle tissue lactate and between oxygen debt and muscle tissue lactate (figure 3). One reason for this rather good relationship may be that our subjects were selected with about the same body weight and physical work capacity. By using bicycle exercise approximately the same muscle mass was engaged in the maximal exercise in all subjects and a concentration figure

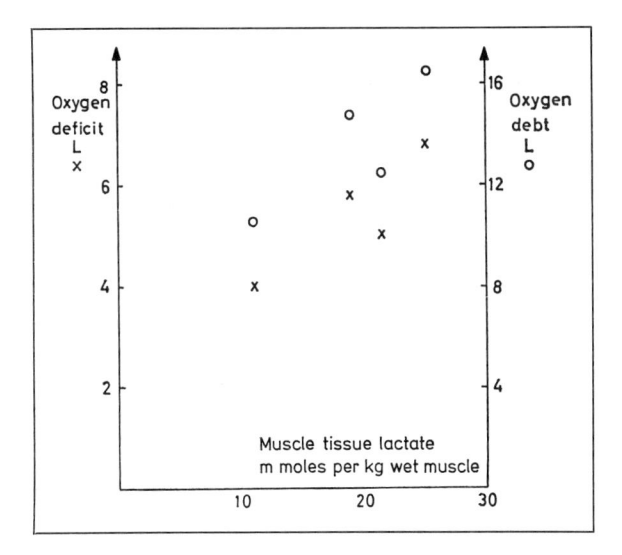

Figure 3. The correlation between oxygen deficit and muscle tissue lactate and between oxygen debt and muscle tissue lactate. Note that the scale for oxygen debt is twice the scale for oxygen deficit.

for the lactate in an exercised muscle then may reflect the oxygen deficit and the oxygen debt.

References

1. ASMUSSEN, E.: Aerobic recovery after anaerobiosis in rest and work. Acta physiol. scand. *11:* 197 (1946).
2. BERGSTRÖM, J.: Scand. J. clin. Lab. Invest. suppl. *68:* (1962).
3. CHRISTENSEN, E. H. and HÖGBERG, P.: The efficiency of anaerobical work. Arbeitsphysiol. *14:* 249–250 (1950).
4. DIAMANT, B.; KARLSSON, J. and SALTIN, B.: Acta physiol. scand. *72:* 383–384 (1968).
5. MARGARIA, R.: Exercise at altitude. Excerpta Medica Foundation (1967).
6. MEYERHOF, O.: Die chemischen Vorgänge im Muskel. *Berlin* (1930).
7. SCHOLZ, R.; SCHMITZ, H.; BÜCHER, TH. und LAMPEN, J. O.: Über die Wirkung von Nystatin auf Bäckerhefe. Biochem. Z. *331:* 71–86 (1959).

Author's address: G. AGNEVIK, Department of Physiology, Gymnastik- och idrottshögskolan, *11433 Stockholm* (Sweden).

Blood Gas Tensions and pH in Brachial Artery, Femoral Vein, and Brachial Vein During Maximal Exercise[1]

L. H. HARTLEY and B. SALTIN

Department of Physiology, Gymnastik- och idrottshögskolan, Stockholm

The object of this experiment was to study blood gases and acid-base balance in various venous and arterial channels during maximal exercise. Three basic types of exercise were used including one cycle load which was just heavy enough to yield maximal oxygen uptake ($\dot{V}_{O_2}$), one very heavy 'supermaximal load' [1], and finally a treadmill maximal oxygen uptake determination [4].

Methods

All subjects were young trained subjects. The lighter maximal cycle load is referred to as 'long maximal' and resulted in exhaustion in 5–10 min. Long maximal was done by five subjects. Of these five, three subjects also did a greater cycle load which resulted in exhaustion in 3 to 5 min, referred to as 'short maximal'. Of those three, two had treadmill maximal studies done also.

All subjects had catheters indwelling in the brachial artery, brachial vein, and femoral vein (inserted in a retrograde direction). During each study samples were drawn always at exhaustion, but before the load had been slowed or stopped. In addition in the long maximal studies blood samples were also taken after 3–4 min of exercise. Cardiac output ($\dot{Q}$) was measured by dye dilution of cardiogreen and $\dot{V}_{O_2}$ was measured by the Douglas bag method [2].

Blood O_2 content determination was made by Van Slyke analysis, and blood O_2 tension was measured on a Clark electrode. The pH was measured on a standard pH electrode.

Results

Cardiac ouptut was less during the short compared to the long maximal on the cycle, but $\dot{V}_{O_2}$ was the same (figure 1). Both $\dot{Q}$ and $\dot{V}_{O_2}$

[1] Supported by grants from The Tri-Centennial Fund of the Bank of Sweden.

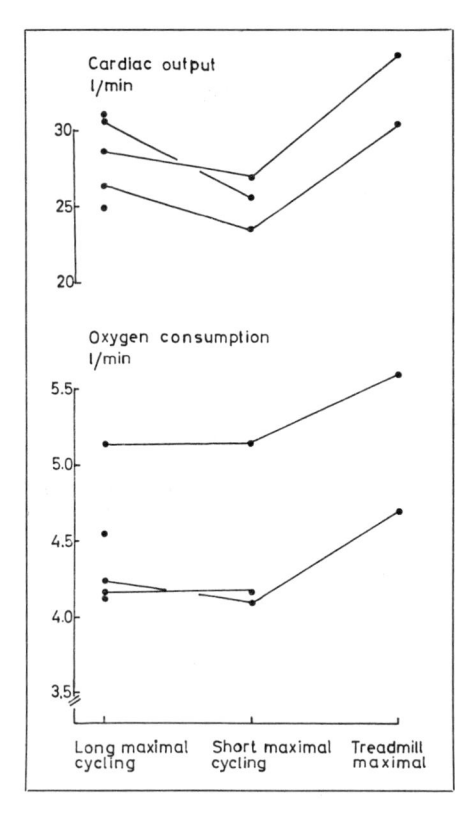

Figure 1. Individual maximal cardiac output and oxygen consumption values. This figure is not a graph but represents the individual values for cardiac output and oxygen consumption. The connecting lines indicate the data in subjects who had either two or three types of maximal exercise studies. Long maximal, short maximal, and treadmill maximal are defined in the text. The maximal cardiac output is least with the short maximal cycle study and greatest with the treadmill maximal test. Oxygen consumption is the same in both types of maximal cycle exercise and greater during the treadmill maximal.

were greater on the treadmill. These hemodynamic and oxygen transport studies are the subject of our other publication [5] and are beyond the scope of this paper. They are mentioned because of the use of calculated systemic arteriovenous O_2 content difference and because of the necessity of using systemic flow in the interpretation.

The systemic arteriovenous oxygen difference is less in the long than in the short maximal cycle studies and is the least of all during maximal treadmill exercise (figure 2). The femoral arteriovenous exercise was also studied (figure 2). Systemic arteriovenous oxygen content difference is considerably

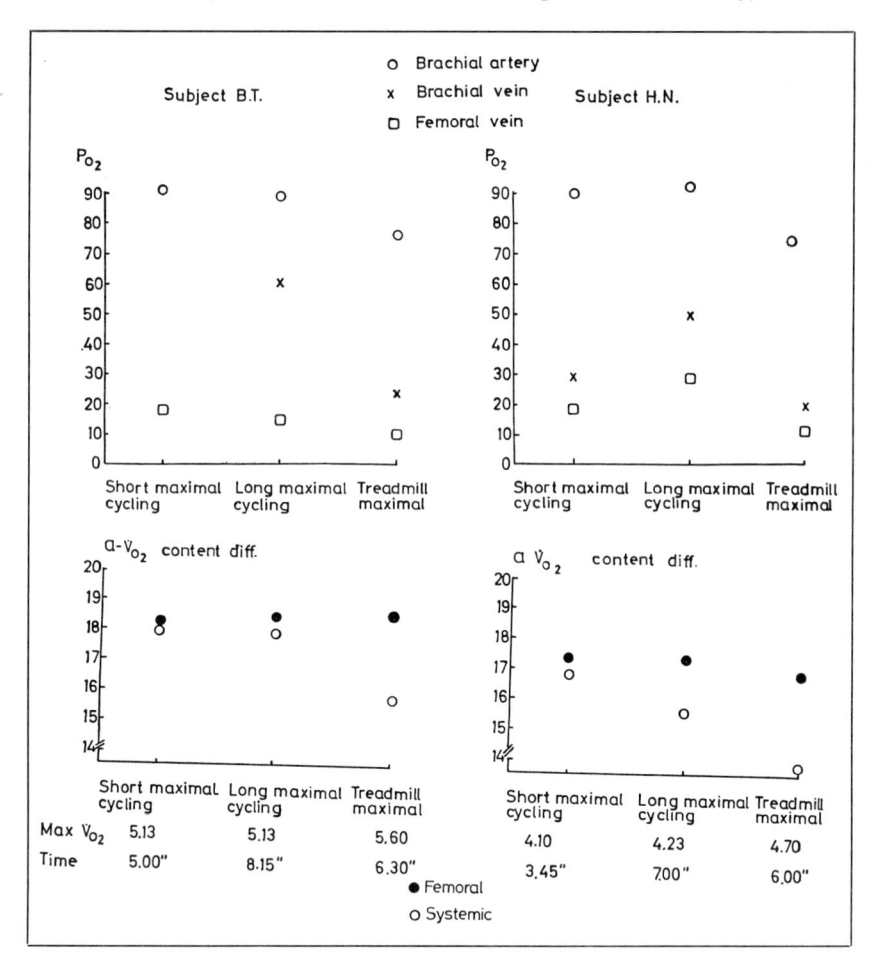

Figure 2. Arteriovenous gas studies during three types of maximal exercise in two individuals. This figure in the upper two panels shows arterial, brachial vein, and femoral vein oxygen tension data in three types of maximal exercise. The symbols are defined at the middle of the top of the figure. They show the lower arterial P_{O_2} during the treadmill maximal and the narrow brachial arteriovenous oxygen difference with long compared to short maximal cycling. The lower panels give arteriovenous oxygen content difference of femoral (closed circles) and systemic (open circles) circuits. The femoral a-v O_2 difference is the same with all types of exercise. During the short maximal cycling exercise the systemic a-v O_2 difference approaches being almost as great as femoral a-v O_2 difference, suggesting the diversion of almost all of the cardiac output to the exercising muscles.

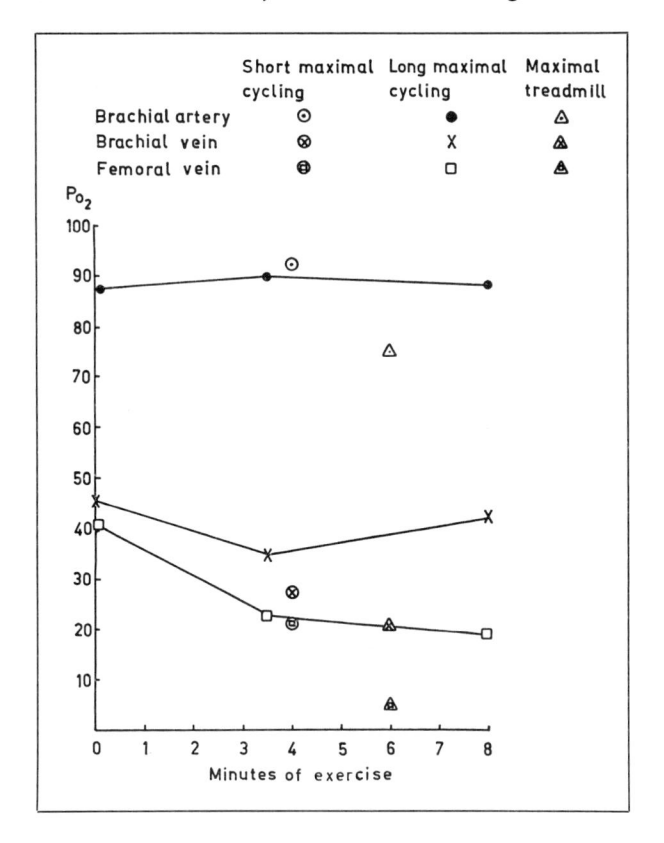

Figure 3. Mean oxygen tension data from brachial artery, brachial vein, and femoral vein during different types of maximal exercise. The ordinate represents P_{O_2} in mm Hg. The abscissa represents minutes of exercise. All data are mean values. The solid lines connect the mean data during the long maximal exercise on the cycle. Circled symbols are short maximal values, and triangle enclosed symbols are treadmill values. The figure shows the lower arterial P_{O_2} on the treadmill (see text). The brachial vein blood P_{O_2} midway in time during the long maximal study is clearly lower than at the end of the exercise period. Short maximal has a slightly lower brachial vein P_{O_2} than long maximal at 3.5 to 4 min, but is markedly lower than long maximal brachial vein P_{O_2} at exhaustion. Femoral vein P_{O_2} is considerably lower on the treadmill than either type of maximal cycle test.

less than femoral arteriovenous oxygen difference during maximal treadmill exercise. On the cycle during long maximal, the systemic arteriovenous oxygen content difference approaches the femoral arteriovenous oxygen content difference and during the short maximal the systemic arteriovenous O_2 difference is almost the same as the femoral. This suggests the cardiac output is almost completely diverted to the exercising muscles in the short maximal.

Interpretation of the blood O_2 tension data requires some special consideration. First the arterial P_{O_2} is lower in the treadmill than in the cycle exercise (figure 3). The reason for this is not entirely clear, but subsequent studies by the authors indicate it may be an artefact due to resistance in the gas collection apparatus at the great ventilations of treadmill exercise. In any event interpretation of the treadmill P_{O_2} studies on the venous side are not entirely comparable to the cycle exercises. Secondly venous P_{O_2} is discussed as a-v O_2 difference, even though it is recognized that differences due to pH, oxygen capacity, and temperature affect the interpretation of tension data as content data. In actual fact pH is very similar in both types of bicycle exercise in brachial vein, and the mean difference in oxygen capacity between the long and short maximal studies is only .7 vol. %, and is not systemically greater in either type of exercise (table I.).

The brachial arteriovenous oxygen tension difference (a-v O_2 t d) at the time of exhaustion during the long maximal load is clearly much narrower than brachial a-v O_2 t d at the time of exhaustion (see figure 2). However if one considers brachial artery a-v O_2 t d in terms of time, the a-v O_2 t d is almost the same at the same time in both short and long maximal and only becomes markedly narrower at exhaustion (figure 3). This suggests at the same time of maximal exercise, the blood flow to the arm is nearly the same regardless of load but with the passage of time flow to the arms increases.

Table I. pH during maximal exercise

	Ba	Bv	Fv
Rest	7.41	7.36	7.36
Long maximal	7.17	7.15	7.06
	7.12–7.25	7.07–7.26	7.01–7.14
Short maximal	7.21	7.11	7.03
	7.16–7.26	7.02–7.26	7.02–7.14
Treadmill	7.22	7.17	7.04
	7.15–7.30	6.98–7.24	7.03–7.05

Abbreviations are as follow: Ba = brachial artery; Bv = brachial vein; Fv = femoral vein. All data are expressed as pH units. The upper figure in each square is the mean value and the lower figures are the range.

The markedly lower femoral vein tension during the treadmill exercise suggests possibly a distribution of the blood to better unload its O_2 supply to the exercising muscle, than is possible during cycle maximal exercise.

Lactate in brachial artery is nearly the same at exhaustion in the short (mean 12.4, range 11.3 to 15.3 mM per l) as in the long maximal loads (mean 13.1, range 10.8 to 14.1 mM per l). It is lower during the treadmill maximal load (mean 11.8, range 9.6 to 14.1 mM per l). Base excess is slightly more negative at exhaustion in long maximal (–17 mEq/l) compared to short maximal (–15 mEq/l), and is least negative at exhaustion on the treadmill (–12 mEq/l). Thus base excess tends to reflect changes in blood lactate.

The pH measurement in arterial blood is in accord with the changes in base excess (table I.). The pH measurements in femoral vein are all considerably lower than arterial blood, but are about the same level in all these types of maximal exercise. Since this pH is determined by both CO_2 locally produced and lactate produced, it does not reflect any clear interpretable change. The differences between brachial vein and brachial artery pH are not understood but indicate poor reflection of arterial pH in brachial vein blood.

Arterial P_{CO_2} is decreased to about the same level in short and long maximal (mean values 29 and 31 mm Hg respectively) and is clearly greater in treadmill (37 mm Hg). These findings are in accord with the degree of metabolic acidosis produced and the lower arterial P_{O_2} during the treadmill study.

Discussion

Earlier studies by REEVES *et al.* [3] showed a gradual convergence of femoral and systemic a-v O_2 differences suggesting a greater percentage of the total blood flow is distributed to the working muscles. The data in this report extends this observation to maximal levels and suggests that during the short maximal study, the combined lower $\dot{Q}$ and great $\dot{V}_{O_2}$ result in a distribution of almost all of the cardiac output to the exercising legs. This may actually deprive other organs and be responsible for the unpleasant sensation experienced by the subjects during a 'supermaximal effort' on the bicycle ergometer.

Brachial blood flow is greater in the long maximal than in the short maximal effort. This can be considered as a result of greater total cardiac output in long maximal, which exceeds flow capabilities to the legs and the excess flow then becomes distributed to other organs including the arms. Against this interpretation is the fact that early in the exercise period the greater flow to the arms does not seem to occur, yet $\dot{Q}$ is essentially the same as at exhaustion [5]. This suggests that the blood is distributed to the skin for temperature regulation at the latter part of the long maximal work. Presumably the very short period of exercise in the short maximal studies is insufficient to accumulate heat enough to influence temperature regulation. Acid base studies indicate similar metabolic acidosis with the short compared to the long maximal studies.

References

1. ÅSTRAND, P.-O. and SALTIN, B.: Oxygen uptake during the first minutes of heavy muscular exercise. J. appl. Physiol. *16:* 971–976 (1961).
2. ÅSTRAND, P.-O.; CUDDY, T. E.; SALTIN, B. and STENBERG, J.: Cardiac output during submaximal and maximal work. J. appl. Physiol. *19:* 268–274 (1964).
3. REEVES, J. T.; GROVER, R. F.; BLOUNT, Jr., S. G. and FILLEY, G. F.: Cardiac output response to standing and treadmill walking. J. appl. Physiol. *16:* 283–288 (1961).
4. SALTIN, B. and ÅSTRAND, P.-O.: Maximal oxygen uptake in athletes. J. appl. Physiol. *23:* 353–358 (1967).
5. SALTIN, B.; HARTLEY, L. H.; EKBLOM, B. and PERNOW, B.: Cardiovascular response to various types of exercise yielding maximal oxygen consumption. (In preparation.)

Author's address: Dr. L. HOWARD HARTLEY, Department of Physiology. Gymnastik- och idrottshögskolan, *11433 Stockholm* (Sweden).

The Relative Value of Stress Indicators, Related to Prediction of Strenuous Athletic (Treadmill) Performance

T. K. CURETON[1]

Physical Fitness Research Laboratory, University of Illinois, Ill.

Introduction

There are several systems for differentiating the effects of stressful athletic performance. This paper is concerned with (1) Changes in stress indicators due to progressive, longitudinal physical training over several months. (2) Acute effects of stressful treadmill work and the interrelationships of several such stress indicators to predict the performance, including the net predictive value of each stress indicator (mainly by Beta weight, and Beta square proportionate analysis [12]. (3) The effect of several systems of work on a variety of hematological measures during one hour of strenuous work, (a) continuously (b) 1 min of work and 1 min rest (c) 2 min of work and 2 min rest (d) 3 min of work and 3 min of rest; with all groups (a) (b)

Hematological indicators	Circulatory-Respiratory	Nervous
lactic acid	brachial pulse wave	T-wave amplitude (highest, precordial)
pyruvic acid	peak RQ in run	
pH	peak RQ in recovery	Heart rate
pCO_2	maximal ventilation (in work)	ICP (after RAAB)
17-OH Ketosteroids	O_2 (peak in run)	EML (after RAAB)
K	O_2 (anaerobic debt)	TP (after RAAB)
Total protein		
Albumin		
Base excess		
Eosinophils		

[1] The several studies have been completed at the University of Illinois, Physical Fitness Research Laboratory, Urbana, Illinois, USA and are only very briefly summarized here. The original studies may be obtained through the library of the University of Illinois (physical education division). The studies have been sponsored and supervised throughout by the author of the paper except in the study of Landry [1968] involving arterial blood by catheterization, the study was carried out in the Medical Research Laboratory of the Canadian government, Ottawa, Canada, by the cooperative help of W/C G.M. FITZGIBBON. The original is a Ph. D. thesis at the University of Illinois (1968) (sponsor: T.K. CURETON).

and (c) and (d) totalling 6000 W for 1 h on bicycle ergometer work. Several such studies having been done, the results are briefly summarized. The several types of stress indicators include hematological indicators, circulatory-respiratory indicators, nervous responses.

The interrelations between these several systems of indicators are relatively unknown. This work seems to be the first to analyze the *net* contribution of each.

Heusner-Cureton Longitudinal Changes Due to Nine Months of Physical Training. In a *single subject* HEUSNER's study [1, 2, 5] demonstrated that in a gradual program of progressive training over seven months, with two months of de-training also following, there was a gradual but steady improvement from pre-season land drills, to water drills, to competition itself in maximal O_2 intake and in all-out treadmill running time (10 min/h, 8.6% grade); and there was immediate reversal toward deterioration to normal values from the fully trained state to the de-trained state in two months. Tests were taken once per month throughout the experiment with a total of 256 measures (indicators) being followed. The subject began at 0.021 l/min/kg and progressed to 0.041 in six months, leveled off in the last month of training, and then deteriorated in the two month period as soon as the daily training was discontinued. The maximal O_2 intake curve was paralleled by the all-out treadmill run time. The *net* O_2 debt in the all-out run test was 6.99 l (10.80 l gross) and increased to 9.43 l (14.28 l gross) in 6–7 months, then retrogressed. These measures were necessary for control in order to study the parallel behaviour of other stress indicators (cardio-vascular, respiratory and hematological). In the first three months the peak working pulse rate went to 196 then reduced (adapted) to 180, then went up again as soon as the training was discontinued to 196 again (the de-trained state). In the 7 months of training the erythrocytes increased 900,000 mm [2] (37 S.S.), increasing the number of RBC in circulation. Thorner found previously that the RBC reduced in strenuous work from 29×10^{-12} to 28.3×10^{-12} g during similar longitudinal training, and this work is in agreement, but the drop was greater in the first four months, with then a gradual return to the normal beginning level. The hemoglobin (Hb) concentration was consistently higher after the treadmill run test than before the run. It was concluded that the training did not increase the quantity of stored Hb but increased the amount in circulation. The Hb/E values agreed with THÖRNER's work, the young erythrocytes increasing during the training but except for a downward shift at the very beginning in the first month, the Hb/E value remained stable throughout the other months. In the run test, however, the Hb/E values were lower after the run than before the run. As the training progressed there was a steady increase in the circulating leucocytes as FARRIS had also indicated [1943]. Most observers have reported an increase in lymphocytes. In our study there was also a steady increase in lymphocytosis, agreeing with THÖRNER [1930] and HERXHEIMER and ERNST [1924]. Our study indicated the WBC increased 3125/mm³ (32 S.S.) from T_1 to T_2 (7 months). Data were also taken on eosinophils, basophils and neutrophils. There was a progressive development of eosinopenia in this subject during the first 7 months, then a reversal. The lymphocyte level is thought to be under direct adrenal cortical control. Training appears to have an effect upon the adrenal cortex. In our subject there was a drop in the total plasma protein both before and after the treadmill run in the first month, then a steady rise throughout the rest of the training, from 8.0 to 8.7 g/100 ml. The pH values indicated almost no change in the first 4 months in resting pH level but after this the pH steadily lowered through the seventh month, then reversed with the close of the training. CURETON [4] reported an association of 0.76 correlation between post-exercise pH and oxygen debt (l/kg,) in 16 subjects [1951]. The relationship is, however, curvilinear and the true relationship is estimated to be higher than this value of 0.76. The pH was lowered by the run in every case, and the longest runs lowered from 7.4 to 6.82. The correlation between the pH after the run and the time of the run was 0.87 (minus). This type of study indicates that stress is reflected in the blood tests. There is much literature to support the eosinophil test if any one test is to be used, and our second choice would be the pH. Comparatively, she blood lactate test is quite unreliable.

Weber-Cureton Study on Relative Value of Several Stress Indicators

WEBER and CURETON [11] reported in 1965 a study on the relative value of several stress indicators, using the causal statistical (net Beta weight square system of SEWELL WRIGHT) [12]. The values obtained, reduced to a 'percentage contribution' comparison were as follows: (30 young male adults from the University population).

Thus, it may be seen that no one stress indicator accounts for the time of the treadmill run in an all-out effort. Seven of these in a multiple regression solution gave the highest multiple R (0.859, S.E. 95.05 s).

Since the total of the *net* percent variance accounted for was only 33.87% it is not possible to account for the stress of the run by these variables

Submaximal Work (on a treadmill, 8.6% grade, 2, 4, 6 mi/h jogs at 7 mi/h):

	Predictive Net Variance
1. Peak Reduction of the Eosinophils (F = 6.07) in the 6-min Run	52.79%
2. Peak Run or Recovery RQ (F = 34.95)	48.05%
4. Immediate Post-Run pH	40.72%
5. Body Weight	51.73%
6. Peak Recovery RQ in the 4 min Run	48.05%
7. Peak Exercise RQ in the All-out Run	47.97%
8. Acid Base Balance (pH) in 4 min Run	40.72%
9. Amplitude of the Post-Exercise Brachial Pulse Wave (1 min after the All-out Treadmill Run)	31.83%
10. Oxygen Intake Capacity (l/min/kg in the 4 min Run, the standard jog)	14.36%

	r	Beta	Beta square	Per Cent Cont.
Peak Eosinophil drop	0.320	0.2746	0.0754	22.26
Peak Gross O_2 Intake (cc/min/kg)	0.657	0.2240	0.0502	14.82
Peak Ventilation in Recovery (l/min/kg)	0.711	0.2682	0.0719	21.23
Peak Exercise RQ	−.444	−.1344	0.0181	5.34
Peak Recovery RQ	−.557	−.1235	0.0153	4.52
Post-Exercise Brachial Pulse Wave Amplitude	.560	.3284	0.1078	31.83
Pulse Wave Change (Pre to Post)	−.478	.0011	0.0000	0.00
			0.3387	100.00

alone. We therefore searched in another area, namely, that of the actual physical ability variables. The results were as follows:

	r	Beta	Beta squared	Net Contribution
Weight	−.657	−.3663	.1342	51.73
Strength/Weight (by dynamometers)	.457	.0949	.0090	3.47
Chinning the Bar	.612	−.0230	.0005	0.19
Dipping	.575	.1394	.0194	7.48
Vertical Jump	.593	.1812	.0328	12.64
Agility Run	−.447	.0598	.0036	1.39
Balance	.577	.2418	.0585	22.55
Standing Broad Jump	.524	.0379	.0014	0.54
			.2594	100.00

R = 0.768   S.E. est. = 119.00

So, the actual physical ability makes a contribution nearly as great as all of the described stress indicators. The performance is due to ability plus disposition to stand stress.

Changes in the ICP, EML and TP

In a very moderate (sub-maximal, non-progressive type of physical training program (such as RAAB's long distance pleasure cyclists or 'cakewalk' performers,) there is a lengthening of the ICP interval, which RAAB [9] has repeatedly claimed is a sharp indicator of the sympatho-adrenergic, tension inducing aspect, influencing the tension built up in the isovolumic (formerly isometric) period of the heart cycle. There is good basis for taking the ICP interval (from the second heart sound to the ejection of the blood from the heart) as a stress indicator. But is has not been known whether this parallels the type of stress indicated by the eosinophils, hormonal blood indicators (adrenaline and epinephrine) or whether the ICP is specific to the heart. We seem to be the first to relate the heart intervals to endurance performance itself, as in an all-out bicycle ride for time. This was done in two experiments at our laboratory by SLONINGER [10] and also by CUNDIFF [3]. Very short, progressive, relatively hard training programs have typically shortened the ICP as contrasted to moderate non-progressive or strength type training programs [8, 9]. Weight training had almost no effect upon the ICP interval but any progressive running type program done over 6 to 26 weeks will shorten it. There is almost no value to the ICP interval of the left ventricle for predicting the time of the ergometer bicycle performance. Moreover, the ICP does not relate well to the eosinopenia or other such measures made in the peripheral blood samples. The EML (Q to first heart sound) is relatively insensitive but both EML and TP (total tension period sum of ICP and EML) will shorten if the training period is hard and relatively short, (1 to 2 months) indicating that adaptation has not occurred. The EML lengthens in sickness and with aging as has been indicated by HYMAN [6]. It is interesting that in our data on 30 male subjects of middle-age (25 to 45 years) that the intercorrelation between ICP and EMP is −.40, so one shortens (EML) and the other may lengthen (ICP) in our most typical progressive training programs. This indicates that they should always be measured separately and not together as TP. The ICP does reflect the stress as experienced right at the heart nerves, and probably is better to reflect the stress upon the heart than the more peripherally measured indicators (eosinophils, O_2 intake or O_2 debt, pH of peripheral blood, etc.). It is an important test of relaxation (lengthened ICP).

Landry-Cureton-Fitzgibbon Study on Hematological Response To Four Types of Ergometer Bicycle Work Patterns

Using continuous recording and sophistocated circulatory-respiratory apparatus, and multiple sampling procedures, LANDRY [7] completed the study of four subjects on four types of work, but with all trials for one hour of work, either continuous or in one of three patterns of 'interval training' work, namely, one minute work and 1 min rest (1 to 1), 2 min work and 2 min rest (2 to 2) and three min work and 3 min rest. In each case the work totalled 6000 W and the rate of the work was adjusted to make this possible. The circulatory-respiratory measures were obtained by means of the Dargatz Magnatest Apparatus (type 510, Hamburg, West Germany). The results of this work are shown in table I:

Table I. Stress responses to four types of work (LANDRY-CURETON-FITZGIBBONS, 1968)

Stress indicator	Continuous type work (Aerobic)	1–1 Interval	2–2 Interval	3–3 Interval
		(no oxygen debt measured)		
O_2 Intake (l/min)	1.67	1.98	2.53	2.73
Lactic acid (mg %)	10.7	33.3	51.8	57.1
Pyruvic acid (mg %)	.78	1.5	1.5	1.3
Base excess (mEq./liter)	−4.3	−5.9	−7.8	−9.1
pH	7.36	7.32	7.31	7.28
pCO_2 (9 mm Hg)	34.1	36.3	33.5	33.5
K (mEq/liter)	4.3	4.9	5.3	5.5
Total Protein (mg %)	7.7	8.0	8.2	8.4
Albumin (g %)	4.7	5.0	5.2	5.3

The results of this experiment indicate:
1. That muscle metabolics bear an excellent witness to the severity of the disturbance and the degree of suffering of the subject during strenuous exertion.
2. The serum profile taken during a continuous hour of work, or in a series of *work* and *rest* intervals reveals functional disturbances in the

metabolites which parallel the distress experienced by the subjects. Such functional disturbances indicate the relative activity of the cells, organs and physiological systems to some real degree.

3. Eight of 12 parameters considered did not differ significantly in the four types if work, namely: Na, Cl, CO_2, alkaline phosphatase, bilirubin, urea and glutamic oxalacetic transaminase.

4. The relative importance of these stress indicators to indicate prediction of performance is not fully worked out as yet.

5. The work performed continuously does not reflect stress results very different from the interval type work at 1–1, 2–2 and 3–3 patterns.

References

1. ADAMS, W. C.: Relationship and possible causal effects of selected variables on treadmill endurance run performance. Res. Quart. *38:* 515–516 (1968).
2. ANDERSON, K. L.; HEUSNER, W. H. and POHNDORF, R. H.: "The progressive effects of athletic training on the red and white blood cells and the total plasma protein", Arbeitsphysiologie *16:* 120–128 (1955).
3. CUNDIFF, D. S.: Training changes in the sympatho-adrenal system determined by cardiac interval hemodynamics, O_2 intake and eosinopenia, Urbana: Ph. D. thesis (unpublished), Physical Education, University of Illinois, p. 188 (1966). (Sponser: T. K. CURETON.)
4. CURETON, T. K.: Physical Fitness of Champion Athletes. 330–341, Urbana: University of Illinois Press (1951).
5. HEUSNER, W. E.: Progressive changes in the physical fitness of an adult male during a season of training for competitive swimming, Urbana, Illinois: Ph. D. thesis (unpublished), Physical Education, University of Illinois, p. 463 (1955). (Sponsor: T. K. CURETON.)
6. HYMAN, A. S.: The Q—to first heart sound interval in athletes at rest and after exercise. J. Sports med. Physical Fitness *4:* 199–203 (Detat., 1964).
7. LANDRY, J. F.: Adaptation of organic functions to continuous and intermittent exercise patterns in four male subjects. Urbana: Ph. D. thesis (unpublished), Physical Education, University of Illinois, p. 149 (1968).
8. LIVERMAN, R. E.: Comparative training effects on simultaneous electrocardiogram, ballistocardiogram and heartograph records, Urbana: Ph. D. thesis (unpublished), Physical Education, University of Illinois, p.126 (1965).
9. RAAB, WILHELM: Training, physical inactivity and the cardiac dynamic cycle. J. Sports med. Physical Fitness *6:* 38–47 (1966).
10. SLONINGER, E. L.: The relationship of stress indicators to pre-ejection cardiac intervals. Urbana: Ph. D. thesis (unpublished), Physical Education, University of Illinois (1966). (Sponsor: T. K. CURETON.)
11. WEBER, H. and CURETON, T. K.: A quantitative study of eosinopenia and other stress indicators, p. 123 in Abstracts of the Research Section, Amer. Ass. Hlth. Physical Education and Recreation, University of Illinois, p. 188 (1966). [Sponsor: T. K. CURETON, Ph. D. thesis by WEBER (1965).]

12. WRIGHT, SEWELL: Correlation and causation, J. agricultural Res. *20:* 562 (Jan. 1921), also, MONROE W. S. and STUIT, D. B.: Correlation analysis as a means of studying contribution of causes, J. of exp. Ed. *3:* 155–165 (1935) and CURETON, T. K.: Endurance of young men, Washington, D. C.: Soc. Res. in Child Development, National Research Council, *X:* Serial No. 40, No. 1, (1945).

Author's address: Dr. T. K. CURETON, Ph. D., D. Sc., F.A.C.S.M., Physical Fitness Research Laboratory, University of *Illinois, Ill.* (USA).

Biochemistry of Exercise.
Medicine and Sport, Vol. 3; pp. 81–88 (Karger, Basel/New York 1969)

The Behaviour of Arterial Blood Gases, Arterial Substrates, pH and Haematocrit in Different Ergometric Work

W. HOLLMANN and K. KASTNER

Institut für Kreislaufforschung und Sportmedizin, Köln

After the determination of normal values for cardiopulmonary function in spiro-ergometric investigations, special interest has focussed on the behaviour of various substrates in the arterial blood in relation to that of blood gases. In view of the difference in ergometric methods of examination it is important to answer the question to what extent different ergometric work can lead to different qualitative and/or quantitative results. Examinations about these questions have been performed by ÅSTRAND, HOLMGREN et al., ASMUSSEN, BOLT, HOLLMANN, VENRATH et al., HARTUNG et al., BROUHA, WYNDHAM et al. and others. The results described in the following report were obtained in 42 healthy male test subjects aged 19 to 31. For details of the methods we must, for reasons of time, refer to a later publication.

The present communication is based on the results of six different test series.

1. Gradually increasing load. Beginning with 6 mkp/sec increasing by 4 mkp/sec each time, duration of work at each load grade 6 min.

2. Constant load of 30 min duration. Load intensity near the so-called endurance limit, individually determined in preliminary tests.

3. Constant work of 30 min duration. Effort intensity above endurance limit (in pseudo-steady state).

4. Constant work of 3–10 min duration with maximal or near-maximal load intensity.

5. Standard test method according to HOLLMANN and VENRATH. Beginning with 3 mkp/sec. After 3 min effort, increase of load intensity by 4 mkp/sec.

6. As 5, but with 16 or 12 vol% O_2 in inspired air.

[1] The examinations have been performed in collaboration with M. HARTUNG, H. VENRATH, W. ISSELHARDT and D. JAENCKNER (see the Monographie: "Über die Atmungsregulation unter Arbeit", von M. HARTUNG et al. (Westdeutscher Buchverlag, Köln 1966).

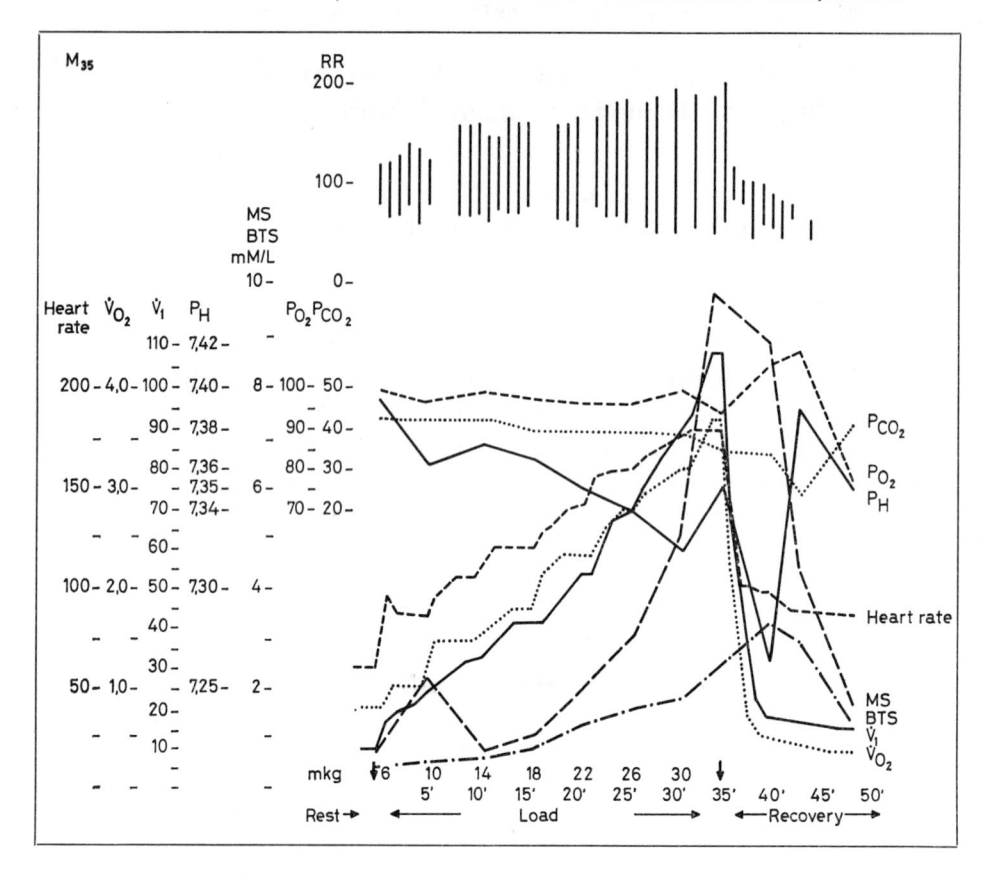

Figure 1. The pattern of ventilation, oxygen intake, arterial substrates and blood gases at rest, during increasing load and in recovery. Subject: G.W., 23 years [with HARTUNG et al.].

Results

1st test series. (Figure 1 – MS means lactic acid, BTS means pyruvic acid.)

PO_2 and SO_2.

In test arrangement 1 a fall of PO_2 or SO_2 occurred in 5 out of 16 persons only towards the end of load. In the remaining subjects there was either no change or a rise.

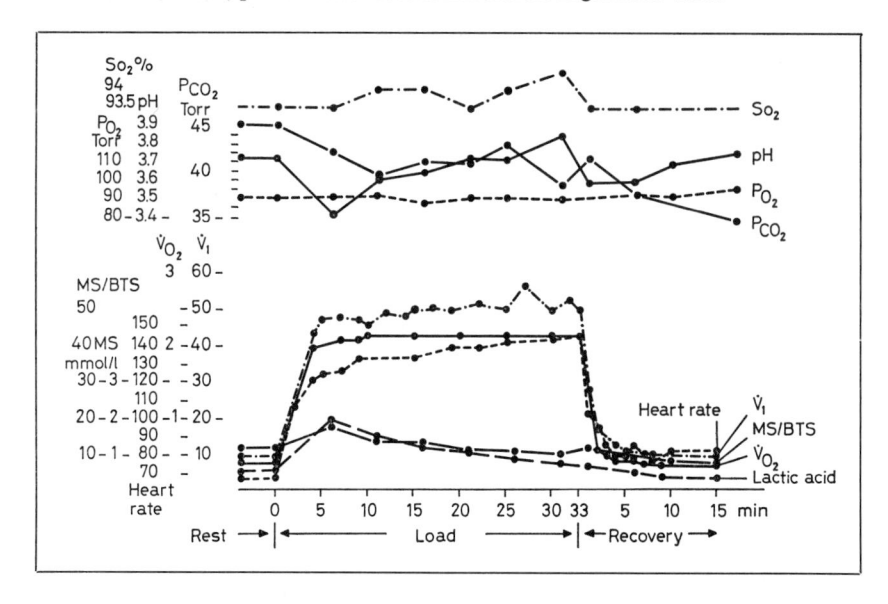

Figure 2. The pattern of ventilation, oxygen intake, arterial substrates and blood gases in rest and during constant load of 30 min duration near endurance limit (16 mkp/sec. corresponding to 49.5% of the maximal oxygen intake ability). Subject: J.A., 24 years [with HARTUNG et al.].

Lactic acid and pyruvic acid

Generally the arterial lactic acid level rose slowly up to an oxygen intake of ca. 1,500 to 1,800 ml per min and increased considerably faster after exceeding this load level. The less efficient subjects showed, at a pulse rate of 180 per min, considerably higher arterial concentrations than the more efficient. During the recovery period there occurred a fall of the lactic acid level immediately on cessation of work.

The pyruvic acid showed a relatively smaller rise. It lagged behind that of lactic acid especially in the higher load grades.

The lactate-pyruvate quotient rose steadily but not in a straight line. In endurance-trained persons there was a fall of the quotient at the start of work. In equal load grades the quotient was higher in untrained subjects than in trained ones. In the first 3 to 5 min of the recovery phase the pyruvate value continued to rise, resulting in a rapid fall of the quotient. This phenomenon was described by HOLLMANN in 1959.

PCO_2 and CCO_2 showed mainly a tendency to fall in the highest

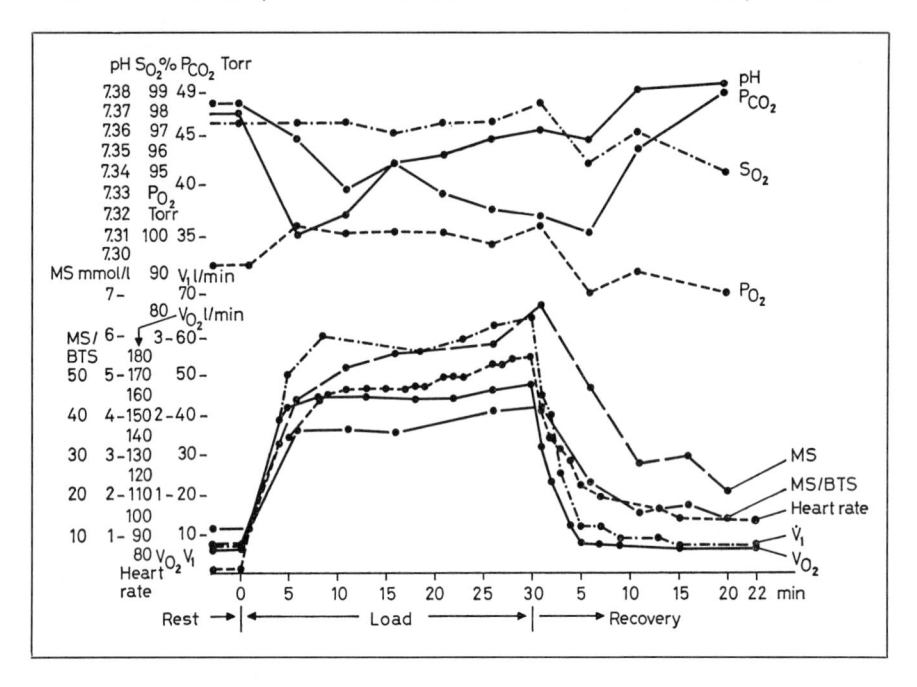

Figure 3. The pattern of ventilation, oxygen intake, arterial substrates and blood gases at rest and during constant load above endurance limit (18 mkp/sec, corresponding to 65% of the maximal oxygen intake ability). Subject: J.N., 22 years [with HARTUNG et al.].

load grades. In all cases an additional reduction of values occurred in the first recovery minutes.

Arterial pH-value

In all subjects a reduction of the pH-value occurred at the start of work. In 7 subjects it later rose again slowly in spite of increasing ergometer load. 11 of the 16 subjects showed a lower pH-value in the first recovery minutes than in the penultimate load grade.

Haematocrit

In all subjects there was a rise in the arterial blood, most marked at the transition from rest to work. In the higher load grades there was a further rise. The maximum occurred in the highest load grade or in the first recovery minutes.

The glucose changes were less uniform. We distinguished three reaction types according to HARTUNG et al. The first showed a progressive decrease of blood sugar values during load, followed by an increase during the recovery period. The second showed an alternating behaviour with fluctuations between fall and rise, followed by a definitive increase during the recovery period. The third showed a progressive blood sugar rise in the various load grades and in the recovery period.

2nd test series (figure 2)

30 min work period with an intensity of 40–50% of aerobic capacity. Start of work always with 6 mkp/sec, rising every minute by 4 mkp/sec until the individually desired load intensity is reached.

PCO_2 and CCO_2 showed in all subjects a fall during load, whereas the PO_2 and SO_2 values during work were above the resting values in all cases.

The arterial lactic acid concentration and the lactate-pyruvate quotient reached their highest values in the 5th work minute and then fell slowly but progressively up to the end of the observation period. The pH-value moved in the same manner. The arterial glucose values in all subjects sank continuously during work. The haematocrit value rose during load.

3rd test series (figure 3)

30 min constant load with 65–70% of maximal oxygen intake. The arterial O_2 partial pressure was above the initial resting value during the whole work period, except in one test subject. The changes in arterial oxygen saturation were not significant and showed a rising tendency under work. PCO_2 decreased considerably in most test subjects. Arterial lactic acid concentration and the lactate-pyruvate quotient were considerably raised in the 5th work minute in all test subjects. During the residual work time it continued to rise in the majority of test subjects. The pH-value fell far below the resting value in the 5th work minute and then rose again up to the 30th min.

Real glucose was reduced at first in the arterial blood but rose again during the last work min. Haematocrit increased considerably in all test subjects during load.

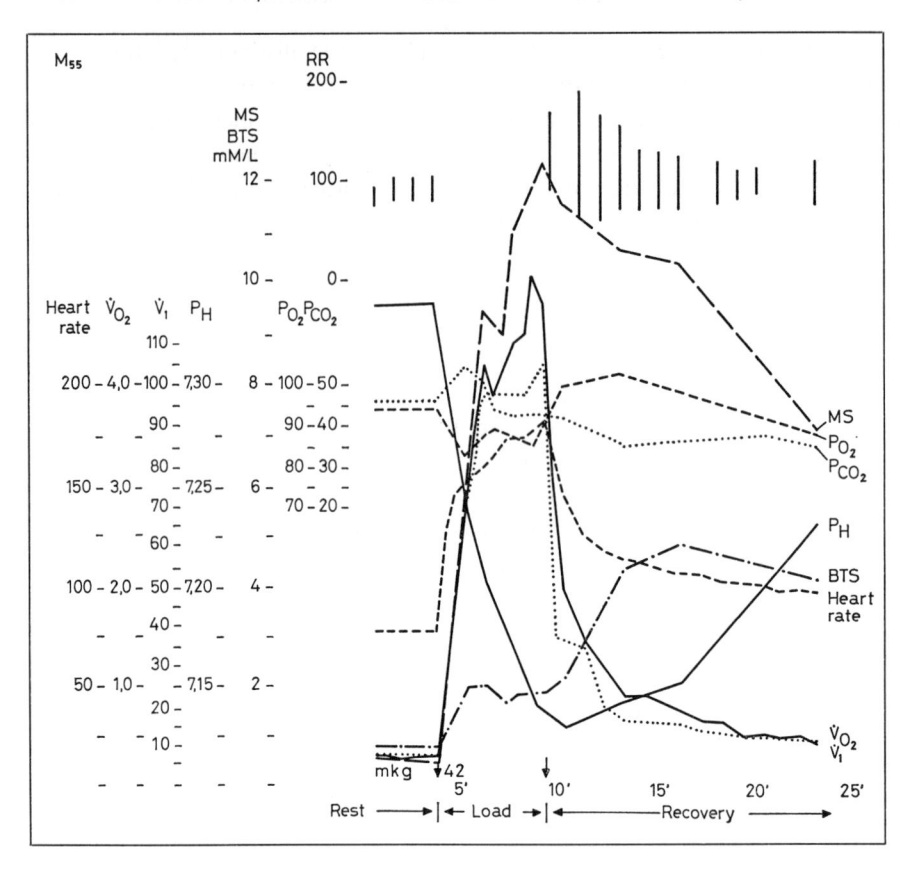

Figure 4. The pattern of ventilation, oxygen intake, arterial substrates and blood gases in rest, during constant work with maximal load intensity (42 mkp/sec) and in recovery. Subject: F.P., 26 years [with HARTUNG et al.].

4th test series (figure 4)

Maximal or near-maximal ergometric load of 3–10 min duration. PO_2 and SO_2 fell, so did the pH-value. The lowest pH was 7.010 and it continued to fall to 7.001 in the 3rd recovery min.

Arterial PCO_2 fell in all test subjects below the resting value as well during work as in the following recovery min. Lactate and lactate-pyruvate quotient rose quickly and reached the highest values obtained by us under normoxia. During the recovery phase pyruvic acid rose again con-

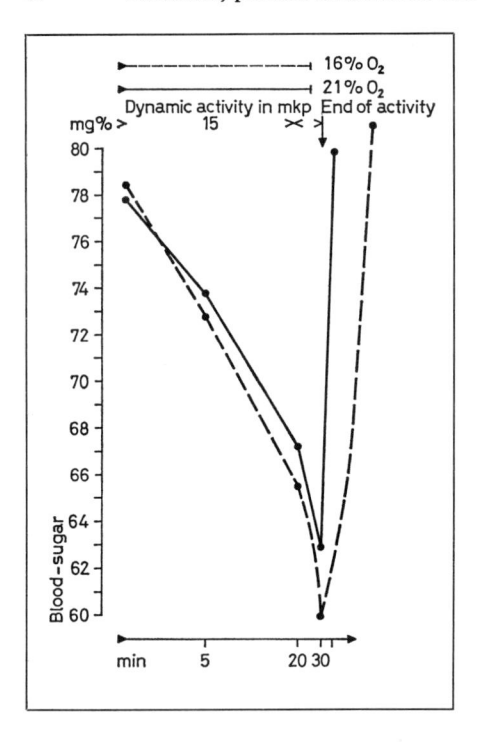

Figure 5. The pattern of glucose during increasing load and in recovery under normoxia and hypoxia.

siderably on cessation of work and showed maximal values between the 10th and 16th recovery min.

5th test series

Standard test method according to HOLLMANN and VENRATH. Tendency and range of the examined criteria agree with the results of the 1st test series.

6th test series (figure 5)

Standard test examinations under 16 and 12 vol% O_2 in the inspired air.

Apart from the initial values, already lowered at rest, there was fundamentally the same tendency under work in all examined criteria as in maximal ergometric work of 5–10 min duration. Only the peak values in maximal work were far exceeded due to hypoxia.

Summary

According to the ergometric test arrangement selected, a different behaviour of the examined blood gases and substrates must be expected not only quantitatively but also qualitatively. Due importance must be attached to this factor in the arrangement of ergometric examination methods.

Authors' address: Prof. Dr. med. W. HOLLMANN and Dr. med. K. KASTNER, Institut für Kreislaufforschung und Sportmedizin, Carl-Diem-Weg, *5 Köln-Müngersdorf* (Germany).

L'acidose métabolique au cours de l'effort musculaire

R. Vanroux

Département de Physiologie respiratoire, Hôpital Civil, Charleroi

On trouve régulièrement, en cours d'effort musculaire, un degré d'acidose métabolique plus ou moins élevé dès le moment où l'on atteint un certain niveau de charge. Ce phénomène est classiquement expliqué par le fait que les cellules musculaires, placées dans des conditions anaérobiques lorsque le débit circulatoire devient insuffisant, libèrent de l'acide lactique en quantité plus ou moins importante dans le torrent circulatoire.

L'objet de cet exposé est de passer en revue les principaux facteurs de variation de ce paramètre en cours d'effort et d'en étudier les répercussions sur la ventilation.

Méthodes utilisées – sujets testés

L'exercice musculaire est effectué sur cyclo-ergomètre (ergostat de Fleisch); la fréquence de pédalage adoptée est habituellement de 60/min. La charge y est croissante régulièrement, de 30 W toutes les trois minutes et les sujets pédalent jusqu'à épuisement; ou bien, dans un autre type d'exercice, la charge y est constante et l'effort imposé est d'une durée moyenne de 20 min.

$\overset{\circ}{V}$, $\overset{\circ}{V}_{O_2}$, $\overset{\circ}{V}_{CO_2}$ sont enregistrés d'une façon continue à l'aide d'un appareil à circuit fermé: le métabographe de Fleisch; la composition du mélange gazeux respiré peut y être modifiée en cours d'expérience.

Des échantillons de sang artériel sont prélevés en cours d'épreuve: on y mesure la PaO_2, la SaO_2, le pH, le CO_2 total (appareil de Van Slyke), l'acide pyruvique et l'acide lactique (méthode enzymatique).

Les sujets testés sont, soit des sujets normaux, sans activité physique particulière, soit des athlètes.

Notation de l'acidose métabolique

Les variations du pH du sang en fonction des modifications du taux des bicarbonates et du CO_2 libre sont exprimées dans la relation

Tableau I.

	Repos	6' à 120 W	3' à 180 W	3' à 240 W	3' à 270 W
pH	7,495	7,45	7,41	7,38	7,36
CO_2 total	57,8 vol.%	56,5 vol.%	53,1 vol.%	48,7 vol.%	47,2 vol.%
Bicarbonates	55,2 vol.%	54 vol.%	50,6 vol.%	46,3 vol.%	44,3 vol.%
$PaCO_2$	38,5 mm Hg	36 mm Hg	37 mm Hg	35,5 mm Hg	37 mm Hg
pH métabolique	7,43	7,42	7,39	7,35	7,335
Acide lactique	16,45 mg%	15,86 mg%	16,45 mg%	25,26 mg%	39,36 mg%
Acide pyruvique	0,68 mg%	1,20 mg%	1,34 mg%	1,47 mg%	1,54 mg%

Tableau II.

	Repos	6' à 120	3' à 180	3' à 240
pH	7,44	7,435	7,415	7,295
CO_2 total	54,7 vol.%	48,7 vol.%	52,1 vol.%	36,4 vol.%
Bicarbonates	52,3 vol.%	46,5 vol.%	49,6 vol.%	34,2 vol.%
$PaCO_2$	35 mm Hg	33 mm Hg	37 mm Hg	33 mm Hg
pH métabolique	7,405	7,37	7,38	7,24
Acide lactique	18,8 mg%	22,32 mg%	28,20 mg%	76,37 mg%
Acide pyruvique	0,30 mg%	0,41 mg%	0,48 mg%	0,68 mg%

Tableau I et II. Evolution de l'acidose métabolique et du taux des lactates au cours d'un effort croissant

d'Henderson-Hasselbach: $pH = pK + \log \dfrac{\text{bicarbonates}}{CO_2 \text{ libre}}$

On conçoit que le pH peut être maintenu constant au cours de l'acidose métabolique, caractérisée par la chute des bicarbonates, dans la mesure où le CO_2 libre diminue proportionnellement, phénomène provoqué par l'hyperventilation que l'acidose déclenche.

On peut chiffrer le pH qui résulterait de cet acidose, s'il n'y avait ce facteur ventilatoire de correction, en maintenant dans l'équation d'Henderson-Hasselbach, au numérateur, le taux des bicarbonates transmis par l'analyse, et en substituant au chiffre du dénominateur la valeur qui correspond à la $PaCO_2$ de base soit 40 mm Hg.

Relation Δ bicarbonates/Δ acide lactique

De l'ensemble des mesures effectuées, on constate que la chute du taux des bicarbonates est, en général, plus importante que l'accroissement du taux des lactates surtout lorsqu'il s'agit d'efforts légers et moyens. Ce n'est qu'à l'occasion d'efforts exhaustifs ou d'efforts réalisés en hypoxie que l'on constate une relation mole à mole de ces deux paramètres.

L'acide lactique n'est d'ailleurs pas le seul métabolite acide à être neutralisé par les bases du sang; en cours d'effort, l'acide pyruvique croît lui aussi; il en est de même des acides intermédiaires du cycle de Krebs et des acides gras.

Mais les lactates prédominent nettement lorsque l'effort est effectué en hypoxie ou au cours d'efforts exhaustifs.

Facteurs de variation de l'acidose métabolique

1. La charge et la durée de l'effort

a) Efforts d'intensité croissante: L'acidose métabolique croît alors de façon exponentielle [Cotes].

Le comportement de tous les sujets testés peut être résumé dans les exemples décrits aux tableaux I et II.

b) Efforts modérés à charge constante tenus en état d'équilibre: à une phase brève d'adaptation de 2 à 5 min, où la ventilation croît, succède un état stable ventilatoire, durant toute la durée de l'épreuve. Le degré d'acidose du sang prélevé 2½ min après le début de l'effort atteint une valeur égale à la moitié environ de ce qu'elle sera au cours de la 5e min de l'effort et est à peu près stable à partir de ce moment durant les 20 min que dure l'exercice. Le taux d'acide lactique suit dans cette condition la même évolution (figure 1). Par contre, lorsqu'il s'agit d'efforts intenses, la ventilation ne cesse de croître; le taux des bicarbonates baisse progressivement, celui des lactates augmente.

Ces deux conditions peuvent être résumées dans les tableaux III et IV.

2. L'aptitude des sujets testés

Quatre groupes de sujets, définis selon leur aptitude (dans ce cas, la puissance maximum supportée, définie comme l'effort maximum tenu en état stable ventilatoire) ont au cours d'un effort de même intensité, 120 W, d'une durée de 20 min, un degré d'acidose métabolique croissant, qui prend des proportions importantes dans le groupe le moins apte, c'est-à-dire là où la PMS est égale à 100 W (figure 2).

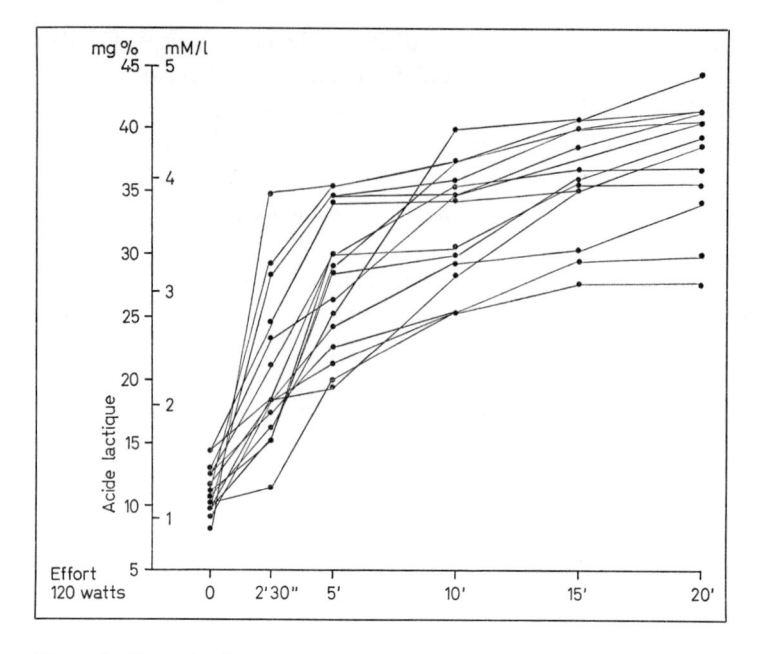

Figure 1. Taux des lactates dans le sang artériel prélevé à la 2½ min, 5e, 10e, 15e, 20e min d'un effort correspondant à peu près à la dépense énergétique maximum en régime stable.

Tableau III. Evolution de l'acidose métabolique et du taux des lactates au cours d'un effort à charge constante

Moment de prélèvement	pH méta.	Bicarb. vol.%	Lact. mg%	Δbic/m mol/l	Δlct/m mol/l
0	7,43	55,83 vol.%	9,98 mg%	–	–
2½	7,385	50,15 vol.%	15,86 mg%	2,55	0,65
5	7,375	48,53 vol.%	29,96 mg%	3,27	2,22
10	7,35	45,29 vol.%	31.13 mg%	4,73	2,35
15	7,35	44,51 vol.%	35,83 mg%	5,08	2,87
20	7,35	44,51 vol.%	35,83 mg%	5,08	2,87

3. Les masses musculaires mises en mouvement

Un effort de 100 W effectué sur cyclo-ergomètre par un sujet normal, réalisé dans des conditions de pédalage normales à l'aide des deux jambes, ou à l'aide d'une seule jambe, entraîne une consommation d'O_2 identique, cependant que la ventilation est nettement plus élevée dans le second cas.

L'acidose métabolique au cours de l'effort musculaire

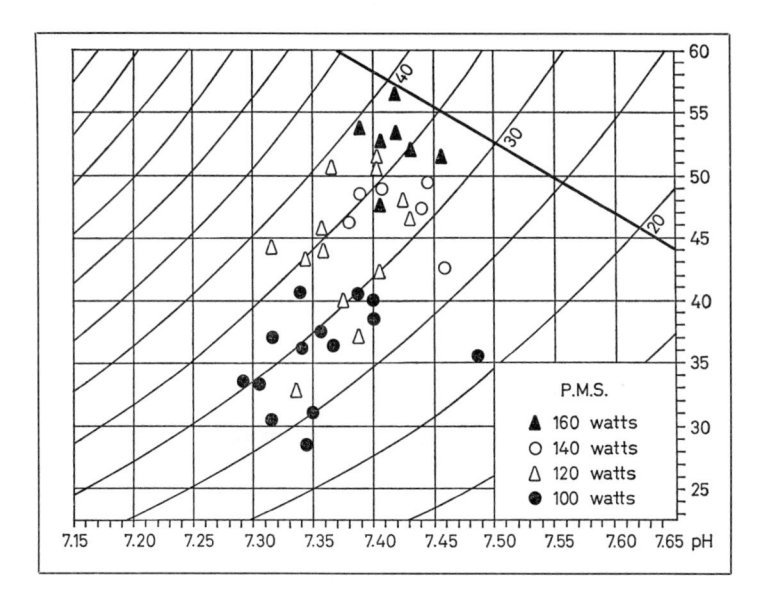

Figure 2. Sur ce schéma de Davenport, expression graphique de l'équation d'Henderson-Hasselbach, sont projetés les points qui définissent le sang artériel prélevé à la 20ᵉ min d'un effort de 120 W. La chute des bicarbonates est très nette dans le groupe constitué des sujets les moins aptes.

Tableau IV. Evolution de l'acidose métabolique et du taux des lactates au cours d'un effort à charge constante

Moment de prélèvement	pH méta.	Bicarb. vol.%	Lact. mg%	Δbic/m mol/l	Δlct/m mol/l
0	7,44	58,35 vol.%	7,63 mg%	–	–
2½	7,385	50,57 vol.%	34,07 mg%	3,49	2,93
5	7,335	44,71 vol.%	35,25 mg%	6,12	3,06
10	7,325	43,67 vol.%	37,01 mg%	6,59	3,26
15	7,315	42,47 vol.%	41,71 mg%	7,13	3,78
20	7,31	41,69 vol.%	44,06 mg%	7,48	4,04

L'acidose métabolique, au cours de cette seconde partie de l'expérience, est plus importante (tableau V); elle peut être interprétée par le fait que l'accroissement du débit circulatoire n'a pas été suffisant pour maintenir en aérobiose le métabolisme des muscles auxquels on a imposé une charge double.

Tableau V. Voir texte.

Conditions d'expérience	pH	CO_2 tot.	Bicarb.	$paCO_2$	pH méta.
Pédalage à l'aide de 2 jambes, 100 W	7,39	53 vol%	50.4 vol%	38 mm Hg	7,375
Pédalage à l'aide d'une jambe, 100 W	7,39	46 vol%	43.9 vol%	30 mm Hg	7,32

4. L'hypoxie

L'acidose métabolique enregistrée au cours d'efforts croissants effectués jusqu'à épuisement par des sujets qui sont placés dans des conditions d'hypoxie sévère (O_2 10%), atteint des degrés élevés; si l'effort est poursuivi dans des conditions d'hyperoxie (O_2 60%), le taux des lactates diminue (seule condition où, au cours de nos expériences, nous avons vu décroître le taux des lactates en cours d'effort) tableau V.

Conséquences de l'acidose métabolique sur les différents paramètres ventilatoires

L'étude simultanée des paramètres ventilatoires et de l'acidose métabolique permet de comprendre l'allure de la courbe de forme asymptotique que prend le débit ventilatoire au cours d'un effort à charge croissante. Pour une charge faible, la ventilation croît uniquement en fonction des besoins métaboliques accrus; à partir d'un certain niveau de charge, l'acidose métabolique apparaît, mais le pH reste stable parce qu'une augmentation supplémentaire de ventilation produit une alcalose respiratoire de compensation; il arrive cependant un moment où le $PaCO_2$ ne se modifie plus dès que l'on atteint les charges limites; l'acidose métabolique continue à croître sans facteur compensatoire désormais.

La liaison est très significative entre le degré d'acidose métabolique et les différents paramètres ventilatoires: l'équivalent ventilatoire, la ventilation alvéolaire et en corollaire la $PaCO_2$.

Elle l'est moins avec le QR qui, en cours d'effort, s'élève et approche de l'unité.

On attribue souvent cet accroissement de QR au fait que les glucides constituent, à l'effort, le combustible de choix; mais il varie également en fonction de l'excès de CO_2 rejeté, dans le but d'assurer, dans la mesure du

Tableau VI. Evolution de l'acidose métabolique et du taux des lactates au cours d'un effort à charge croissante réalisé dans des conditions d'hypoxie

Moment de prélèvement		pH méta.	Bicarb. vol.%	Lact. mg%	Δbic/m mol/l	Δlct/m mol/l
Repos		7,42	51,58 vol.%	16,45 mg%	–	–
60 W 3'	hypoxie 10%	7,40	49,52 vol.%	20,56 mg%	0,92	0,45
90 W 3'		7,38	46,26 vol.%	30,55 mg%	2,38	1,56
120 W 3'		7,335	42,29 vol.%	49,35 mg%	4,17	3,65
150 W 3'		7,315	34,07 vol.%	84,60 mg%	7,86	7,57
150 W 6' O2 60%		7,325	42,76 vol.%	50,52 mg%	3,96	3,78

possible, l'homéostasie du pH. On peut, en recalculant le QR sur la base d'une $PaCO_2$ égale à 40 mm Hg, définir la part métabolique.

Conclusions

En première approximation, on peut considérer que dans la plupart des cas, le facteur circulatoire est l'élément prépondérant qui assigne une limite à l'effort musculaire. S'il est défaillant, l'acide lactique est libéré car les conditions anaérobiques de métabolisme apparaissent et s'aggravent; la ventilation doit dès lors faire face à un nouvel impératif: assurer l'homéostasie du pH. La gêne respiratoire qui apparaît, dès que l'on atteint un certain débit ventilatoire, mettra finalement un terme à l'exercice musculaire.

Bibliographie

BATES and CHRISTIE: Respiratory function in disease (Saunders, Philadelphia 1964).
COMROE, J. H.: Physiology of respiration (Year Book Medical Publishers, Chicago 1966).
COTES, J. E.: Lung function (Blackwell, Oxford 1965).
DAVENPORT, H. W.: The ABC of acid-base chemistry, 4th ed., University of Chicago, 1958.
HUCKABEE, W. E.: Relationship of pyruvate and lactate during anaerobic metabolism. II. Exercise and formation of oxygen debt. J. clin. Invest. *37:* 255–263 (1958).
KARPOVICH, P. V.: Physiology of muscular exercise, 6th ed. (Saunders, Philadelphia 1965).
PIVOTEAU, C.: L'équilibre acido-basique en physio-pathologie respiratoire. Thèse Université de Nancy, Faculté de Paris, 1958.
SELKURT, E.: Physiology. Second Edition, Boston.
VANROUX, R.: L'effort musculaire; in OLIVIER, H. R., Traité de biologie appliquée, vol. IV, 1969.

Adresse de l'auteur: Dr RAYMOND VANROUX, 8, rue d'Angleterre, *Charleroi* (Belgique).

Quelques modifications hématochimiques causées par le travail musculaire chez des sujets d'âge moyen

G. C. Topi, L. Gandolfo d'Alessandro et G. Piovano

Istituto di Medicina dello Sport, Roma

Dans le cadre des recherches visant à étudier les modifications hématochimiques déterminées par les différents types de travail musculaire chez des catégories différentes de sujets (athlètes et sujets non athlétiques d'âges divers) nous avons étudié le comportement de la glycémie, de la pyruvicémie, de la lactacidémie, de la cholestérolémie et des acides gras totaux dans le sérum d'un groupe de sujets non entraînés, soumis au travail au cyclo-ergomètre.

Nous avons pris en considération six sujets âgés de 30 à 50 ans, exerçant des professions libérales, non entraînés, un peu trop lourds, à diète mixte équilibrée, présentant des valeurs normales, à jeun, des paramètres considérés.

Le travail musculaire a été réalisé au cyclo-ergomètre (Elema-Schollander avec contrôle électronique de la charge) préparé pour une charge de 565 kg-m/min. Etant donné que les sujets ne devaient pas atteindre un état de fatigue, le travail a été effectué par périodes variant de 15 à 30 min, le travail extérieur total étant de 5 250 à 16 950 kg-m.

En même temps, l'on a effectué, pendant toute la durée de chaque expérience, les relevés du volume respiratoire, de la consommation de O_2, de la production de CO_2, en utilisant un appareil de Hartmann-Brown modifié, à circuit ouvert. Les prélèvements de sang ont été effectués d'abord avant l'effort (après 30 min de repos absolu), puis aussitôt après l'effort et enfin après 30 min de repos.

La glycémie a été déterminée sur le sang total par la méthode du «glucose vrai» de Hugget et Nixon; la pyruvicémie par la méthode enzymatique de Bücher, la lactacidémie par la méthode de Scholtz et al., la cholestérolémie par la méthode de Bloor et Knudson modifiée, les acides gras totaux du sérum par la méthode de Rappaport.

Les résultats sont rapportés au tableau I.

Comme on peut le remarquer d'après le tableau, la glycémie a présenté presque constamment une faible réduction au terme du travail, et une tendance à remonter vers les valeurs de base après la phase de repos.

Tableau I.

Cas	Temps	Glycémie mg%	Pyruvicémie mg%	Lactacidémie mg%	Cholestérolémie mg%	Acides gras mg%
1	A	96	0,49	17,19	190	371
	B	81	0,66	53,12	176	389
	C	89	0,44	2,06	164	154
2	A	104	0,33	6,25	165	–
	B	94	0,39	10,00	190	–
	C	104	0,64	3,25	141	–
3	A	110	0,78	10,50	159	311
	B	90	1,34	30,56	203	354
	C	88	0,79	11,50	182	354
4	A	112	1,38	13,25	186	241
	B	92	1,46	14,19	190	302
	C	98	0,82	13,12	125	207
5	A	116	0,88	13,19	251	475
	B	87	0,98	18,44	281	492
	C	103	0,69	11,69	245	328
6	A	95	0,88	3,25	252	1 089
	B	98	1,31	15,44	218	771
	C	92	1,20	5,31	216	881

A = repos; B = aussitôt après l'effort; C = après 30 min de repos.

Ces résultats s'accordent avec les données de la littérature; en effet, d'après la plupart des auteurs, un effort bref, intense, principalement anaérobie implique, au terme du travail, une hyperglycémie, alors qu'un effort principalement aérobie mais demandant un certain effort musculaire et d'une durée suffisante entraîne une diminution de la glycémie. Dans les deux cas, pendant la phase de repos après l'effort, il y a tendance au retour aux valeurs de base.

La pyruvicémie a montré une augmentation, parfois faible, mais constante, au terme du travail, et par la suite une diminution. La lactacidémie a présenté un comportement semblable. Les modifications observées, augmentation après l'effort et recouvrement, parfois incomplet, à la 30ᵉ min de repos, calquent, quant à leur importance, les modifications bien connues dans la littérature, provoquées par des efforts d'intensité et de durée moyennes, donc principalement aérobies.

Dans le travail principalement anaérobie, l'augmentation de l'acide lactique après l'effort est bien supérieure.

La cholestérolémie est augmentée d'une façon inconstante au terme du travail, présentant cependant dans tous les cas une diminution après la période de recouvrement, par rapport aux valeurs initiales. A l'heure actuelle une explication exhaustive du phénomène ne peut être donnée; d'ailleurs, la littérature l'a déjà signalée.

Les acides gras totaux du sérum n'ont pas démontré un comportement univoque, bien qu'une diminution par rapport aux valeurs initiales se soit vérifiée chez quatre sujets, au terme de l'observation, comme plusieurs AA. l'ont déjà remarqué pour les triglycérides et les NEFA.

L'accumulation de données nouvelles sur les modifications métaboliques provoquées par le travail musculaire dans ses différentes formes rend de plus en plus nécessaire et intéressante une étude corrélative des différentes sections du métabolisme intermédiaire intéressées, qui permettrait aussi de déterminer les rapports avec les variations quantitatives et qualitatives des paramètres respiratoires.

Adresse des auteurs: Prof. G. C. Topi, Dr L. Gandolfo d'Alessandro et Dr G. Piovano, Istituto di Medicina dello Sport, *Roma* (Italie).

II. Carbohydrate and Lipid Metabolisms

Metabolism of Lipids in Blood and Tissues during Exercise

S. O. FRÖBERG

King Gustaf V's Research Institute, Stockholm

Since the discovery of the plasma FFA as a metabolically active substance [22], studies have appeared on their role in the energy generation during exercise. With the introduction of isotopes and improved technics it became evident that also other sources than the circulating plasma FFA was available for oxidation. In 1965 available data on the plasma FFA metabolism during exercise were reviewed [14]. Interest was focused on circulating as well as locally stored esterified fatty acids as possible sources for long fatty acids available in the energy metabolism during exercise. Such sources have been summarized in table I. A discussion of the effect of exercise and physical training on plasma and tissue lipids will be presented.

Plasma Lipid Transport System

During conditions with increased demands on the energy metabolism, such as exercise, the supply of substrate for combustion must also be increased. Fatty acids for oxidation may be delivered from plasma by either of the three major lipid transport classes.

Free fatty acid (FFA). In the beginning of exercise the plasma FFA concentration first falls [3] then increases [9]. The fall is due to an increased efflux from plasma [10, 26, 35] and the following increase probably due to an increased mobilisation of FA from the adipose tissue (AT) [27, 36]. This is suggested from the concomitant increase in the plasma concentration of glycerol [11, 27]. The uptake of FA by muscle is proportional to the amount perfused per unit time. Therefore, the initially increased efflux probably is the consequence of the altered hemodynamics when exercise starts [10]. Similarly the post-exercise increase in the plasma FFA concentration is due to a greater inflow to than outflow from plasma as a consequence of reduced blood flow through the muscles. Hormonal, nervous and nutritional factors are involved in the mobilisation of FA [56]. Of the many factors discussed in this mobilisation of FFA during exercise the sympathetic nervous system is

Table I. Possible sources for long-chain fatty acid supply to muscle oxidative metabolism

---

Plasma Lipid Transport System
    Chylomicrons
    Lipoproteins
    Free fatty acids
Intracellular Lipid Pools
    Triglycerides
    Phospholipids
    Other?
Extracellular Lipid Pools
    Adipose tissue between muscle fibers

---

probably the most important [36]. This is based on the fact that the activity of the sympathetic nervous system is increased during exercise [62, 63] and catecholamines are potent stimulators of the FFA mobilisation from the AT *in vitro* [33] and *in vivo* [32, 46, 59].

HAVEL et al. have performed experiments designed to quantitate the amount of plasma FFA that was oxidized during exercise in fasting men [36]. They infused C^{14} labelled palmitic acid in exercising men and determined the label appearing in the CO_2 of expired air. On the assumption that C^{14} labelled palmitic acid is representative for the metabolism of the plasma FFA in general it was found that less than 50 % of the expired CO_2 was derived from immediate oxidation of plasma FFA. Since the RQ was about 0.75 this suggests that plasma FFA did not account for all lipids oxidized during exercise.

Lipoproteins. Other plasma sources for fatty acid are the TG rich lipoproteins in plasma. The most important is probably the endogenously TG synthesised in the liver (very low density fraction = VLD). The VLD is believed to transport endogenous fatty acids to peripheral tissues [37]. Few studies are available on the lipoproteins during exercise and the knowledge about their metabolism under this condition is poor. Studies in man have shown that the VLD fraction of the lipoproteins was reduced after exercise for several hours [13]. Although this lipoprotein fraction contains a great amount of TG the cholesterol content is small. Therefore, the cholesterol concentration of plasma will be fairly unchanged after prolonged acute exercise [13]. In another study we followed the concentration of plasma lipids during a ten day period of low caloric intake with exercise [16]. In this study the TG concentration of plasma declined until the third day and then remained constant. Also in this study the decrease was the result of lowered TG concentration in the VLD fraction. Fasting itself has been reported not to depress the plasma TG concentration [44, 58]. Therefore it is probable that the exercise was responsible for the observed decrease. In this study also the cholesterol concentration of plasma decreased. The major part of the cholesterol content of plasma is found in the low density (LD) lipoprotein fraction. The observed decrease was due to progressively lowered amounts of cholesterol in this lipoprotein class. The reason for this decrease, however, is not clear. Exercise per se [13, 25, 40, 43, 49, 60] or fasting [24, 44, 48] has been reported not to decrease the plasma cholesterol concentration. During training, however, with a concomitant weight decrease as was also observed in this study, the cholesterol concentration of plasma seems to fall [31, 40, 57].

Possible mechanisms involved in the regulation of the plasma TG metabolism during exercise has been discussed earlier [13]. One factor of importance is the vascular lipoprotein lipase system which hydrolysis circulating TG and the liberated fatty acids (TGFA) can then be taken up by tissues for further metabolism. The activity of this enzyme system has also been reported to increase in myocardium as well as in skeletal muscle during exercise [53]. Most quantitative studies on circulating TG have been performed on isolated perfused hearts. Thus it has been shown that the TG in the perfusate are rapidly hydrolysed and that the TGFA are readily extracted and oxidized [19, 20, 34, 45]. HAVEL et al. studied the oxidative metabolism in leg tissues during bicycle exercise in man. It was found that about ten percent of the oxidized FA was derived from TG circulating in the plasma [38].

Chylomicra. The chylomicra are produced in the gastrointestinal tract and introduced into the blood through the thoracic duct. The fat particles are then transported to different tissues for deposition or utilisation. Previous studies have shown that the alimentary lipemia after a fat rich meal is reduced by exercise [52]. However, no studies are available on the time course or which mechanisms are involved in the effect of exercise on the lowered TG concentration.

The removal of exogenous TG can be characterized by two constants K1 and K2 [12]. K1 describes a zero order reaction for the elimination of TG above a certain concentration, normaly around 1 mmole per l. Below this concentration the elimination is proportional to the concentration. K2 thus describes a first order reaction.

We studied the effect of exercise on the alimentary lipemia by infusing a fat emulsion in man during exercise. The kinetics for the elimination of the fat emulsion from the blood is almost identical to those of chylomicra in man [35] and dog [12]. After one hour of exercise (about 800 km per min) we found no increase in the elimination of the fat emulsion from the plasma. The K1 remained unchanged and the K2 tended to decrease during exercise. Therefore exercise was without effect on the concentration of the circulating chylomicra.

In another type of study young male subjects were fed a standardized fat meal. Exercise started 30 min after the ingestion of the fat and lasted for 60 min. The alimentary lipemia was followed during exercise and rest (table II). The TG concentration was found to be reduced during exercise. After exercise, however, no difference was observed in the lipemia between resting and exercised subjects.

These studies indicate that exercise depressed the rate of entry of chylomicra from the gastrointestinal tract to the blood. When the exogenous TG, e.g. chylomicra, were analysed by the K1 and K2 technic it was found that this concentration was also lowered by exercise. This finding combined with the study on the elimination of infused exogenous TG during exercise support the idea that exercise reduces the inflow of TG from the gut rather than increases their outflow to different tissues.

Tissue TG and Energy Metabolism

Fatty acids may also be taken from local pools of esterified fatty acids – extracellular or intracellular. These pools have been synthetised when the availability of substrate is good and may serve as reservoirs from which energy could be obtained when demands exceeds supplies via the blood. The possible role of these pools in the energy metabolism will be briefly discussed.

Diafragma incubated in substrate free medium respired at an RQ of about 0.70 [61]. Under similar conditions the amount of esterified FA decreased [51]. Perfusion of hearts with substrate free media was followed by a decrease in the endogenous TG content of myocardium [21, 54]. If adrenalin was added to the perfusate the glycerol concentration of the medium increased [18]. This indicates an increased hydrolysis of the myocardial TG. Concomitant with this the oxygen consumption increased [18] which suggest enhanced oxidation of endogenous TGFA. These studies

Table II. Effect of exercise on the concentration of total and exogenous (chylomicron) triglycerides in plasma

Time, min		0	60	90	120	210	330
Total triglycerides, mmole/l	Rest n = 10	0.78 ± 0.09	1.08 ± 0.09	1.72 ± 0.20	2.01 ± 0.17	2.05 ± 0.19	1.17 ± 0.13
	Exercise n = 5	0.76 ± 0.04	0.96 ± 0.09	1.25 ± 0.08	1.82 ± 0.16	2.32 ± 0.18	1.29 ± 0.14
Exogenous triglycerides, mmole/l	Rest n = 10	0.03 ± 0.01	0.05 ± 0.01	0.29 ± 0.06	0.44 ± 0.09	0.37 ± 0.06	0.08 ± 0.02
	Exercise n = 5	0.04 ± 0.01	0.03 ± 0.01	0.08 ± 0.03	0.26 ± 0.09	0.44 ± 0.07	0.06 ± 0.03

Mean value ± standard error of the mean. Standardized fat meal (1 g/kg) was given at zero time. Ten subjects rested comfortably during the whole study, five exercised at moderate work loads for 1 h from 30 to 90 min. Exogenous (chylomicron) triglycerides were determined by the polyvinyl pyrrolidone technique of Gordis [cf. 35]. (From CARLSON, EKELUND, FRÖBERG and HALLBERG, unpublished data.)

indicate that diafragma as well as myocardium utilized local TG pools in the energy metabolism.

From analysis of data on blood lipids during forearm exercise [1] and treadmill running [36] it has been suggested that more than 25% of the energy expenditure was derived from muscle lipids. However, no direct studies are available on the metabolism of muscle lipids in man during exercise. We have started such studies and also used rats to get information on the effect of the lipids of myocardium and liver. I will start with a discussion of our findings in the rat.

Striated muscle contains two main types of fibres, the red and the white ones. Histochemical studies [5, 23, 50] have shown differences in the enzyme pattern and myoglobin concentration between these fibres. This may indicate differences in the rate of metabolism of lipids, which has been shown for carbohydrates in vitro [2, 4, 7]. Therefore, we wanted to study the lipid metabolism in the different types of muscle fibres separately. The two muscle types were readily isolated from the gastrocnemius muscle of the rat. The blood content as well as the concentration of phospholipids and cholesterol, probably mainly structural elements of cellular membranes, was found to be higher in red than white muscle type [28]. The higher activity of oxidative enzymes combined with the finding of higher concentration of phospholipids and cholesterol in red muscle may indicate a higher mitochondrial density. Furthermore, the higher blood and myoglobin content of red than white muscle indicate that red muscle is better equipped for oxygen transport. Together this suggests that red muscle has a higher oxidative potential for lipids than white muscle. This is also in accordance with the observation that the TG concentration of red muscle type was depressed after 60 min in moist air at room temperature unlike that of the white [28].

It is of interest in this context that administration of nicotinic acid to fasting rats was followed by a decreased TG concentration of myocardium as well as red muscle but no change was observed in the white muscle tissue [15]. A concomitant decrease in liver as well as plasma TG concentration was also observed. This was probably due to a decreased synthesis of TG in the liver consequent upon the reduction of available plasma FFA. Since the flow of FFA to tissues such as myocardium and skeletal muscle also was reduced, these tissues probably had to draw upon their own sources of endogenously stored substrate for the energy metabolism.

Available studies on the effect of physical activity on muscle TG have been performed with electrically induced muscle contraction on anaes-

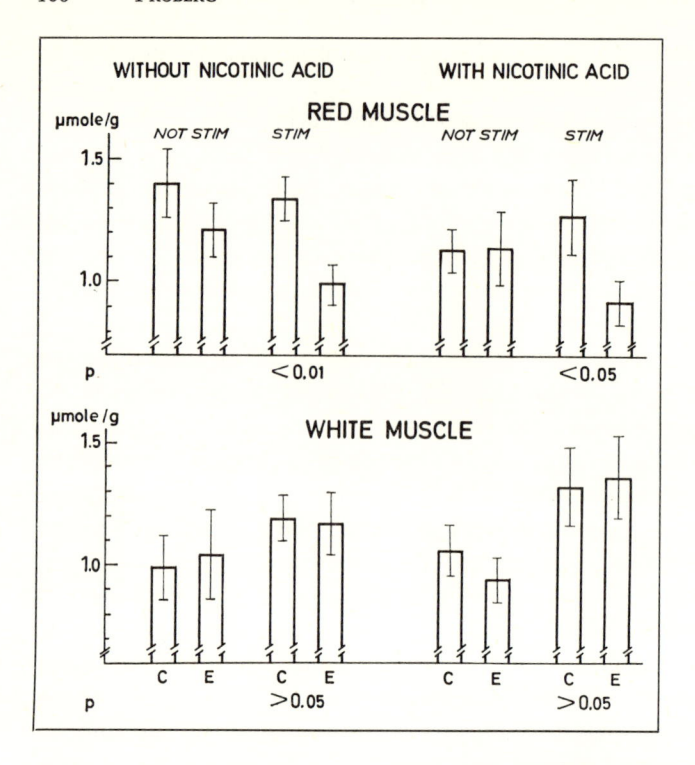

Figure 1. Effect of electrical stimulation on the triglyceride concentration of red and white muscle in fasted rats. Nicotinic acid was administered subcutaneously, 250 mg per kg body weight. The rats were anaesthetised with pentobarbital given intraperitoneally, 50 mg per kg body weight. Exercise against a resistance of 50 g, was induced by electrical stimulation through the right sciatic nerve frequency: 5 impulses per s, voltage: 0.5–1.0 V. (P denotes degree of stutistical difference between exercised and nonexercised muscle tissue.) (Unpublished results: S. O. Fröberg, R. Gross.)

thetized animals. No decrease was found in the TG concentration [8, 29, 47]. We found that the TG concentration of red muscle tissue decreased with about 35% after stimulation. No change was found in the white muscle tissue (figure 1). This suggests an increased rate of oxidation of endogenous TG in the red muscle tissue. No change occurred in the concentration of cholesterol which suggests that the water content of the muscle tissue was probably unchanged after exercise (unpublished results). The effect of exercise on the muscle TG concentration was not changed after inhibition of the mobilisation of FFA from the adipose tissue by nicotinic acid.

In another type of experiment rats were exercised by running. Exercise of untrained rats for three hours was followed by depressed con-

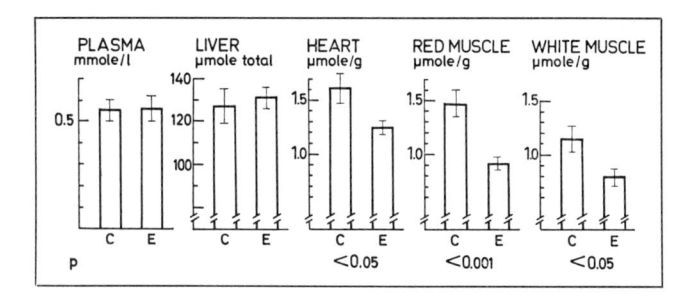

Figure 2. Effect of acute exercise on the triglyceride concentration of plasma, myocardium, red and white skeletal muscle. The total liver content of TG triglycerides is also given. Freely fed male rats, 2 months old, run for 3 h on an endless belt at a speed of 33 cm per second. (C = control, E = exercised rats. P indicates the difference between control and exercised animals.) (Unpublished results: L. A. CARLSON, S. O. FRÖBERG.)

Table IV. Effect of exercise on muscle triglycerides and glycogen concentration in man

Glycerides μmole per gram (N = 15)			Glycogen mg per gram (N = 10)		
Before exercise	After exercise	Indiv. diff. before-after	Before exercise	After exercise	Indiv. diff. before-after
9.01 ± 0.90	7.55 ± 0.69 > 0.05	1.46 ± 1.06 > 0.05	10.9 ± 1.0	3.2 ± 1.0 < 0.001	7.7 ± 1.1 < 0.001

Effect of acute exercise on the concentration of triglycerides and glycogen in the femoral muscle of man. The RQ, not shown in the table, was close to 0.9 during the study. (Unpublished results: L.-G. EKELUND, S. O. FRÖBERG.)

centration of TG in red and white muscle as well as of the myocardium (figure 2) but no change occurred in the plasma TG concentration or in the total liver TG content. In rats trained by running for two months before the experiment three hours of exercise was followed by a decrease in the red muscle as well as in the plasma TG concentration (table III). However, we found no decrease in the TG concentration of either white muscle or of the myocardium or of the total content of the liver TG.

The lack of decrease in the liver TG content suggests that the lowered plasma TG concentration after exercise in trained rats was not due to a decrease in the liver TG production but rather to an increased outflow of TGFA to the muscles e.g. the fractional turn over rate may have increased and thus the oxidation of plasma TG. Turnover studies on plasma and TG would add information on this question.

Table III. Effect of training and acute exercise on plasma and tissue triglycerides

		Plasma mmole/l C	T	T+E	Liver μmoles total C	T	T+E	Heart μmole/g C	T	T+E	Red muscle μmole/g C	T	T+E	White muscle μmole/g C	T	T+E
1	M	0.87	0.80	0.43	102	70	93	2.54	1.66	1.64	1.50	1.19	0.92	1.46	0.92	0.84
	SEM	0.07	0.04	0.05	8	4	6	0.24	0.08	0.07	0.12	0.09	0.10	0.11	0.07	0.07
	n	14	15	12	15	15	15	15	15	15	14	13	14	15	15	15
	P	>0.05	<0.001		<0.001	<0.005		<0.01	>0.05		<0.05	<0.05		<0.01	>0.05	
2	M	0.97	1.01	0.60	116	117	124	2.04	1.74	1.60	1.71	1.40	1.28	1.88	1.53	1.60
	SEM	0.06	0.08	0.04	7	6	6	0.22	0.12	0.17	0.13	0.07	0.08	0.16	0.14	0.12
	n	14	14	15	15	15	15	15	15	15	14	15	15	15	15	15
	P	>0.05	<0.001		>0.05	>0.05		>0.05	>0.05		<0.05	>0.5		>0.05	>0.05	

1) 33 cm per second   2) 25 cm per second

Effect of training and acute exercise of trained, fed, young rats on the concentration of triglycerides in plasma, myocardium, red and white skeletal muscle. The total liver triglyceride content is also given. Two different training intensities were used. In the two experiments the rats were acutely exercised at the training speed. (C = control, T = trained, T+E = trained and acutely exercised animals. P denotes difference between C and T and between T and T+E.)
(Unpublished results: L. A. CARLSON, S. O. FRÖBERG.)

We have also begun studies on the effect of exercise on skeletal muscle of man. The muscle tissue is collected by a previously described biopsy technic [6]. After bicycle exercise to exhaustion (about 100 min at a starting pulse rate of 140) we found no decrease in the TG concentration of the femoral muscle of fasting male subjects (table IV). However, the RQ was around 0.9 and concommitant determination of muscle glycogen showed a marked decrease after exercise. This is in accordance with previous findings in man under similar experimental conditions [39]. These workers found a close relationship between utilized glycogen and combusted carbohydrate. Therefore, the high RQ and the marked decrease in glycogen concentration indicated mainly carbohydrate metabolism and the tissue TG probably contributed only to a minor part in the energy metabolism during this short time of fairly heavy exercise.

Tissue TG, age and Physical Training

It was suggested that training might exert an influence upon factors involved in the regulation of plasma lipids during acute exercise. From table III it is seen that the TG concentration of myocardium, red and white muscle and also of the total liver content of TG was reduced after training *per se*, if vigorous enough. No effect, however, was observed on the plasma TG concentration. This may indicate that physical training was followed by

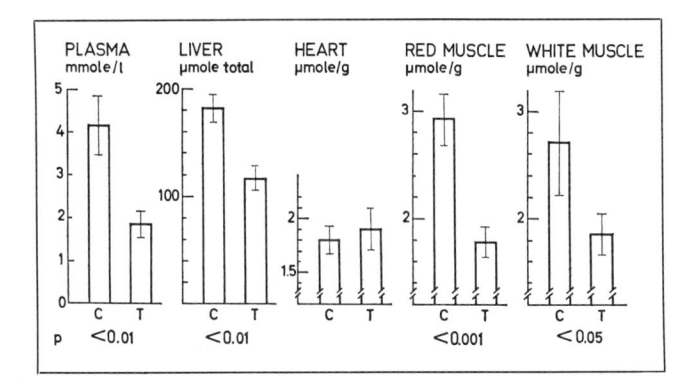

Figure 3. Effect of physical training on the concentration of triglycerides in plasma, myocardium, red and white skeletal muscle. The total TG content of liver is also given. Male rats 12–13 months old run on an endless belt for 3 h daily, 5 days a week for 4 weeks at a speed of 33 cm per second. (C = control, T = trained. P denotes the difference between trained and untrained animals.) (To be published: L. A. CARLSON, S. O. FRÖBERG.)

effects on the intracellular metabolism of TG. The mechanism for this is not known, but there are evidence suggesting an increase in the oxidative capacity after physical training. Thus it has been observed that the myoglobin concentration [55] as well as the activity of oxidizing enzymes of muscle mitochondria [41] is increased after physical training in the rat.

The association between elevated levels of blood lipids in plasma and coronary heart disease has stimulated a growing interest on factors that decrease the plasma lipids. In a recent study we found that the concentration of plasma lipids increased with age in the rat in a similar way to that in man [17]. Also the skeletal muscle TG level increased with age in the rats. Figure 3 shows the effect of training on plasma and tissue TG in elderly rats. The decrease in the TG content of all tissues with the exception of the myocardium and also of the plasma TG concentration indicate that changes in the metabolism of circulating as well as of local TG after physical training occurred also in elderly rats.

Summary

Lipids are oxidized by muscle tissue during exercise. Two major routes of supply of fatty acids for this oxidation were discussed – transport via blood plasma and from local pools. The effect of exercise on the three main components of the plasma lipid transport system – chylomicrons, lipoproteins and free fatty acids – was reviewed; exercise effects all three. Data from experiments on rat indicated that the fractional turn over rate of plasma TG might have been increased after training. Local pools of TG in contractile tissues were decreased after acute exercise in untrained rats suggesting increased rate of oxidation. Training *per se* reduced the local pools of TG in liver and contractile tissues and changed the responce of acute exercise on these pools in myocardium and white muscle. In elderly rats the TG concentration was lowered by training in plasma, liver, red and white muscle but not in myocardium.

References

1. ANDRES, R.; CADER, G. and ZIERLER, L. K.: The quantitatively minor role of carbohydrate in oxidative metabolism by skeletal muscle in intact man in the basal state. Measurements of oxygen and glucose uptake and carbon dioxide and lactate production in the forearm. J. Clin. Invest. *35:* 671–682 (1956).
2. BÄR, U. and BLANCHAER, M. C.: Glycogen and CO_2 production from glucose and lactate by red and white skeletal muscle. Amer. J. Physiol. *209:* 905–909 (1965).
3. BASU, A.; PASSMORE, R. and STRONG, J. A.: The effect of exercise on the level of nonesterified fatty acids in the blood. Quart. J. exp. Physiol. *45:* 312–317 (1960).
4. BEATTY, C. H.; PETERSON, R. D. and BOCEK, R. M.: Metabolism of red and white muscle fiber groups. Amer. J. Physiol. *204:* 939–942 (1963).

5. BEATTY, C. H.; BASINGER, G. M.; DULLY, C. C. and BOCEK, R. M.: Comparison of red and white voluntary skeletal muscles of several species of primates. J. Histochem. cytochem. *14:* 590–600 (1966).
6. BERGSTRÖM, J.: Muscle electrolytes in man. Scand. J. clin. Lab. Invest. Suppl. *68* (1962).
7. BOCEK, R. M.; PETERSON, R. D. and BEATTY, C. H.: Glycogen metabolism in red and white muscle. Amer. J. Physiol. *210:* 1101–1107 (1966).
8. BUCHWALD, K. W. and CORI, C. F.: Influence of repeated contractions of muscle on its lipid content. Proc. Soc. exp. Biol., N.Y. *28:* 737–740 (1930–31).
9. CARLSON, L. A. and PERNOW, B.: Studies on blood lipids during exercise. Arterial and venous plasma concentrations of unesterified fatty acids. J. lab. clin. Med. *53:* 833–841 (1959).
10. CARLSON, L. A. and PERNOW, B.: Studies on blood lipids during exercise. The arterial plasma free fatty acid concentration during and after exercise and its regulation. J. lab. clin. Med. *58:* 673–681 (1961).
11. CARLSON, L. A.; EKELUND, L.-G. and ORÖ, L.: Studies on blood lipids during exercise. IV. Arterial concentration of plasma free fatty acids and glycerol during and after prolonged exercise in normal men. J. lab. clin. Med. *61:* 724–729 (1963).
12. CARLSON, L. A. and HALLBERGER, D.: Studies on the elimination of exogenous lipids from the blood stream. The kinetics of the elimination of a fat emulsion and of chylomicrons in the dog after a single injection. Acta physiol. scand. *59:* 52–61 (1963).
13. CARLSON, L. A. and MOSSFELDT, F.: Acute effects of prolonged, heavy exercise on the concentration of plasma lipids and lipoproteins in man. Acta physiol. scand. *62:* 51–59 (1964).
14. CARLSON, L. A.; BOBERG, J. and HÖGSTEDT, B.: Some physiological and clinical implications of lipid metabolism from adipose tissue. Handbook of physiology. Adipose tissue. Washington, D.C. 1965. Amer. physiol. Soc., sect. 5, chapt. 63, pp. 625–644.
15. CARLSON, L. A.; FRÖBERG, S. O. and NYE, E. R.: Acute effects of nicotinic acid on plasma, liver, heart and muscle lipids. Nicotinic acid in the rat II. Acta med. scand. *180:* 571–579 (1966).
16. CARLSON, L. A. and FRÖBERG, S. O.: Blood lipid and glucose levels during a ten-day period of low-caloric intake and exercise in man. Metabolism *16:* 624–634, 1967.
17. CARLSON, L. A.; FRÖBERG, S. O. and NYE, E. R.: Effect of age on blood tissue lipid levels in the male rat. Gerontologia *14:* 65–79 (1968).
18. CHALLONER, D. R. and STEINBERG, D.: Metabolic effect of epinephrine on the QO_2 of the arrested isolated perfused rat heart. Nature *205:* 602–603 (1965).
19. CRASS, M. F. III and MENG, H. C.: The removal and metabolism of chylomicron triglycerides by the isolated perfused rat heart. The role of a heparin released lipase. Biochim. biophys. Acta *125:* 106–117 (1966).
20. DELCHER, H. K.; FRIED, M. and SHIPP, J. C.: Metabolism of lipoprotein lipid in the isolated perfused rat heart. Biochim. biophys. Acta *106:* 10–18 (1965).
21. DENTON, R. M. and RANDLE, P. J.: Concentrations of glycerides and phospholipids in rat heart and gastrocnemius muscles. Biochem. J. *104:* 416–422 (1967).
22. DOLE, V. P.: A relation between nonesterified fatty acids in plasma and the metabolism of glucose. J. clin. Invest. *35:* 150–154 (1956).
23. DUBOWITZ, U. and PEARSE, A. G. E.: A comparative histochemical study of oxidative enzymes and phosphorylase activity in skeletal muscle. Histochemie *2:* 105–117 (1960).

24. ENDE, N.: Starvation studies. With special reference to cholesterol. Amer. J. clin. Nutrit. *11:* 270–280 (1962).
25. FITZGERALD, O.; HEFFERNAN, A. and MCFARLANE, R.: Serum lipids and physical activity in normal subjects. Clin. Sci. *28:* 83–89 (1965).
26. FRIEDBERG, S. J.; HARLAN, W. R.; TROUT, D. L. and ESTES, E. H., Jr.: The effect of exercise on the concentration and turnover of plasma nonesterified fatty acids. J. clin. Invest. *39:* 215–220 (1960).
27. FRIEDBERG, S. J.; SHER, P. B.; BOGDONOF, M. D. and ESTES, E. H., Jr.: Changes in emotional state and in plasma free fatty acid metabolism during exercise. J. Lipid Res. *4:* 34–38 (1963).
28. FRÖBERG, S. O.: Determination of muscle lipids. Biochim. biophys. Acta *144:* 83–93 (1967).
29. GEMILL, C. L.: The effect of stimulation on the fat and carbohydrate content of the gastrocnemius muscle in the phlorizinized rat. Bull. Johns Hopkin's Hosp. *66:* 71–89 (1940).
31. GOLDING, L.: The effect of physical training upon total serum cholesterol levels. Res. Quart. *32:* 499–506 (1961).
32. GORDON, R. S., Jr., and CHERKES, A.: Unesterified fatty acid in human blood plasma. J. clin. Invest. *35:* 206–212 (1956).
33. GORDON, R. B. Jr., and CHERKES, A.: Production of unesterified fatty acids from isolated adipose tissue incubated *in vitro*. Proc. Soc. exp. Biol., N.Y. *97:* 150–151 (1958).
34. GOUSIOS, A.; FELTS, J. M. and HAVEL, R. J.: The metabolism of serum triglycerides and free fatty acids by the myocardium. Metabolism *12:* 75–80 (1963).
35. HALLBERG, D.: Studies on the elimination of exogenous lipids from the blood stream. The kinetics for the elimination of chylomicrons studied by a single intravenous injection in man. Acta physiol. scand. *65:* 279–284 (1965).
36. HAVEL, R. J.; NAIMARK, A. and BORCHGREVINK, C. F.: Turnover rate and oxidation of free fatty acids in the blood plasma in man during exercise. Studies during continuous infusion of palmitate -1-C^{14}. J. clin. Invest. *42:* 1054–1063 (1963).
37. HAVEL, R. J.: Metabolism of chylomicrons and very low-density lipoproteins. Handbook of physiol. Adipose tissue, Washington, D.C. 1965. Amer. physiol. Soc. sect. 5, chapt. 50, pp. 499–507.
38. HAVEL, R. J.; PERNOW, B. and JONES, N.: Uptake and release of free fatty acids and other metabolites in the legs of exercising men. J. appl. Physiol. *23:* 90–96 (1967).
39. HERMANSEN, L.; HULTMAN, E. and SALTIN, B.: Muscle glycogen during prolonged severe exercise. Acta physiol. scand. *71:* 129–139 (1967).
40. HOLLOSZY, J. O.; SKINNER, I. S.; TORO, G. and CURETON, T. K.: Effect of a six month program of endurance exercise on the serum lipids of middle aged men. Amer. J. Cardiol, *14:* 753–760 (1964).
41. HOLLOSZY, J. O.: Effects of exercise on mitochondrial oxygen uptake and respiratory enzyme activity in skeletal muscle. J. biol. Chem. *242:* 2278–2282 (1967).
42. ISSEKUTZ, B., Jr.; MILLER, H. J.; PAUL, P. and RODAHL, K.: Source of fat oxidation in exercising dog. Amer. J. Physiol. *207:* 583–589 (1964).
43. JOHNSON, T.; WONG, H.; SHIM, R.; LIU, B. and HALL, A.: The influence of exercise on serum cholesterol, phospholipids and electrophoretic serum patterns of protein in college swimmers. Fed. Proc. *18:* 77 (1959).
44. KARTIN, B. L.; MAN, E. B.; WINKLER, A. W. and PETERS, J. P.: Blood ketones

and serum lipids in starvation and water deprivation. J. clin. Invest. *23:* 824–835 (1944).

45. KREISBERG, R. A.: Effect of diabetes and starvation on myocardial triglyceride and free fatty acid utilization. Amer. J. Physiol. *210:* 379–383 (1966).
46. LAURELL, S. and CHRISTENSON, B.: Effect of a single dose of some hormones on plasma unesterified fatty acid (UFA). Acta physiol. scand. *44:* 248–254 (1958).
47. MASORO, E. J.; ROWELL, L. B.; MCDONALD, R. M. and STEIERT, B.: Skeletal muscle lipids. II Nonutilization of intracellular lipid esters as an energy source for contractile activity. J. biol. Chem. *241:* 2626–2634 (1966).
48. MIETTINEN, M.: Effect of fasting on serum lipoproteins. Ann. Med. Intern. Fenn. *51:* 169–172 (1962).
49. MONTOYE, H.; VAN HUSS, W.; BREWER, W.; JONES, E.; OHLSON, M.; MAHONEY, E. and OLSON, H.: The effect of exercise on blood cholesterol in middle aged men. Amer. J. clin. Nutrit. *7:* 139–145 (1959).
50. NACHMIAS, N. T. and PADYKULA, H. A.: A histochemical study of normal and denervated red and white muscles of the rat. J. biophys. biochim. Cyt. *4:* 47–54 (1958).
51. NEPTUNE, E. M., Jr.; SUDDUTH, H. C.; FOREMAN, D. R. and FASH, F. J.: Phospholipid and triglyceride metabolism of excised rat diafragma and the role of these lipids in fatty acid oxidation and uptake. J. Lipid Res. *1:* 229-230 (1960).
52. NIKKILÄ, E. A. and KONTTINEN, A.: Effect of physical activity of postprandial levels of fats in serum. Lancet *i:* 1151–1154 (1962).
53. NIKKILÄ, E. A.; TORSTI, P. and PENTTILÄ, O.: The effect of exercise on lipoprotein lipase activity of rat heart, adipose tissue and skeletal muscle. Metabolism *12:* 863–865 (1963).
54. OLSON, R. E. and HOESCHEN, R. J.: Utilization of endogenous lipid by the isolated perfused rat heart. Biochem. J. *103:* 796–801 (1967).
55. PATTENGALE, P. K. and HOLLOSZY, J. O.: Augmentation of skeletal muscle myoglobin by a program of treadmill running. Amer. J. Physiol. *213:* 783–785 (1967).
56. RENOLD, A. E. and CAHILL, G. F., Jr. (editors): Metabolism of adipose tissue: a summary. Handbook of physiol. Adipose tissue, Washington, D.C. 1965. Amer. physiol. Soc., sect. 5., pp. 483–490.
57. ROCHELLE, R. H.: Blood plasma changes during a physical training program. Res. Quart. *32:* 538–550 (1961).
58. RUBIN, L. and ALADJEM, F.: Serum lipoprotein changes during fasting in man. Amer. J. Physiol. *178:* 263–266.
59. SCHOTZ, M. C. and PAGE, J. H.: Effect of norepinephrine and epinephrine on nonesterified fatty acid concentration in plasma. Proc. Soc. exp. Biol., N.Y. *101:* 624–626 (1959).
60. TAYLOR, H. L.; ANDERSON, J. T. and KEYS, A.: Effect on serum lipids of 1,300 calories of daily walking. Fed. Proc. *16:* 128 (1957).
61. TUERKISCHER, E. and WERTHEIMER, E.: The *in vitro* synthesis of glycogen in the diafragmes of normal and alloxan diabetic rats. Biochem. J. *42:* 603–609 (1948).
62. VENSALU, A.: Studies on adrenaline and noradrenaline in human plasma. Acta physiol. scand. *49* (suppl. 173): 1–123 (1960).
63. VON EULER, U. S. and HELLNER, S.: Excretion of noradrenaline and adrenaline in muscular work. Acta physiol. scand. *33* (suppl. 118): 10–16 (1955).

Author's address: Dr. S. O. FRÖBERG, King Gustav V's Research Institute, *Stockholm* (Sweden).

Influence of Muscular Exercise on Glucose Regulation

V. Conard, H. Brunnengraber, R. Vanroux,
A. Deschaepdrijver, E. Moermans and J. R. M. Franckson

Department of Physio-pathology and department of Clinical Chemistry, University of Brussels, Department of Pneumology, Hospital of Charleroi, and Institute of Pharmacology and Therapeutics, University of Ghent

Abstract

The influence of muscular exercise on the glucose regulation has been investigated in 70 normal subjects and 25 diabetic patients who wera submitted by groups to various dynamic tests. Exercise was performed on e bicycle ergometer (80–100 W during 20–45 min).

Exercise induced but small variations in the level of blood-sugar: in untrained sedentary people (medical students) a mean drop of 10% was recorded whereas in manual workers, the concentration remained fairly stable. These minute changes sharply contrast with the deep modifications occurring both in glucose production and utilization rates.

In a first group of experiments, glucose utilization rate was measured following intravenous injection of a glucose load (0.33 g/kg body weight). This procedure entails a sharp rise in the plasma glucose concentration (up to 250 mg/100 ml) which stops or dramatically reduces the liver glucose output, making it possible to isolate the uptake process. This technique applied to 30 normal subjects and 20 diabetic patients treated with long-acting insulin revealed in both groups a marked enhancement of the glucose uptake rate during the performance of exercise and the ensuing hour.

Labelled glucose turnover studies were made in 19 normal subjects. Due to the importance and earliness of recycling phenomena, the single injection technique had to be rejected. Following procedure was used: a first tracer of glucose-1-^{14}C (5–10 μC) was injected 70 min before exercise for basal estimation and a second one (15–30 μC), at the onset of exercise; at the end of the 45 min exercise 50 μC of glucose-6-^{14}C were injected to characterize the post-effort state. Some experiments were carried out under mild hyperglycaemia (140–170 mg/100 ml) induced by glucose infusion at variable rates.

Labelled glucose catabolic rate increased from 1.2%/min to 3.4%/min during exercise and remained at a mean value of 2.2%/min during the first hour of the post-exercise period. Rapid adaptation of the liver glucose supply to the changes in tissue uptake rate resulted in minute variations in plasma glucose-^{12}C concentration. Hypoglycaemia did not appear as the signal for enhanced glucose release, since prolonged glucose infusion did not prevent the marked increase in hepatic production; even under this hyperglycaemic condition recycling of glucose-1-^{14}C during the first hour following the arrest of exercise represented 20% of the pre-injected amounts.

Insulin is not responsible for the augmentation of the glucose utilization rate. In none of the 16 experiments performed either under fasting condition or under glucose infusion, did exercise modify the plasmatic level of immunoreactive insulin. Constant infusions of ^{125}I-insulin (0.2 atom iodine per mole) performed in 7 normal subjects, revealed a 17% reduction of the metabolic clearance of insulin without change in the size of extracellular compartment during and after exercise. Reduction in the catabolic rate of slightly labelled insulin associated with stability of the plasma insulin level throughout the experiment strongly suggests a decrease in endogenous insulin secretion.

Variable in magnitude from one individual to another a systematic rise in plasma catecholamines was recorded in 10 experiments, the peak occurring during the exercise or the post-exercise. Here also hypoglycaemia was not involved in the trigger mechanism since the phenomenon was observed under hyperglycaemic condition (glucose infusion).

Cortisol and growth hormone did not seem to play a major role in the modifications of the glucose regulation induced by muscular exercise.

Author's address: Dr. V. CONARD, Department of Physio-Pathology, University of Brussels, *Brussels* (Belgium).

Biochemistry of Exercise.
Medicine and Sport, Vol. 3; pp. 116–121 (Karger, Basel/New York 1969)

Alterations in Human Skeletal Muscle Lipid Composition and Metabolism Induced by Physical Conditioning[1]

T. E. MORGAN[2], F. A. SHORT[3], and L. A. COBB[2]

Department o Medicine, University of Washington, School of Medicine, Seattle, Wash.

The observations in humans reported by COBB et al. [2] suggest that physical training induces adaptive changes in muscle which alter its response to exercise. Animal studies on the effect of training and exercise yield variable results which may depend on species, age of animal, diet or duration of training or exercise. To limit these variables we have studied human volunteers who trained the quadriceps muscle of one thigh by daily isotonic exercise, the opposite leg serving as an untrained control.

Methods

The program of physical conditioning employed has been described by COBB et al. [2]. In this program one leg fitted with a weighted boot was exercised to exhaustion daily for 4 to 6 weeks. At the end of the training period the vastus lateralis of both control and trained legs was biopsied under local anesthesia without epinephrine. The biopsy samples were carefully cleaned of fascia, blood and adipose tissue and weighed. Aliquots of muscle were taken for *in vitro* studies and determination of dry weight. The remaining muscle was homogenized and extracted twice with chloroform-methanol [10]. Lipid extracts were subjected to duplicate analysis of total phospholipid, phosphatidyl choline (lecithin), cholesterol and triglyceride [10]. Triglyceride was determined by two methods: first, by glycerol liberated by periodate oxidation [4] and, second, by the infrared method of MASORO et al. [9].

Results and Discussion

Results of lipid analyses are given in figure 1. There was considerable variation in values obtained between experimental subjects but the

[1] Supported by U.S. Public Health Service Grants Nr. HE-02354, HE-07478.
[2] Drs. MORGAN and COBB are recipients of PHS Research Career Development Awards 5K3 HE-7268 and 5K3 HE-4570.
[3] Dr. SHORT was supported by PHS Postdoctoral Fellowship Nr. 1-F2-HE23, 403-01A1.

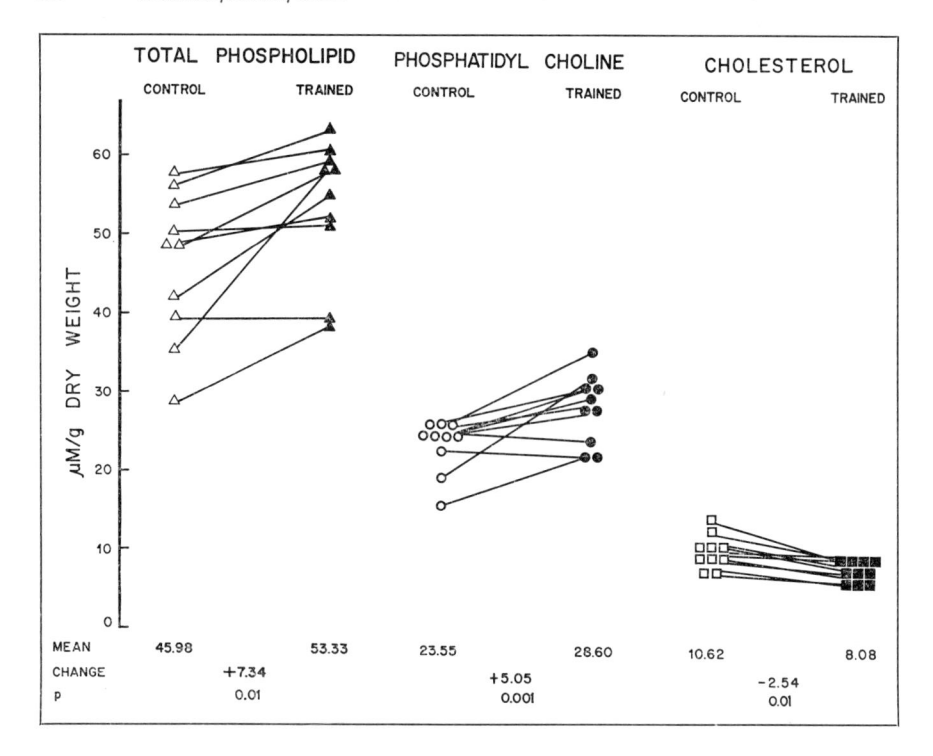

Figure 1. Lipid analyses of control and conditioned vastus lateralis. Open figures (△, ○, □) indicate control values; solid figures (▲, ●, ■), conditioned muscles. Lines connect values from same subject.

least variance was noted when results were expressed per gram dry weight. The experimental design partially compensates for this variance since, from each subject, paired biopsies were taken from control and conditioned legs. Tests of statistical significance were based upon these paired samples and differences were significant at the 0.01 level or less for all results reported.

Total phospholipid increased in 9 of 10 subjects (figure 1) and there was a mean increase of 7.3 micromoles phospholipid per gram dry muscle weight. Phosphatidyl choline (lecithin) also increased in 8 of 10 subjects with a mean change of 5 micromoles per gram dry weight and highly significant results. In contrast to the increased phospholipid values muscle cholesterol decreased in all subjects. The mean decrease in cholesterol was 2.54 micromoles cholesterol per gram dry weight or 24 per cent. Figure 1 also shows the normal range of variation encountered and emphasizes the

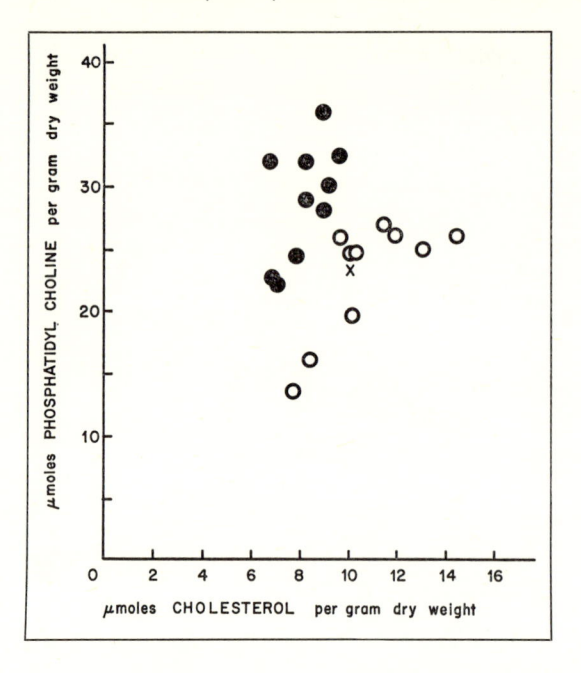

Figure 2. Alterations in vastus lateralis lipid content induced by physical conditioning. Open circles (○) indicate control values; solid circles (●), conditioned muscle. The symbol × indicates the average ratio cholesterol:phosphatidyl choline obtained in 3 untrained subjects from whose muscle subcellular fractions were also obtained.

danger of comparisons between individuals and especially between studies in various laboratories.

Figure 2 compares the effect of exercise training on two cell membrane lipids – phosphatidyl choline and cholesterol. The ratio phosphatidyl choline to cholesterol was calculated for controls and for trained legs. The results indicate two clearly different groups even when pairing is ignored. Mitochondria are rich in phospholipids and poor in cholesterol [7], therefore, the analytical data suggest that an increase in mitochondria might have occurred as a response to training. To study this possibility lipid analyses were performed on cell fractions prepared from human muscle homogenates by differential centrifugation. Cell fractions were prepared by the method of MARINETTI *et al.* [8] and extracted by the same methods reported in this study. The phosphatidyl choline:cholesterol ratio was then calculated for each fraction (table I). Whole muscle homogenate had a ratio of 2.30;

Table I. Lipid analyses of isolated muscle cell fractions[1]

	Cholesterol	Phospholipid	Phosphatidyl Choline	μM Phosphatidyl Choline / μM Cholesterol
	(μM/g dry wt muscle)	(μM/g dry wt muscle)	(μM/g dry wt muscle)	
Whole cell homogenate	10.1	42.5	23.2	2.30
Nuclei, myofibrils, etc.	7.2	21.5	11.2	1.57
Mitochondria	1.2	7.0	3.1	2.55
Microsomes	2.0	8.6	4.5	2.25
Supernatant	1.5	2.8	1.7	0.88

[1] Cell fractions were prepared as described in text after the general method of MARINETTI et al. [8]. Values are means of duplicates from 5.0 g samples obtained from the quadriceps muscle of three male subjects.

it was exceeded only by the mitochondrial ratio of 2.55. All other fractions – nuclei, myofibrils, microsomes and supernatant – had lower values. These results indicate that a rise in phosphatidyl choline:cholesterol ratio might be expected from an increase in mitochondrial size or number. These results in man agree with the electron micrographic data obtained in rats by GOLLNICK and KING [3] and mitochondrial enzyme and protein data of HOLLOSCZY [5].

Our studies also have produced information on the intracellular lipid stores of triglyceride. Fatty acids stored as intracellular triglyceride have been repeatedly suggested as sources for energy for muscle contraction [1, 6, 11]. There appears, however, to be some doubt as to the actual levels of intracellular triglyceride present in muscle. For example, MASORO finds very low muscle triglyceride which is not changed by exercise [9] but others find higher levels which fall after exercise [11]. We also found low levels of triglycerides (figure 3) in 5 control (untrained) muscle biopsies but higher levels in the trained legs in all individuals. Calculation of the energy available from 'intracellular' lipid stores indicates that the trained muscle ac-

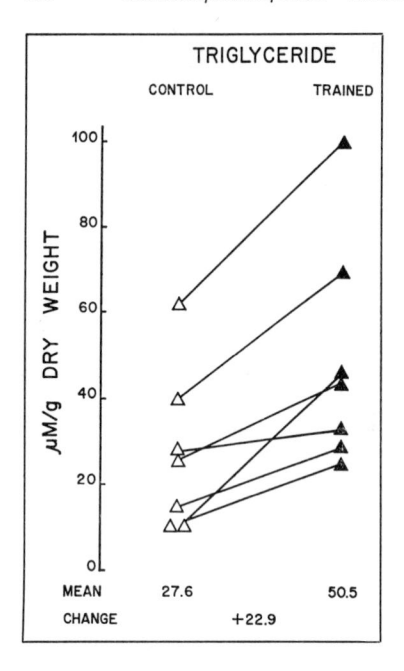

Figure 3. Triglyceride content of control and conditioned vastus lateralis. Open triangles (△) indicate control values; solid triangles (▲), conditioned muscle. Lines connect values from same subject.

quired an average 3.6 calories/100 g wet weight addition to stores which ranged from 0.2 to 27 cal/100 g wet weight in the control, untrained muscle. The data in the present study show a wide range of values for 'intracellular' triglycerides in both the control and trained muscles. So great is this variation that interpretation of the results is hazardous; however, all subjects studied showed a net increase in triglyceride in the trained muscle as compared to the control. We emphasize, however, that apparent alterations in intracellular triglyceride stores may be due to contamination by adipose tissue incompletely removed in spite of our best efforts.

Summary

We have studied the effect of 4 to 6 weeks of quadriceps training on concentration of total phospholipid, phosphatidyl choline, cholesterol and triglyceride in the trained and contralateral untrained vastus lateralis of 10 normal men. Phospholipid, phosphatidyl choline and triglyceride concentrations were higher in trained muscle but cholesterol was lower. In each subject the phosphatidyl choline:cholesterol ratio was higher in the trained muscles. Cell fractions prepared from human muscle showed a high phosphatidyl choline: cholesterol ratio for mitochondria. The observed changes in phosphatidyl choline and cholesterol were compatible with increased mitochondrial size or number and decreased cell cholesterol. Triglyceride content was variable but was also consistently greater in trained muscle.

References

1. FRÖBERG, S. O.: Metabolism of lipids in blood and tissues during exercise. Biochemistry of Exercise. Medicine and Sport, Vol. 3, pp. 100–113 (Karger, Basel/New York 1969).
2. COBB, L. A.; SHORT, F. A. and SMITH, P. H.: Inhibition of lactate production in exercised trained muscle. Biochemistry of Exercise (unpublished).
3. GOLLNICK, P. D. and KING, D. W.: The immediate and chronic effect of exercise on the number and structure of skeletal muscle mitochondria. Biochemistry of Exercise. Medicine and Sport, Vol. 3, pp. 239–244 (Karger, Basel/New York 1969).
4. HANAHAN, D. J. and OLLEY, J. N.: Chemical nature of monophosphoinositides. J. biol. Chem. *231:* 813–828 (1958).
5. HOLLOSCZY, J. O.: Biochemical adaptations in muscle. J. biol. Chem. *242:* 2278–2282 (1967).
6. ISSEKUTZ, B.; MILLER, H. I.; PAUL, P. and RODAHL, K.: Source of fat oxidation in exercising dogs. Amer. J. Physiol. *207:* 583–588 (1964).
7. MAJERUS, P. W. and VAGELOS, P. R.: Fatty acid biosynthesis and the role of acyl carrier protein; in PAOLETTI and KRITCHEVSKY's Advances in Lipid Research. vol. 5, p. 16 (Academic Press, New York 1967).
8. MARINETTI, G. V.; ERBLAND, J. and STOTZ, E.: Phosphatides of pig heart cell fractions. J. biol. Chem. *233:* 562–565 (1958).
9. MASORO, E. J.; ROWELL, L. B.; MACDONALD, R. M. and STEIERT, B.: Skeletal Muscle Lipids. II. Nonutilization of intracellular lipid esters as an energy source for contractile activity. J. biol. Chem. *241:* 2626–2634 (1966).
10. MORGAN, T. E. and EDMUNDS, L. H.: Pulmonary artery occlusion. III. Biochemical alterations. J. appl. Physiol. *22:* 1012–1016 (1967).
11. NEPTUNE, E. M.; SUDDUTH, H. C. and FOREMAN, D. R.: Labile fatty acids of rat diaphragm muscle and their possible role as a major endogenous substrate for maintenance of respiration. J. biol. Chem. *234:* 1659–1664 (1959).

Authors' address: T. E. MORGAN, M.D., F. A. SHORT, M.D. and L. A. COBB, M.D. University of Washington, School of Medicine, *Seattle, Wash. 98105* (USA).

Influence of Exercise Training on In Vitro Metabolism of Glucose and Fatty Acid by Human Skeletal Muscle[1]

F. A. SHORT[2], L. A. COBB[3], and T. E. MORGAN[3]

Department of Medicine, University of Washington School of Medicine and King County Hospital, Seattle, Wash.

Introduction

Alterations of myoglobin [2] and lipid [6] concentrations induced by training in human skeletal muscle have been reported in this symposium. This report describes studies of glycogen concentration and the metabolism *in vitro* of trained and untrained human skeletal muscle.

Six normal male prison volunteers trained the quadriceps muscle of one leg as previously described [2].

24 to 48 h after completion of the exercise training, biopsies of the vastus lateralis of each leg were obtained under local anesthesia. The muscle was transferred to normal saline and cleaned of fat and fascia. A portion was weighed and digested for measurement of glycogen concentration, and fibers approximately 1 mm in diameter were teased away and collected in Krebs Ringer bicarbonate buffer (KRB) gassed with 5% CO_2–95% O_2 to maintain pH 7.4. Groups of 3 to 4 fibers (100 to 150 mg) were then blotted lightly, weighed, and distributed into flasks containing 3.0 ml of KRB containing the following substrates:

1. Glucose, 1 mg/ml and UL C^{14} glucose, 0.1 µc/ml (New England Nuclear Corp., Specific Activity 0.1 mc/5.5 mg).

2. Albumin, 6.02 gm% (Armour crystalized bovine plasma albumin), fatty acid (FA) 0.68 mM, and 9, 10 H^3 palmitic acid, 4.0 µc/ml (New England Nuclear Corp., Specific Activity 200 mc/mM).

3. Glucose, C^{14} glucose, albumin, FA and H^3 palmitate in the concentrations of media 1 and 2.

Except for the relatively small amount of added H^3 palmitate, the

---

[1] Supported by U.S. Public Health Service Grants No. HE-02354 and HE-07478.

[2] Dr. SHORT was supported by PHS Postdoctoral Fellowship No. 1-F2-HE23, 403-01A1.

[3] Drs. COBB and MORGAN are recipients of PHS Research Career Development Awards 5K3-HE-4570 and 5K3-HE-7268.

FA was that native to the albumin, and was determined by the method of Trout et al. [9].

The flasks were stoppered, gassed, and incubated with shaking for two hours. The incubation was terminated by addition of HCl to the medium. CO_2 was trapped in Hyamine® (Packard Instrument Company) introduced into a cup suspended within the flask, and media was analyzed for concentrations of glucose [8], pyruvate [7], lactate [1] and FA [9]. C^{14} lactate was separated by paper chromatography and located by radioautography. Glycogen was done by the method of Good et al. [4]. Liquid scintillation counting of glucose, glycogen, lactate and CO_2 was used to determine the distribution of C^{14} glucose.

Results and Discussion

Table I shows paired glycogen concentrations in vastus lateralis of the 6 subjects. The paired differences are highly significant, and demonstrate that the effect is localized to the exercised muscle. These data indicate that the increased glycogen concentration found by Hultman [5] in muscle following depletion of glycogen by strenuous work persists after several weeks of daily exercise.

Glucose incorporation into glycogen *in vitro*, while small in relation to the total glycogen concentration, was stimulated in trained muscle in the

Table I. Muscle glycogen concentration

	mg/g Wet weight untrained	trained	Tr.-Un.[1]	mg/g Dry weight untrained	trained	Tr.-Un.[1]
STE	10.2	13.6	3.4	39.7	66.7	27.0
WAT	13.7	19.8	6.1	56.2	83.4	27.2
RUS	14.7	20.0	5.3	58.6	81.5	22.9
HUN	9.3	14.6	5.3	47.2	84.6	37.4
BLA	10.8	15.0	4.2	39.5	62.0	22.5
BRO	16.0	23.2	7.2	75.1	116.0	40.9
Mean	12.4	17.7	5.3	52.7	82.4	29.7
Standard Error of Mean			0.5			2.9
p[2]			<0.001			<0.001

[1] Difference, Trained-Untrained.
[2] Student's t test of paired observations.

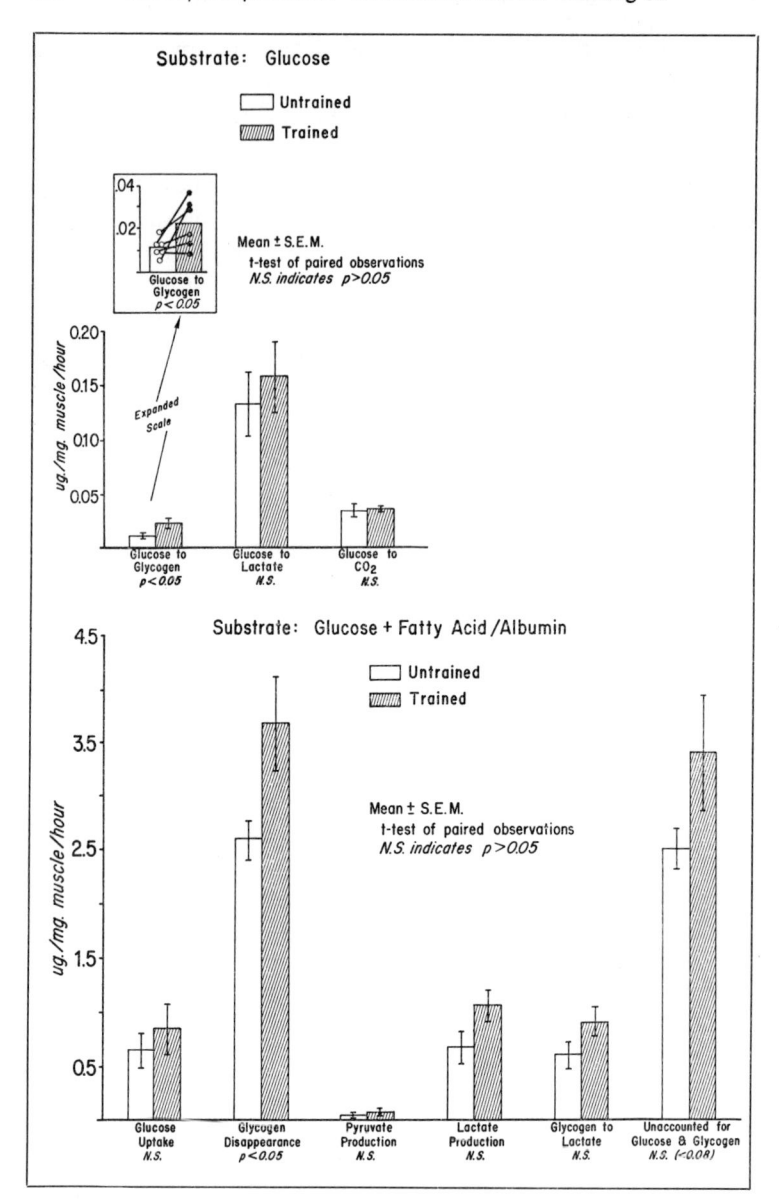

Figure 1. Effect of exercise training on *in vitro* metabolism of skeletal muscle.

1a. C[14] glucose distribution. Expanded scale shows values for untrained and trained muscle of each subject joined by a line.

1b. Glucose and glycogen metabolism.

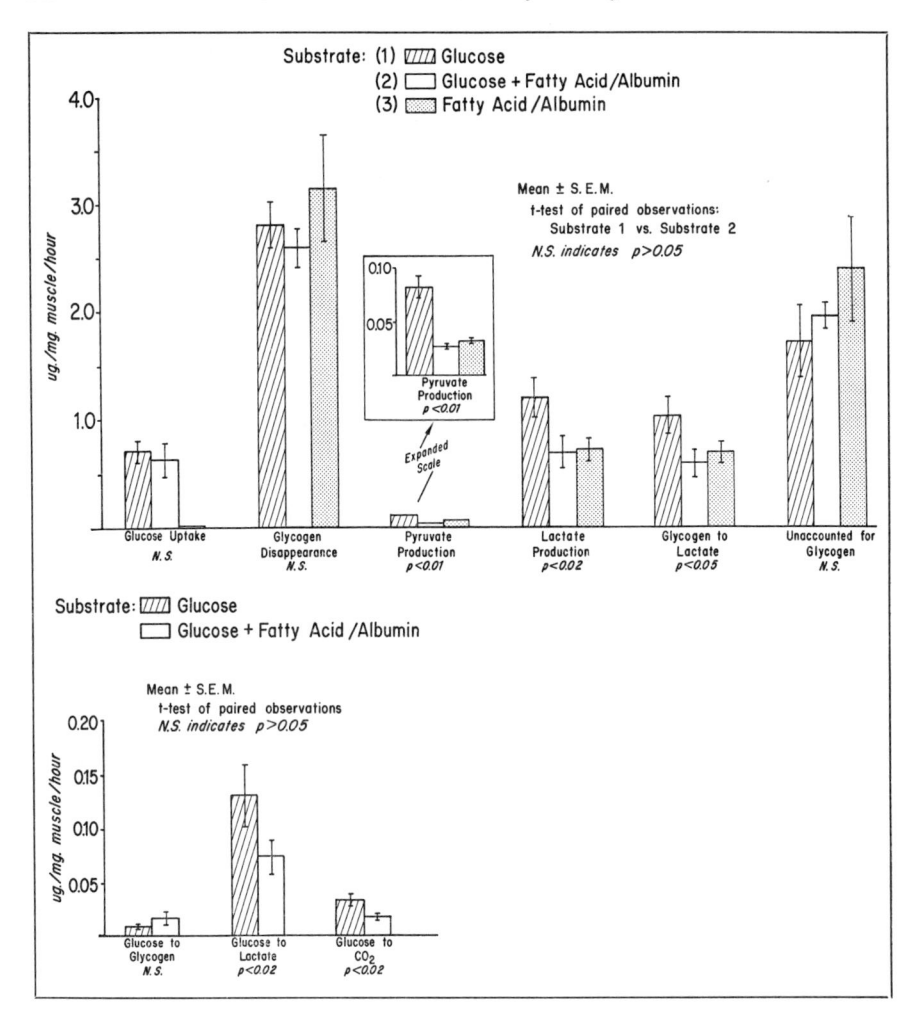

Figure 2. Effect of media substrate on *in vitro* metabolism of untrained muscle.
2a. Glucose and glycogen metabolism.
2b. C[14] glucose distribution.

flasks containing only glucose as substrate (figure 1a). The fact that the trained muscle demonstrated increased incorporation of glucose into glycogen *in vitro*, in spite of the higher glycogen concentration in this muscle, suggests that such muscle has the capacity to synthesize not simply an increased total amount of glycogen, but to synthesize it at an increased rate.

The presence of FA-albumin in glucose containing medium did not affect glucose uptake or glycogen disappearance in normal, untrained skeletal muscle, but significantly decreased production of lactate and pyruvate (figure 2a) and incorporation of C^{14} glucose into lactate and CO_2 (figure 2b). This differs from the data of GARLAND et al. [3] for rat diaphragm. They reported a decreased rate of glycolysis (glucose uptake plus glycogen breakdown), without change in the production of pyruvate and lactate in albumin-palmitic acid containing medium, and showed that oxidation of $2C^{14}$ pyruvate to $C^{14}O_2$ was impaired in the presence of this substrate, with shunting of pyruvate to lactate.

It appears from our data that FA-albumin inhibits glycolysis at some point between glucose-6-phosphate and pyruvate. It is apparent that the amount of glycogen converted to lactate is significantly reduced in the presence of this substrate, and that there tends to be a larger amount of glycogen unaccounted for in these flasks than in those containing only glucose. Some of this glycogen is converted to CO_2 or to intermediates between pyruvate and CO_2. If oxidation to CO_2 of glucose originating from glycogen is inhibited to the same degree by FA-albumin as is C^{14} glucose, a still larger amount of glycogen is unaccounted for in the FA-albumin containing flasks. The unaccounted for glucose moieties of glycogen could re-enter glycogen synthesis, enter the pentose cycle, or accumulate as glycolytic intermediates. Of these intermediates, dihydroxyacetone phosphate can be reduced to alpha-glycerophosphate, which is able to enter mitochondria. This alpha-glycerophosphate shuttle can provide a mechanism for oxidation of cytoplasmic DPNH, but it is interesting to speculate that this shunt, occurring to a greater extent in the muscle exposed to FA-albumin than to glucose alone, might also provide a source of phosphatidic acid for synthesis of triglyceride and phosphatides.

Disappearance of glycogen during incubation was greater in the trained than untrained muscle in all media, although this effect was most clearly significant in the FA-albumin exposed muscle (figure 1b). In addition, when the glycogen and glucose not accounted for are combined, there tends to be more unaccounted for in the trained than untrained muscle (figure 1b) (t = 2.29, p <0.08). Our observation that phosphatidyl choline and triglyceride concentrations are significantly increased in trained muscle [6] supports the postulate that augmentation of synthesis of these lipids may occur, and that alpha-glycerophosphate generated by glycolysis may provide the necessary phosphatidic acid.

Uptake of FA was not affected by the presence of glucose in the medium or by training.

In conclusion, addition of FA-albumin to glucose as substrate for human skeletal muscle *in vitro* does not affect glucose uptake or glycogen breakdown but does inhibit the formation of pyruvate, lactate, and glucose oxidation to CO_2. Glucose incorporation into glycogen is stimulated in the trained muscle, most notably in that exposed only to glucose as substrate, demonstrating the capacity to synthesize glycogen at an increased rate as well as to store it. We propose that the addition of FA-albumin to glucose as substrate may divert alpha-glycerophosphate into mitochondria for synthesis of triglyceride and phospholipid, and that this occurrence is stimulated by training.

References

1. BARKER, S.B. and SUMMERSON, W.H.: The colorimetric determination of lactic acid in biological material. J. biol. Chem. *138:* 535–554 (1941).
2. COBB, L.A., SHORT, F.A. and SMITH, P.H.: Inhibition of lactate production in exercised trained muscle Biochemistry of Exercise (unpublished).
3. GARLAND, P.B., NEWSHOLME, E.A. and RANDLE, P.J.: Regulation of glucose uptake by muscle. 9. Effects of fatty acids and ketone bodies, and of alloxan-diabetes and starvation, on pyruvate metabolism and on lactate/pyruvate and L-glycerol 3 phosphate/dihydroxyacetone phosphate concentration ratios in rat heart and rat diaphragm muscles. Biochem. J. *93:* 665–678 (1964).
4. GOOD, C.A., KRAMER, H. and Somogyi, M.: The determination of glycogen. J. biol. Chem. *100:* 485–491 (1933).
5. HULTMAN, E.: Studies on muscle metabolism of glycogen and active phosphate in man with special reference to exercise and diet. Scand. J. clin. Lab. Invest. *19:* Suppl. 94 (1967).
6. MORGAN, T.E., SHORT, F.A. and COBB, L.A.: Alterations in human skeletal muscle lipid composition and metabolism induced by physical conditioning Biochemistry of Exercise. Medicine and Sport, Vol. 3, pp. 116–121 (Karger, Basel/New York 1969).
7. SEGAL, S., BLAIR, A.E. and WYNGAARDEN, J.B.: An enzymatic spectrophotometric method for the determination of pyruvic acid in blood. J. lab. clin. Med. *48:* 137–143 (1956).
8. Technicon Auto Analyzer Methodology, Method File N-2b, Technicon Instruments Corporation, Chauncey, New York (1965).
9. TROUT, D.L., ESTES, E.H., Jr., and FRIEDBERG, S.J.: Titration of free fatty acids of plasma: a study of current methods and a new modification. J. Lipid Res. *1:* 199–202 (1960).

Authors' address: Dr. F.A. SHORT, Dr. LEONARD A. COBB and Dr. THOMAS E. MORGAN, Department of Medicine, University of Washington School of Medicine and King County Hospital, *Seattle, Wash. 98104* (USA).

Oxidation of Free Fatty Acids by Skeletal Muscle During Rest, Electrical Stimulation and Administration of 2,4-dinitrophenol[1]

J. J. Spitzer

Dept. of Physiology and Biophysics, Hahnemann Medical College, Philadelphia, Pa.

Since the demonstration of the ability of skeletal muscle to oxidize free fatty acids (FFA) under *in vivo* conditions [1, 3, 8], a number of studies have been concerned with the contribution of FFA to the energy metabolism of skeletal muscle [2, 4, 6, 9], mostly during exercise. Much less information is available concerning the metabolism of the resting skeletal muscle under *in vivo* conditions. The aim of the present study was to compare the uptake and oxidation of FFA by skeletal muscle in the same animal during rest, direct electrical stimulation and the infusion of 2,4-dinitrophenol (DNP).

Materials and Methods

Four male, mongrel dogs weighing approximately 20 kg were employed in these studies. The animals were anesthetized with Nembutal. A constant intravenous infusion of $1-C^{14}$ palmitic and $9-10H^3$-oleic acid was administered in the form of FFA as described previously [7]. The FFA infusion was preceded by a 10 min infusion of $50\mu c$ of $NaHC^{14}O_3$ to facilitate the equilibration of the tissue bicarbonate pools. Blood flow measurements in the right profunda femoris veins were carried out as described previously [5]. Simultaneous arterial and venous (from the profunda femoris veins) blood samples were removed at regular intervals. No anticoagulant was used in the animals. FFA, glucose, lactate, CO_2 and $C^{14}O_2$ were determined by the methods used in previous studies [8]. Direct electrical stimulation of the thigh muscles was performed for 30 min by applying 8 V, at a frequency of 6/sec and for a duration of 20 msec. DNP was infused in intravenously for 50 min at the rate of 2.5 mg/min.

[1] Supported by a grant from the American Heart Association, Inc.

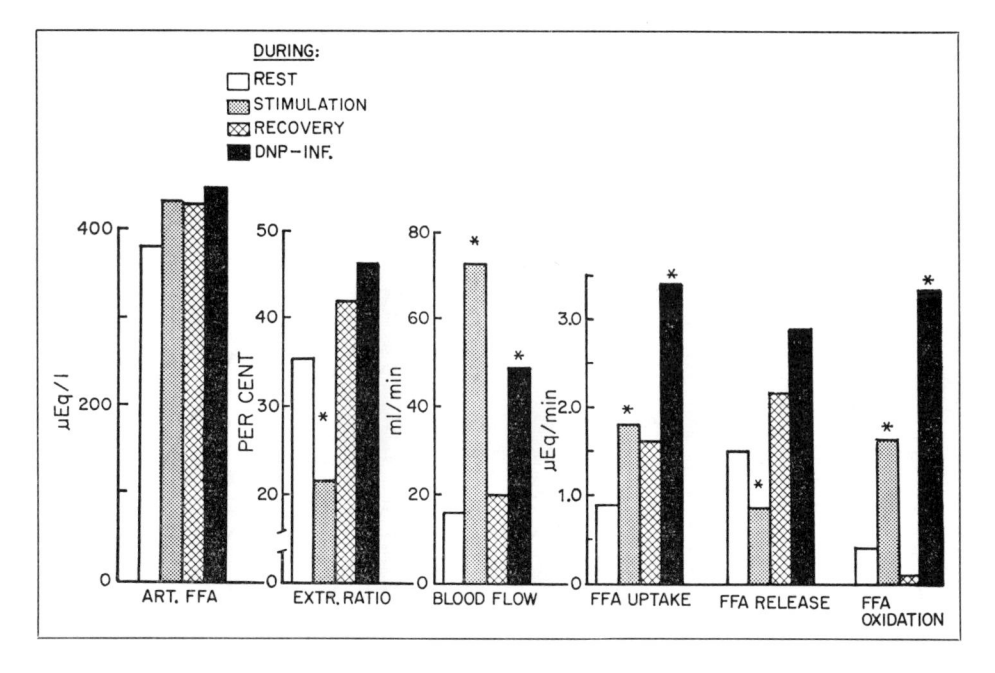

Figure 1. Changes in skeletal muscle metabolism during electrical stimulation and DNP administration. *=change is significant at p <0.05 level.

Results and Discussion

As shown in figure 1, the arterial FFA concentration was not altered significantly during the four phases of the experiment. During electrical stimulation and during the administration of DNP, blood flow through the muscles increased considerably. During stimulation, with the increased FFA supply (due to the increased blood flow) a smaller fraction of the arterial FFA was removed by the muscles, as indicated by the diminished extraction ratio $\left(\frac{A-V}{A} \times 100\right)$. This was not the case during DNP infusion. FFA uptake, however, was significantly elevated during both hypermetabolic states due to the increased blood flow. Oxidation of FFA to CO_2 by the area under study was also greatly increased by either muscle stimulation or DNP administration.

Electrical stimulation of the thigh muscles did not alter the total FFA flux in these dogs (figure 2). DNP infusion resulted in the expected increase in this parameter.

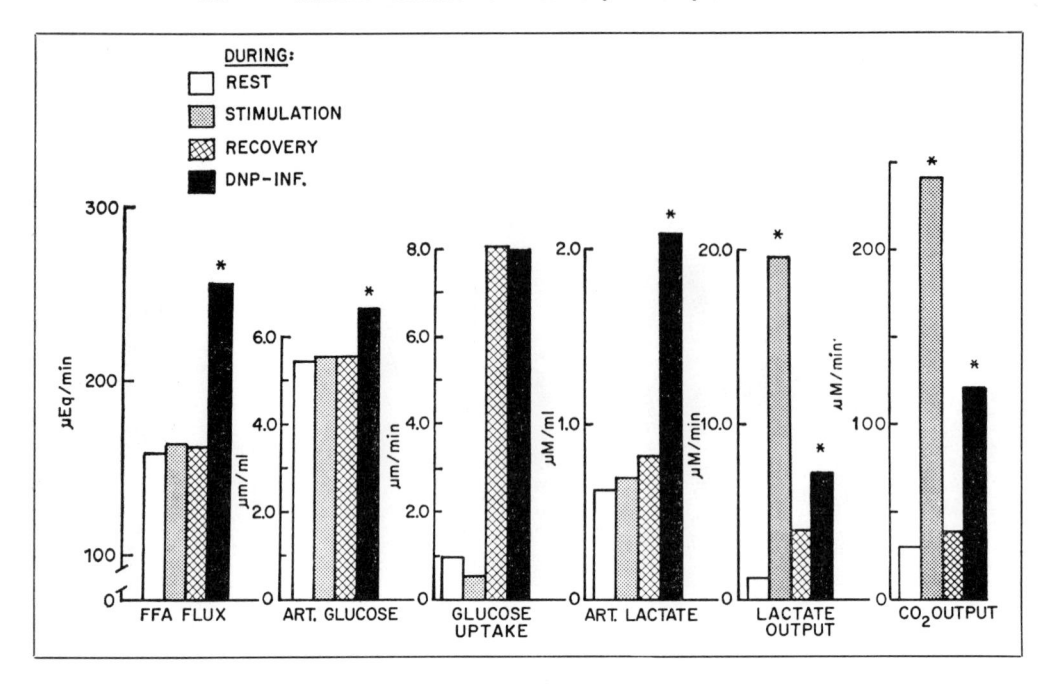

Figure 2. Changes in skeletal muscle metabolism during electrical stimulation and DNP administration.

Neither arterial glucose nor lactate concentration changed during stimulation (figure 2). Both were elevated by DNP infusion. Glucose uptake was not changed by the experimental procedures, while lactate and CO_2 output showed the expected elevations.

On the average the ratio of the oxidized FFA to the removed FFA was 45% during rest, 82% during stimulation, 8% during recovery and 99% during DNP infusion. Of the amount of CO_2 produced by the muscle 31% could be attributed to FFA oxidation during rest, 23% during stimulation, 17% during recovery and 33% during DNP infusion. The rest of the CO_2 presumably arose from carbohydrate oxidation.

References

1. ANDRES, R.; CADER, G. and ZIERLER, K.L.: The Quantitatively minor role of carbohydrate in oxidative metabolism by skeletal muscle in intact man in the basal state. J. Clin. Invest. *35:* 671–682 (1956).

2. Carlson, A. and Pernow, B.: Studies on Blood Lipids During Exercise. J. lab. clin. Med. *58*: 673–681 (1961).
3. Friedberg, S.J. and Estes, E.H.: Direct evidence for the oxidation of free fatty acids by peripheral tissues. J. Clin. Invest. *41:* 677–681 (1962).
4. Havel, R.J.; Pernow, B. and Jones, N.L.: Uptake and release of free fatty acids and other metabolites in the legs of exercising men. J. Appl. Physiol. *23:* 90–99 (1967).
5. Issekutz, B. and Spitzer, J.J.: Uptake of free fatty acids by skeletal muscle during stimulation. Proc. Soc. exper. Biol. Med. *105:* 21–23 (1960)
6. Miller, H.I.; Issekutz, B., Jr., and Rodahl, K.: Effect of exercise on the metabolism of fatty acids in the dog. Amer. J. Physiol. *205:* 167–172 (1963).
7. Scott, J.C.; Gold, M.; Bechtel, A.A. and Spitzer, J.J.: Metabolism of 2,4-dinitrophenol on myocardial metabolism and hemodynamics. Metabolism *17:* 370–376 (1968).
8. Spitzer, J.J. and Gold, M.: Free fatty acid metabolism by skeletal muscle. Am. J. Physiol. *206:* 159–163 (1964).
9. Spitzer, J.J. and Gold, M.: Studies on the metabolism of free fatty acids in diabetic and fasting dogs. Ann. N.Y. Acad. Sci. *131:* 235–249 (1965).

Author's address: John J. Spitzer, M.D., Professor of Physiology, 1114 Bobst Building 235 North 15 Street, *Philadelphia*, Pa. (USA).

The Influence of the Form of Exercise on the Arterial Concentrations of Glucose, Lactate, Pyruvate, and Free Fatty Acids

D. KEPPLER, J. KEUL and E. DOLL

Medizinische Universitätsklinik Freiburg i. Br.

To compare the influence of different types of work on arterial substrate levels, we used exercise in the supine position on a bicycle ergometer. Glucose, lactate and pyruvate were determined enzymatically [2, 3, 5] in the arterial blood and free fatty acids were measured by titration in the

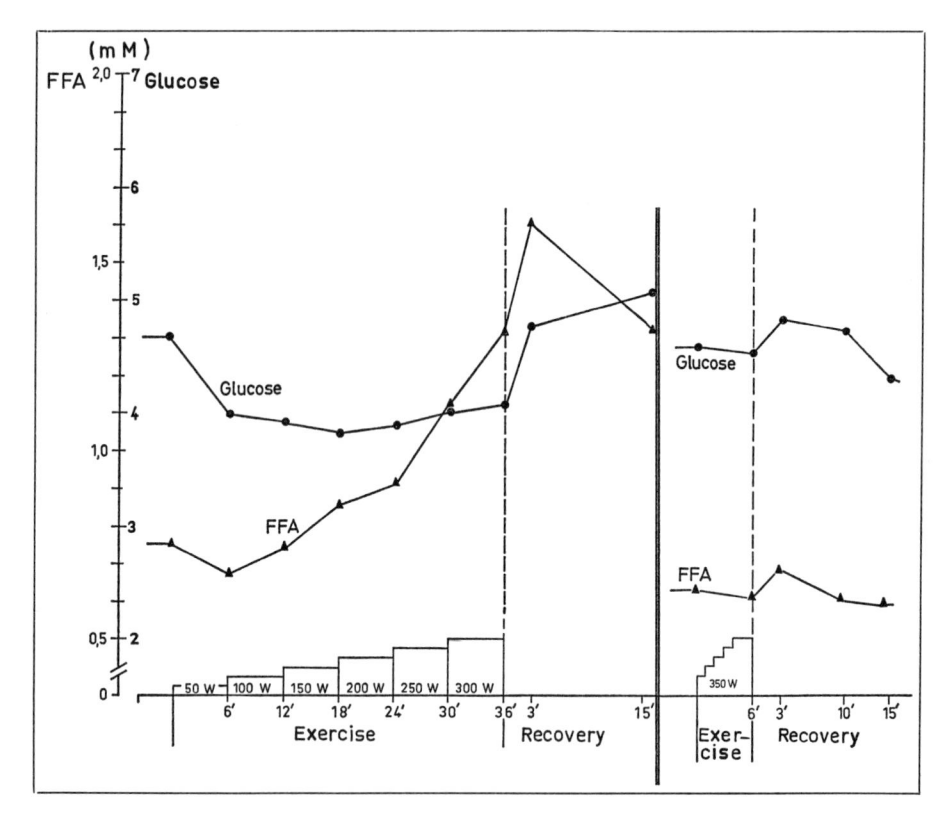

Figure 1. Arterial glucose (m moles/l blood) and free fatty acids (m moles/l plasma) during steady state and *vita maxima* exercise in athletes (N=12).

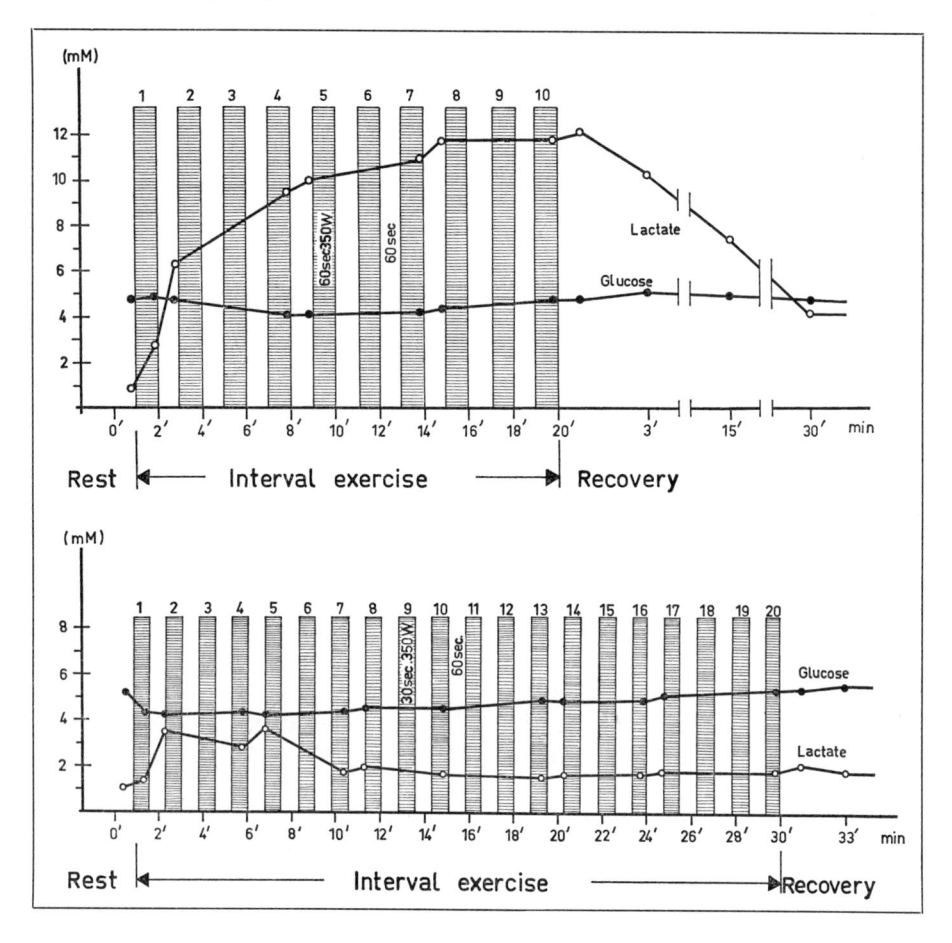

Figure 2. Arterial lactate and glucose (m moles/l) during interval exercise of athletes on the bicycle ergometer at 350 W. Top: 10 times 60 sec of work and 60 sec recovery. Bottom: 20 times 30 sec of work and 60 sec for recovery.

arterial plasma [9]. These metabolites were studied in 56 male athletes and 14 students under the following conditions:

1. Exercise according to the principle of the relative steady state with an uninterrupted series of work loads, starting at 50 W and increasing every 6 min by 50 W.

2. Exercise under *vita maxima* conditions for about 6 min with a maximal work load of 350 W. One group had been working with a submaximal load of 50 and 100 W immediately before starting *vita maxima* exercise.

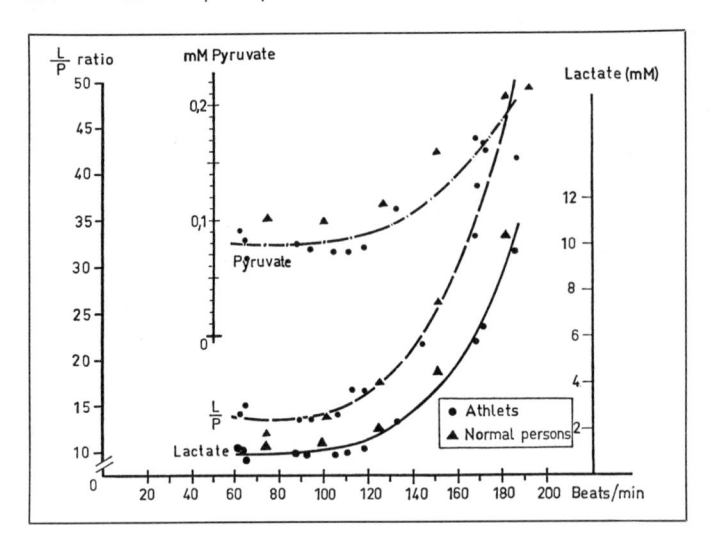

Figure 3. Arterial lactate, pyruvate (m moles/l) and lactate/pyruvate ratio in athletes (N=36) and untrained students (N=14) during exercise-type 1) and 2) in their correlation with the heart rate.

3. Interval exercise with 350 W was done either in 10 work periods of 60 sec, or in 20 work periods of 30 sec with 60 sec for recovery in both types.

The significant increase of the free fatty acids seen during steady state exercise was not observed during the brief *vita maxima* exercise (figure 1).

The well known decrease in blood glucose is only seen during exercise of longer duration. This is in agreement with studies showing that the breakdown of muscle glycogen plays the major role in energy supply to contracting skeletal muscle during short-term work [7], whereas the utilisation of blood glucose is low under these conditions. The arterial glucose and free fatty acid concentrations remain unchanged also during interval exercise with work periods of 30 and 60 sec (figure 2).

A considerable increase in arterial lactate was observed during all types of exercise that we studied, except during interval exercise with work periods of only 30 sec. Interval exercise with 60-sec work periods, however, induced the highest lactate concentrations that we measured in athletes. This difference may be due to two points. (1) During 30 sec the total lactate production is relatively small, due to the time course of phosphorylase

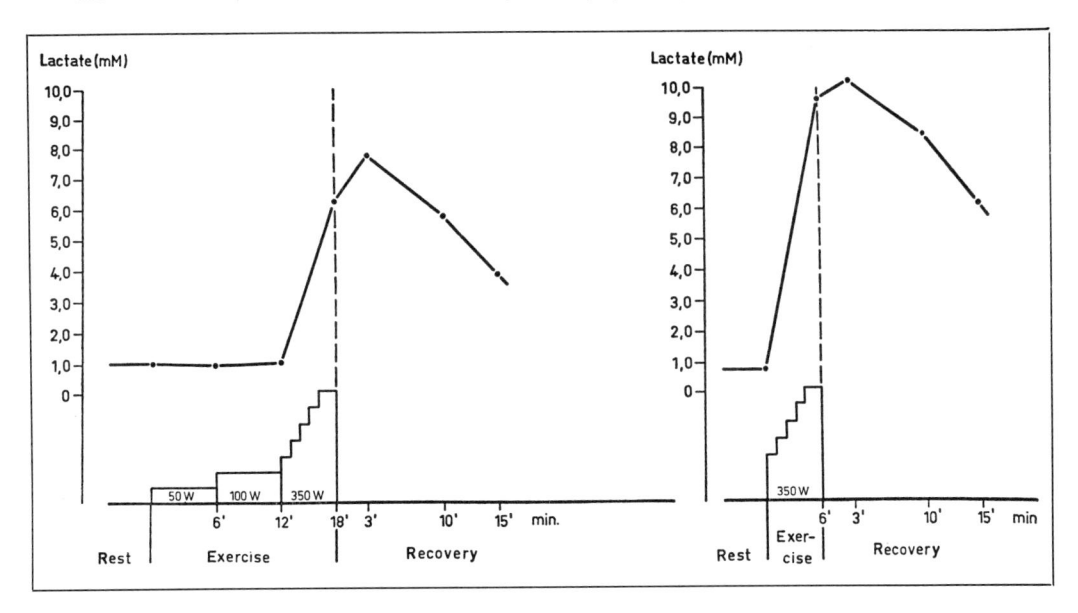

Figure 4. Arterial lactate concentration (mM) during *vita maxima* exercise with and without preceeding submaximal work and during recovery.

activation [4]. (2) The breakdown of phosphorylcreatine plays a major role in energy production during a short-term work period [6]. During the 60-sec work periods, however, muscle glycogenolysis seems to be maximally activated and surpassing the mitochondrial capacity for pyruvate oxidation. This is indicated by the extremely high lactate output from working skeletal muscles, seen in the measurement of arterio-femoralvenous differences [8].

Although work of high intensity was done during the 30-sec interval exercise, only a small increase in the lactate concentration was observed (figure 2) [1]. So one factor necessary for lactate increase during exercise is a work time of more than 30 sec. On the other hand there was no significant lactate increase in athletes or non-athletes during submaximal exercise at 50 and 100 W, indicating that intensity of work is important as well. For this reason arterial lactate and pyruvate concentrations were plotted against the heart rate as a measure for the relative work intensity. Increases are not seen below a heart rate of 120/min (figure 3).

In one group of 36 athletes we compared the arterial metabolites during *vita maxima* exercise with and without a period of submaximal work immediately before *vita maxima* exercise (figure 4). At the end of both types of work the concentrations of glucose and free fatty acids do not differ significantly. However the lactate concentration is significantly higher (∼50%) if no submaximal work was done before. With respect to the correlation between arterial lactate and heart rate, it may be mentioned that the heart rate was also higher if no submaximal work was done beforehand. These findings may explain some of the favourable effects of the so-called 'warming up' before athletic performance.

References

1. ÅSTRAND, I.; ÅSTRAND, P. O.; CHRISTENSEN, E. H. and HEDMAN, R.: Myohemoglobin as an oxygen store in man. Acta physiol. scand. *48:* 454–460 (1960).
2. BERGMEYER, H. U. und BERNT, E.: D-Glucosebestimmung mit Glucoseoxydase und Peroxydase, in: H. U. Bergmeyer's Meth. der enzymat. Anal. (Verlag Chemie, Weinheim 1962).
3. BÜCHER, TH.; CZOK, R.; LAMPRECHT, W. und LATZKO, E.: Pyruvat in: H. U. Bergmeyer's Meth. der enzymat. Anal. (Verlag Chemie, Weinheim 1962).
4. DANFORTH, W. H. and HELMREICH, E.: Regulation of glycolysis in muscle. I. The conversion of phosphorylase b to phosphorylase a in frog sartorius muscle. J. biol. Chem. *239:* 3133 (1964).
5. HOHORST, H. J.: L-(+)-Lactat, Bestimmung mit Lactatdehydrogenase und DPN, in: H. U. Bergmeyer's Meth. der enzymat. Anal. (Verlag Chemie, Weinheim 1962).
6. HULTMAN, E.; BERGSTRÖM, J. and MCLENNAN ANDERSON, N.: Breakdown and resynthesis of phosphorylcreatine and adenosine triphosphate in connection with muscular work in man. Scand. J. clin. Lab. Invest. *19:* 56–66 (1967).
7. HULTMAN, E.: Studies on muscle metabolism of glycogen and active phosphate in man with special reference to exercise and diet. Scand. J. clin. Lab. Invest. Suppl. *94:* 19, 1–63 (1967).
8. KEUL, J.; DOLL, E. und KEPPLER, D.: Zum Stoffwechsel des Skelettmuskels. I. Glucose, Lactat, Pyruvat und freie Fettsäuren im arteriellen und venösen Blut der arbeitenden Muskulatur bei Hochleistungssportlern. Pflügers Arch. ges. Physiol. *301:* 198–213 (1968).
9. TROUT, D. L.; ESTES, E. H., Jr., and FRIEDBERG, S. J.: Titration of free fatty acids of plasma, a study of current methods and a new modification. J. Lipid. Res. *1:* 199 (1960).

Authors' addresses: Dr. D. KEPPLER, Biochemisches Inst. der Universität, Hermann-Herder-Str. 7, *78 Freiburg i. Br.* (Germany). Doz. Dr. J. KEUL and Doz. Dr. E. DOLL, Medizinische Univ.-Klinik, Hugstetterstr. 55, *78 Freiburg i. Br.* (Germany).

The Effect of Age and Various Motor Activity on Fat Content, Lipoproteinase Activity and Experimental Necrosis in the Rat Heart

J. PAŘÍZKOVÁ

Adaptation to increased physical activity changes not only the fat proportion in the body, but also the metabolic activity of adipose tissue, as was proved previously in an experimental model [PAŘÍZKOVÁ and STAŇKOVÁ, 1964; PAŘÍZKOVÁ, 1965]. The character of changes is dependent not only on the intensity of physical activity, but also the life period when physical activity was changed as shown previously [PAŘÍZKOVÁ and STAŇKOVÁ, 1967]. There was a question whether also other parameters of fat metabolism in other tissues can be modified by changing physical activity – especially heart muscle, and in what relation these changes can be to experimental heart necrosis after isoprotenerol.

Adipose Tissue Proportion and Metabolic Activity after Increased or Reduced Motor Activity in Different Ages

The fat proportion in the organism of male rats with increased physical activity (i.e. daily run on a tread-mill) was significantly lower than that of controls with limited motor activity (kept in small cages), mean body weight having been the same. When comparing mean values of fat proportion, significantly higher values in limited growing rats were proved not only in comparison with the running, but also the control rats, which was not shown in adults. Further comparison showed general increase of total fat proportion with increasing age; running animals from older groups had always the same fat proportion as control rats from younger groups.

Spontaneous release of free fatty acids (FFA) from adipose tissue *in vitro* was always higher in running animals; release of FFA after various doses of adrenaline as an important mobilising factor was higher in running animals too. During growth this difference was significant, however, between running and limited rats only, but in adults between running and the other two groups, which did not differ significantly. Limited physical activity was no more an important stimulus in adult age from this point of view, as

Table I.

		HEART				
		WEIGHT mg	WEIGHTmg/100g WEIGHT	WEIGHT/100g LBM	% FAT	LIPOPROTEINE-LIPASE ACTIVITY
A) YOUNG	x̄	358,60	351,9	375,5	2,62	11,54
n = 10	SD	41,02	35,2	36,0	0,30	2,72
B) RUNNING	x̄	808,25	264,6	282,9	2,58	13,37
n = 12	SD	98,34	14,69	17,0	0,57	2,07
C) CONTROLS 1.	x̄	815,5	257,11	279,6	2,85	10,1
n = 9	SD	94,38	22,99	21,1	0,50	3,06
D) RUNNING + LIMITED	x̄	818,90	260,1	276,5	2,84	8,67
n = 10	SD	85,21	27,20	32,1	0,37	1,09
E) CONTROLS 2.	x̄	781,8	245,6	276,7	3,05	17,83
n = 8	SD	133,6	22,2	22,9	0,34	2,91
F) LIMITED	x̄	807,50	252,0	283,2	3,41	13,57
n = 12	SD	99,0	20,9	21,6	0,75	3,50

it was during growth. It seems therefore that in growth period the limitation of physical activity is a more significant stimulus resulting in increased fat proportion and lower FFA release, and *vice versa* in the adult, when, on the contrary, only increased motor activity causes changes in fat metabolism – the decrease in fat proportion and increase of FFA release [PAŘÍZKOVÁ and STAŇKOVÁ, 1964, 1967].

Lipoproteinase (LPL) Activity and Fat Content in Heart and Skeletal Muscles in Rats of Different Motor Activity and Age

Corresponding results in lipoproteinase activity in heart and skeletal muscles were proved; CRASS [1966] showed that the release of LPL after heparin correlates with uptake and oxidation of FFA in the heart. In male rats 195 days old, only significantly decreased LPL activity [CHERKES and GORDON, 1957] in the heart was proved in animals with limited motor activity in comparison with other groups. A daily run on a tread-mill for 60 min starting after weaning did not influence significantly LPL activity

Table II.

		ANTERIOR TIBIALIS MUSCLE				
		WEIGHT 100 mg	WEIGHT mg/100g WEIGHT	WEIGHT mg/100g W LBM	% FAT	LIPOPROTEINE-LIPASE ACTIVITY
A) YOUNG n = 10	x̄ SD	184,0 27,1	178,4 11,1	191,1 12,0	1,87 0,37	3,05 0,61
B) RUNNING n = 12	x̄ SD	517,0 82,36	168,0 10,0	179,4 8,6	1,67 0,47	2,39 0,50
C) CONTROLS 1. n = 9	x̄ SD	540,4 57,0	170,2 9,65	186,1 10,2	1,49 0,26	2,08 1,16
D) RUNNING +LIMITED n = 10	x̄ SD	546,1 80,7	171,6 7,3	184,4 5,6	1,72 0,47	1,98 0,40
E) CONTROLS 2. n = 8	x̄ SD	533,5 64,4	168,3 8,0	186,1 8,7	1,63 0,44	3,13 0,54
F) LIMITED n = 12	x̄ SD	526,7 4,04	164,7 10,3	185,2 26,8	2,71 1,39	1,29 0,48

in the liver, heart, anterior tibialis and soleus muscles. – Changes in total fat proportions etc. were the same as mentioned above [PAŘÍZKOVÁ et al., 1966].

In further experiments LPL activity was tested in male rats running daily 90 min from 35th till 160th day of life. Weights of the hearts did not differ (table I) except according to age both absolutely and in relation to total or lean body weight. Proportion of fat in heart muscle was not different neither according to age nor to motor activity. LPL activity was highest in running (by 32%) and growing rats (by 14%) in comparison with controls. In animals limited in motor activity since weaning LPL activity was decreased by 24% in comparison with the corresponding control group, and in those with motor activity limited since adult age after previous daily run by 15% approximately.

Mean absolute weight of anterior tibialis muscle (a dynamic one) differed only according to age. Relative weights as well as proportion of fat were the same (table II). LPL activity was significantly higher in growing animals only in comparison with adult controls and those rats limited since

Table III.

| | | WEIGHT mg | SOLEUS MUSCLE ||||
			WEIGHT mg/100 g WEIGHT	WEIGHT/100g LBM	% FAT	LIPOPROTEINE - LIPASE ACTIVITY
A) YOUNG	x̄	41,8	40,8	43,5	2,81	12,30
n = 10	SD	7,6	5,8	5,7	0,58	3,18
B) RUNNING	x̄	149,0	48,6	51,8	2,22	8,11
n = 12	SD	31,0	8,1	8,8	0,79	1,93
C) CONTROLS 1.	x̄	114,2	36,0	39,1	1,87	4,38
n = 9	SD	18,7	1,7	1,7	0,47	1,01
D) RUNNING + LIMITED	x̄	106,1	33,4	36,8	2,09	5,46
n = 10	SD	20,0	5,3	4,6	0,50	0,63
E) CONTROLS 2.	x̄	125,2	39,3	43,5	3,15	4,08
n = 8	SD	22,5	3,9	5,0	0,88	1,31
F) LIMITED	x̄	112,6	25,3	39,6	2,70	4,23
n = 12	SD	22,1	6,3	6,6	0,86	1,33

adult age. But reduction in motor activity since weaning lowered significantly LPL activity in the tibialis anterior in comparison with controls; the mean value was only 41% of that of the corresponding controls.

The soleus muscle (a postural one) seems to be more sensitive to motor activity changes: its absolute and relative weights were significantly higher in running animals. Reduction of motor activity, however, did not influence its weight significantly. Proportion of fat was influenced only by age, having been highest in growing animals in which LPL activity was highest too. LPL activity in the soleus muscle of running animals was also significantly higher in comparison with control and limited animals by 85% approximately. Reduction of motor activity did not influence LPL activity in the soleus muscle, which is probably caused by the different functions of the muscles in question [PAŘÍZKOVÁ and KOUTECKÝ, 1968].

It is possible to conclude that organism of animals adapted to long-term daily run contains a lower proportion of adipose tissue, which is moreover metabolically more active, i.e. is able to release more FFA both spontaneously and after adrenaline. This is in connection with higher LPL activity in heart and skeletal muscles; from these selected points of view an organism adapted to increased motor activity resembles a young growing organism.

Experimental Heart Necrosis in Male Rats of Different Age and Physical Activity

In young and light male rats heart necrosis after application of isoprotenerol is always less marked, and also spontaneous mortality is much lower than in adult animals with increased body weight. Further analysis showed that the most important factor is not the total body weight, but fat proportion, which is significantly lower in young growing animals

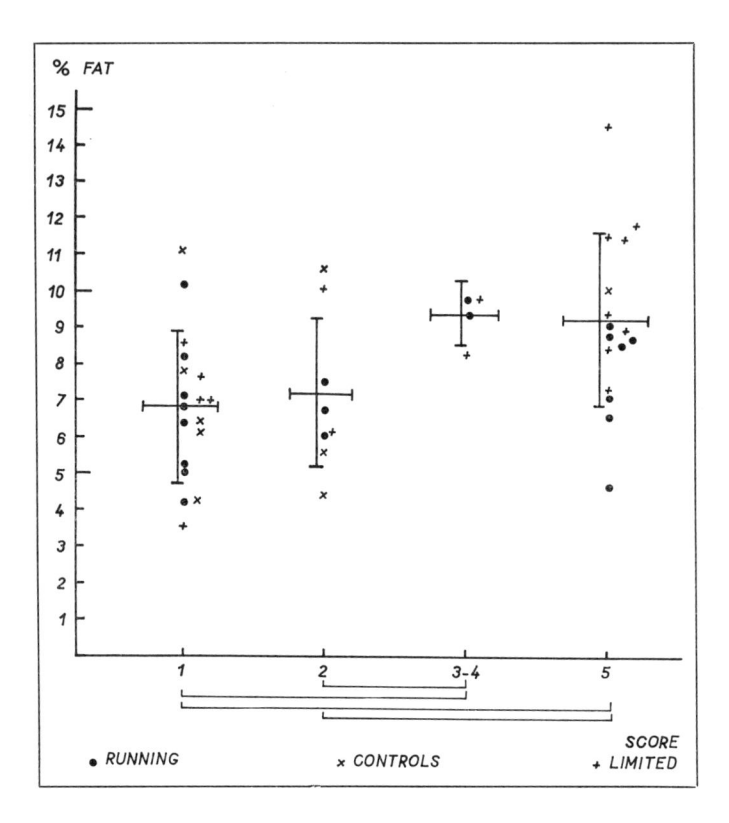

Figure 1.

[FALTOVÁ; PAŘÍZKOVÁ and POUPA, 1968]. When in running and limited animals the cardiotoxicity of isoprotenerol was tested in five series of experiments in male rats, no significant differences between mentioned groups (i.e. running, control and limited) were found when the change in motor activity was of shorter duration, and was studied in relatively young animals (i.e. starting from 21st, 35th or 55th day of life till 100–125th day of life), and the resulting difference in body fat proportion was 2–3% only. On the other hand, when surviving animals with lightest grade of heart necrosis (score 1) with those which died spontaneously were compared, a significantly higher fat proportion was found in those which died spontaneously (5) [PAŘÍZKOVÁ and FALTOVÁ, 1968]. This applied both for the comparison of younger and older, and for active and inactive animals (figure 1). However, when run on a tread-mill was performed daily from the 21st to the 204th day of live, more marked differences in death rate as well as heart necrosis were proved (30% in running to 70% in controls). Animals which were active during such a long period were markedly lighter and less fat in comparison with controls. But the cardiotoxicity of isoprotenerol was not entirely dependent on physical activity, as limited animals which were also lighter than controls had a correspondingly lower death rate. It seems therefore that the cardiotoxicity of isoprotenerol is not directly related to motor activity, but is more dependent on total body weight and fat proportion which could be changed by various factors influencing energetic turnover such as motor activity, diet [BALASZ et al., 1962], etc.

References

1. BALASZ, T.; SAHASRABUDHE, M. R. and GRICE, H. C.: The influence of excess body fat in the cardiotoxicity of isoprotenerol in rats. Toxicol. appl. Pharmacol. *4:* 613–618 (1962).
2. CRASS, M. F. and MENG, H. C.: The removal and metabolism of chylomicron triglycerides by the isolated perfused rat heart; the role of a heparin-released lipase. Biochim. biophys. Acta *125:* 1 (1966).
3. CHERKES, A. and GORDON, R. S., Jr.: The liberation of lipoprotein lipase by heparin from adipose tissue in vitro. J. Lipid. Res. *1:* 97–104 (1957).
4. FALTOVÁ, E.; PAŘÍZKOVÁ, J. and POUPA, O.: The influence of age and early nutrition on cardiotoxicity of isoprotenerol of rats in relation to body fat proportion (in press).
5. PAŘÍZKOVÁ, J. and STAŇKOVÁ, L.: Influence of physical activity on a tread-mill on the metabolism of adipose tissue in rats. Brit. J. Nutr. *18:* 325–332 (1964).
6. PAŘÍZKOVÁ, J.: Physical activity and body composition. 1st ed., p. 161–176. Symposia of the Society for the study of Human Biology, vol. VII. Human body composition. Ed. by JOSEF BROŽEK (Pergamon Press, 1965).

7. PAŘÍZKOVÁ, J.; STAŇKOVÁ, L.; FÁBRY, P. and KOUTECKÝ, Z.: Liberation from and uptake of non-esterified fatty acids into adipose tissue of rats with different work output. Physiol. bohemoslov. *15:* 31–37 (1966).
8. PAŘÍZKOVÁ, J.; KOUTECKÝ, Z. and STAŇKOVÁ, L.: Fat content and lipoproteine lipase activity in muscles of male rats with increased or reduced motor activity. Physiol. bohemoslov. *15:* 237–243 (1966).
9. PAŘÍZKOVÁ, J. and STAŇKOVÁ, L.: Release of free fatty acids from adipose tissue *in vitro* after adrenaline in relation to the total body fat in rats of different age and different physical activity. Nutr. Diet. *9:* 43–55 (1967).
10. PAŘÍZKOVÁ, J. and KOUTECKÝ, Z.: The influence of age and various physical activity on relative weights, fat content and lipoproteinase activity of internal organs, heart and skeletal muscles. Physiol. bohemoslov. *17:* 179–189 (1968).
11. PAŘÍZKOVÁ, J. and FALTOVÁ, E.: The relationship of motor activity and body fat proportion to cardiotoxic effect of isoprotenerol in male rats of different ages (in press).

Author's address: Dr. J. PAŘÍZKOVÁ, Vút, Ujezd 450, *Praha 1* (Czechoslovakia).

Comparative Investigations on the Daily Rhythm of Blood Glucose after Rest, after Exhaustive Interval Exercise, and after Exhaustive Continuous Exercise[1]

J.-P. Kosiek, U. Kersting, F. Küsters and E. J. Klaus

Institute of Sports Medicine of Münster University (Director: Prof. E. J. Klaus)

Biological rhythms as the characteristic time structure of biological processes represent a dynamic regularity. This knowledge has gained practical importance for sports or occupational physiology, with regard to optimum readiness for training and performance at the different times of the day and according to the pertinent rhythm. It is also of interest to see in how far physical stress influences the course of the daily rhythm. Numerous studies on the daily rhythm of blood glucose are known from literature [3, 4, 5, 6, 7, 8, 9, 10, 11, 13, 14, 16, 17, 18], however, the results and their interpretation show many contradictions.

In our series of experiments we formed groups of 20 healthy male athletes aged from 18 to 28 years. Capillary blood was taken every hour for 24 hours. We observed the daily rhythm of the blood glucose after preceding bedrest (group I), after 4 hours exhaustive interval exercise on the ergometer (group II) and after two times 40 min of exhaustive continuous ergometer-exercise within 4 hours (group III). The trial subjects were in bed during the experiment. After every withdrawal of blood they got a constant rhythm-diet according to Menzel [12]. The total amount of calories of this diet per trial subject and per experiment amounted for group I to 2,000 cal., for group II to 2,700 cal., and for group III to 3,000 cal. No food or fluids whatsoever were given besides this rhythm-diet. Blood glucose was determined according to the enzymatic method by means of glucose peroxydase [2], three determinations were made of each blood sample. The experiments were conducted in a room especially equipped for this purpose with climatic conditions, which were felt to be pleasant. All trial subjects felt well during and after termination of the experiment.

In group I the daily curves of the blood glucose show a range of fluctuation of the mean daily values between 100.2 mg% and 126.7 mg% and of the 'amplitudes' (defined as double, mean square deviation from each mean daily value) from 15.4 mg% to 26.6 mg%; they have mainly a 12 hourly periodicity besides 6 curves with an 8 hourly periodicity. In group II a 12

[1] This work was supported by the Kuratorium für Sportmedizinische Forschung.

Table I. Mean values of the daily mean levels, the 'amplitudes' and the times of the highest and lowest blood-glucose concentrations

	Mean daily level (mg%)	Mean "amplitude" (mg%)	1. max (h ± hrs)	Times of the day of the 1. min (h ± hrs)	2. max (h ± hrs)	2. min (h ± hrs)
Group I (n = 14)	109.8 ± 16.9	19.8 ± 6.8	2.00 ± 1.5	9.30 ± 1.5	14.30 ± 2.5	19.30 ± 1.5
Group II (n = 16)	94.0 ± 19.4	32.1 ± 12.6	0.30 ± 3	6.00 ± 4	12.30 ± 4.5	16.00 ± 4
Group III (n = 16)	93.6 ± 20.3	28.5 ± 15.3	4.30 ± 1.5	11.30 ± 3.5	16.00 ± 4	21.00 ± 3

hourly rhythm predominates besides 4 curves with 8 hourly or 24 hourly periodicity. The mean daily values of the individual experiments vary from 74.6 mg% to 112.0 mg% and the 'amplitudes' from 20.4 mg% to 54.1 mg%. The daily fluctuations of group III in 16 cases follow a marked 12 hourly rhythm, while 4 daily curves again show an 8 hourly or 24 hourly periodicity. The mean daily values of this group III fluctuate between 73.2 mg% and 110.4 mg%, the 'amplitudes' between 21.0 mg% and 44.2 mg%. The daily fluctuations of the blood glucose thus are greater after preceding exercise than after preceding rest.

The phase position of the biphasic individual curves shows the individual differences known from former studies of rhythm [11], but the accumulated occurrence of corresponding extremes within the three groups is within such narrow limits, that they can be assigned reliably to the different times of the day. Table I shows in confrontation, at what times both the *maxima* and the *minima* of the biphasic curves occur accumulatedly in the individual groups. Even though a nocturnal main maximum and a secondary maximum in the afternoon are found congruently in all three groups, a phase-shifting of the daily rhythm of the blood glucose after preceding extreme physical exercise is shown as compared to the course of the curves after rest. In none of the three groups a statistically significant correlation could be computed between the height of the daily level and the occurrence of the extremes at the different times of the day, or between the height of the daily level and the extent of the daily fluctuation, as described occasionally in former studies of rhythm.

In order to be independent of the individual phase differences we established – before forming the sum curves – a graphic balance of the

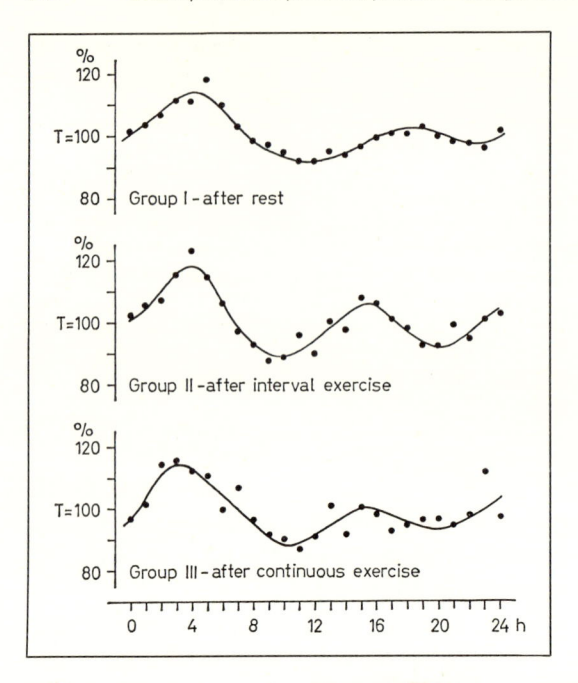

Figure 1. Sum curves of the 24-hours-blood glucose rhythm after graphic balance of the phase-differences, expressed in p.c. values of the daily mean values.

phase differences according to BERGES [1]. Therefore, the sum curves of the daily rhythm of the blood glucose of each group – as shown in figure 1 – understandably no longer can be assigned to certain times of the day.

It can be shown that after exhaustive interval or continuous exercise the daily rhythm of the blood glucose is not blurred or eliminated in its existence, but rather becomes more marked with regard to the extent of the daily fluctuations. This clearer marking of the rhythm might be due to the fact, that the exhausting physical exercise results in a more extensive, stress-caused synchronization of the metabolic mechanisms interfering in the blood glucose regulation.

References

1. BERGES, D.: Elektromyographische Untersuchungen an Sportlern zur Frage einer Tagesrhythmik der Muskelaktivität. Med. Diss. Münster/W. (1957); Int. Z. Physiol. *17:* 57 (1958).

2. BERGMEYER, H. U. und BERNT, E.: Bestimmung der D-Glukose mit Glukose-Oxydase und Peroxydase. In: Bergmeyer, H. U.: Methoden der enzymatischen Analyse. Verlag Chemie, Weinheim/Bergstr. (1962).
3. BROCKMANN, G.: Enzymatische Blutzuckerbestimmung im Nüchternzustand bei Ruhe zur Tagesrhythmik beim Sportler. Med. Diss. Münster/W. (1966).
4. DIENST, C. und WINTER, B.: Schlaf, Blutzucker und Säurebasenhaushalt. Z. klin. Med. *133:* 91 (1938).
5. HATLEHOL, R.: Blood sugar studies. Section III: Paradoxical rise of blood sugar concentration in diabetes mellitus. Acta med. Scand. Suppl. *8:* 211 (1924).
6. HOPMANN, R.: Insulinbehandlung unter Berücksichtigung des 24-Stunden-Rhythmus des Diabetes mellitus. Acta med. Scand. Suppl. *108:* 143 (1940).
7. JORES, A.: Physiologie und Pathologie der 24-Stunden-Rhythmik des Menschen. Ergebn. inn. Med. *48:* 574 (1935).
8. KALKOFEN, G.-L.: Einfluss des Nebennierenhormons 11-Desoxycorticosteron und des chemisch verwandten Follikelhormons auf die Periodik des Blutzuckers. Med. Diss. Hamburg (1952).
9. KOSIEK, J.-P.: Untersuchungen zur Frage einer Tagesrhythmik der Blutzuckerkonzentration unter dem Einfluss stündlicher Nahrungszufuhr bei Sportlern. Med. Diss. Münster/W. (1966).
10. KRASNJANSKIJ, L. M.: Die Tagesschwankungen des Blutzuckergehaltes beim Menschen. Biochem. Zschr. *205:* 180 (1929).
11. LANGE, H. und SCHLOSS, J.: Über das Verhalten des Blutzuckers in der Nacht und in den Morgenstunden. Arch. exp. Path. Pharmakol. *139:* 274 (1929).
12. MENZEL, W.: Menschliche Tag-Nacht-Rhythmik und Schichtarbeit. Schwabe & Co., Basel/Stuttgart (1962).
13. MENZEL, W. und OTHLINGHAUS, I.: Inversion des Blutzuckertagesrhythmus durch Percorten. Dtsch. med. Wschr. *73:* 326 (1948).
14. MÖLLERSTRÖM, J. und ULLMARK, R.: Der Einfluss von Muskelarbeit auf den Blutzucker während verschiedener Phasen der rhythmischen Leberfunktion. Acta med. Scand. Suppl. *108:* 132 (1940).
15. REINDELL, H.; ROSKAMM, H. und GERSCHLER, W.: Das Intervalltraining. Barth, München (1962).
16. SACHSE, P.: Gleichzeitige Untersuchungen der 24-Stunden-Schwankungen des Blutzuckers und Blutdrucks beim Menschen. Med. Diss. Düsseldorf (1937).
17. TRIMBLE, H. C. and MADDOCK, S. J.: The fluctuations of the capillary blood sugar in normal young men during 24-hour period, including a discussion in the effect of sleep and of mild exercise. J. biol. Chem. *81:* 595 (1929).
18. VOGEL, G.: Über tageszeitliche Blutzuckerschwankungen. Z. ges. inn. Med. *3:* 606 (1948).

Author's address: Dr. med. J.-P. KOSIEK, Institute of Sports Medicine of Münster University, Horstmarer Landweg 39, *44 Münster* (Germany).

The Effect of Two Types of Physical Strain During Summer and Winter on Cholesterolemia in Young People

JOSEF DOLEŽEL

Institute of Sports Medicine of Palacky University, Olomouc

The cholesterol level in blood serum is considered to be one of the factors which influences the onset and development of arteriosclerosis. That is the reason why different possibilities of lowering the cholesterolemia are being examined.

Method and Results

In winter 1967 I observed how one weeks ski-training would influence the cholesterolemia in 60 medical students both men and women aged 19–20. It was a basic training in downhill runs which lasted 5 hours a day. All students ate during this week three times a day the same food in a restaurant.

The blood samples for the determination of cholesterolemia were collected on the first and last (i.e. 6th) day of the training always in the morning before breakfast.

The cholesterol levels found at the beginning of the programme were relatively high, higher than described for this age group by KEYS et al. [6] and by RATH et al. [8].

Table I shows the mean values of cholesterolemia in men and women and in the whole group before and after winter training. Before training the average value of cholesterolemia in women was significantly higher than the average value in men. The significant decrease of the cholesterol level was observed both in men and women.

Further observations were carried out in 19–20-year-old students of medicine during the summer training programme. 94 examined men and women took their meals in the camp so that the quantity of food was practically unlimited. The scheme of this summer training included water sports, tourism and ball games.

The blood samples for the determination of cholesterolemia were again collected on the first and last (i.e. 10th) day of the training, always in

Table I. Mean cholesterolemia values in winter in mg%

	Women	Men	Men and women
n	25	35	60
Before training	236±45	214±53	223±52
After training	165±36	156±37	160±37
p	<0.0005	<0.0005	<0.0005

Table II. Mean cholesterolemia values in summer in mg%

	Women	Men	Men and women
n	38	56	94
Before training	197±21	189±19	192±20
After training	228±19	190±18	206±28
p	<0.0005	>0.05	<0.0005

the morning before breakfast. The average cholesterolemia in men and women and of the whole group are presented in table II. At the end of this training there was a significant increase of cholesterolemia in the whole group. The increase of cholesterolemia was especially remarkable in women and influenced considerably the statistical results of the evaluation of the whole group. The increase of cholesterolemia in men was not significant.

18 men in the above mentioned observation had been already examined during the winter ski-training; in all of them a marked decrease of cholesterolemia had been found at that time. At the end of the summer training, however, there was a mild increase of cholesterolemia (though statistically insignificant), from the average value 185 mg% to 189 mg%.

All examined subjects belong to slim or muscular type of body configuration.

The method of HORÁK et al. [5] was used to assay the cholesterolemia. This method gives the same results as the method of PEARSON et al. [7].

Discussion

There was a great dispersion of values at the beginning of the winter training which could have been caused by different ways of living (and different food and its quantity) before this training. In 15 subjects (i.e. 25%) cholesterolemia was higher than 260 mg%. It must be kept in mind that the people in question belong to those who in older age most often suffer from the ischemic cardiac disease in our country as observed BALOGH [1]. Already the studies of medicine have the character of sedentary occupation with a lot of psychic stress and in the job of a physician these features become still more pronounced.

The decrease of cholesterolemia was found in 88% of examined subjects and made 72 mg% in the average. Such a marked and prompt depressive effect of physical training was described by CARLSON and FRÖBERG [4] in people who had fasted during a ten days' march. The mean cholesterolemia value at the beginning of the summer training was lower than at the beginning of the winter training. The seasonal variations of cholesterolemia, influence of the temperature and other climatic factors should be taken into consideration.

The cholesterol levels behaved differently during the winter and summer training. It is interesting that cholesterolemia increased in 87% of women by an average amount of 36 mg%, whereas only in 57% of men by an average of 15 mg% during the summer training. It seems that women manifest a tendency to higher cholesterolemia. This tendency was also observed in comparison with men during the fasting period by BLOOM *et al.* [2].

The fact that during the summer training the meals were practically unlimited, whereas during the winter programme they did not surpass a normal restaurant-meal may be one of the factors which account for the different behaviour of cholesterolemia. Another factor might be the character of the physical exercise in question. During the skiing training in downhill runs, no violent mobilization of the reserves of energy was required, and the increased output of energy was extended to a relatively great part of the day. During the summer training, however, there were very often the exercises of maximal or submaximal intensity which required a great mobilization of the energetic sources.

The terms physical training, training programme etc. may differ considerably and this is probably the reason why numerous authors have observed remarkable decrease of cholesterolemia after a certain training programme, whereas other authors did not find any changes. The effect of physical exercises will surely depend upon the kind and intensity of the exercise and to a certain degree also upon the efficiency and health conditions of the examined subjects as CAMPBELL and LUMSDEN [3] tried to demonstrate.

Summary

The marked decrease of cholesterolemia in 60 medical students of both sexes from mean value 223 mg% to 160 mg% was observed during a week's winter skiing programme.

Not so marked, but significant increase of cholesterolemia from 192 mg% to 206 mg% was observed in 94 medical students during the summer training programme (water sports, tourism, ball games).

In women there is a tendency to higher cholesterol values.

Different changes of cholesterolemia after exercises under various conditions are discussed.

References

1. BALOGH, J.: Nekolik zajímavych statistickych údaju o vyskytu akutního infarktu u zamestnancu. Prakt. Lék. *42:* 355–357 (1962).
2. BLOOM, W. L.; AZAR, G. and CLARK, J. E.: Electrolyte and lipid metabolism of lean fasting men and women. Metabolism *15:* 401–408 (1966).
3. CAMPBELL, D. E. and LUMSDEN, T. B.: Serum cholesterol concentrations during physical training and during subsequent detraining. Amer. J. med. Sci. *253:* 155–161 (1967).
4. CARLSON, L. A. and FRÖBERG, S. O.: Blood lipid and glucose levels during a ten-day period of low calorie intake and exercise in man. Metabolism *16:* 624–634 (1967).
5. HORÁK, M.; JÍCHA, J. and VOTRUBA, M.: Stanovení cholesterolu a jeho esteru ultramikrometodou. Prakt. Lék. *46:* 710–712 (1966).
6. KEYS, A.; MICKELSEN, O.; MILLER, E.; HAYES, E. and TODD, R.: The concentration of cholesterol in the blood serum of normal men and its relation to age. J. clin. Invest. *29:* 1347 (1950).
7. PEARSON, S.; STERN, S. and McGAVACK, T.: A rapid, accurate method for determination of total cholesterol in serum. Analyt. Chem. *25:* 813–814 (1953).
8. RATH, R.; VAVŘÍNKOVÁ, H.; PETRÁSEK, R. and MAŠEK, J.: Relationship between the ratio of body fat and plasma levels of cholesterol, esterified fatty acids, triglycerides and blood pressure values in men and women with different body weights. Rev. czech. Med. *13:* 106–123 (1967).

Author's address: JOSEF DOLEŽEL, M. D., Institute of Sports Medicine of Palacky University, I. P. Pavlova 6, *Olomouc* (Czechoslovakia).

Changes in Cholesterol Serum Levels after Spiroergometric Examinations in Children

Z. Jirka and J. Doležel

Institut of Sports Medicine (Head: MUDr. Z. Jirka, CSc), Medical Faculty of the Palacky University, Olomouc

The question of cholesterol serum level changes after physical activity is still open. Immediately after effort the cholesterol in the serum increases [3]. Most examinations concern adults; we haven't found any data on changes in children. This fact has lead us to this research, in which we follow the immediate influence of one single effort on cholesterol serum level in twelve-year-old children.

Spiroergometric examinations with two grades of submaximal load (250 and 500 mkp/min) joined with examinations of maximal oxygen consumption were performed to enable comparison of the results obtained with common indicators of physical fitness. Examinations were always performed in the morning, the venous blood before effort was obtained after 15 min rest, and in the first minute after effort [method see 2]. We examined 93 children (47 boys and 46 girls) completely. The choice of children was not incidental. All examined children were very good at 300 m run: they were chosen from 400 pupils. In all cases of differences, changes or correlations of the mentioned values are statistically significant ($p < 0.05$); all other findings are supposed to be equal or without correlations.

Serum cholesterol levels in boys and girls differ (table I). At rest they are higher in girls. Rath [4] found higher levels in adult women. Our previous study in twenty-year-old women revealed higher serum cholesterol levels too. Increased cholesterol serum levels were found in persons with higher amounts of depot fat [4]. Our girls weighed more than the boys and their depot fat was higher even at the same rate of lean body mass.

After work serum cholesterol levels were higher in boys inspite of the same effort in boys and girls, where the same maximal oxygen intake, working capacity and serum lactic acid levels were found. The increase in serum cholesterol may, according to Stocker [7] be produced by mere alteration of attitude from lying to standing. This increase correlates with haematocrit changes and is therefore due to haemoconcentration. On the other hand there seems to be a firm binding of serum cholesterol to albumin [1]. Therefore we followed changes of haematocrit in both groups and we did

Table I. Mean values, standard deviations and significance

Mean values	in	boys	girls	p
cholesterol before effort	mg%	139.8±14.9	145.8±18.2	p<0.02
cholesterol after effort	mg%	166.9±23.1	156.9±11.5	p<0.01
change of the cholesterol	%	20.8±10.8	7.8± 6.0	p<0.01
weight	kg	39.0± 4.5	42.5± 7.3	p<0.02
height	cm	151.6± 5.6	154.6± 5.7	p<0.05
depot fat	%	10.2± 2.04	19.4± 3.27	p<0.001
coefficient of slenderness	–	9.17± 1.74	4.59± 1.05	p<0.001
$\dot{V}O_2$ max	ml	1787 ± 251	1741 ± 348	p>0.05
PWC max	mkp/min	712 ± 131	692 ± 146	p>0.05
PWC 170	mkp/min	539 ± 140	467 ± 262	p>0.05
puls rate max	pro min	193.4± 7.5	196.0± 30	p>0.05
blood lactate before effort	mg%	19.4± 2.2	19.1± 2.2	p>0.05
blood lactate after effort	mg%	66.7± 9.0	65.9± 7.6	p>0.05
haematocrit before effort	%	39.6± 2.3	40.1± 1.5	p>0.05
haematocrit after effort	%	44.2± 1.8	43.6± 1.6	p>0.05
lean body mass	kg	35.1± 3.78	34.2± 4.6	p>0.05

not find any correlations in serum cholesterol levels and haematocrit changes in boys, inspite of their higher increase of serum cholesterol. In girls this correlation was found at the limit of significance (r = 0.39).

From our findings in boys there is an evidence of correlation in cholesterol serum levels at rest and after effort and in amounts of depot fat. There we analysed and correlated lean body mass and amounts of depot fat in kg $\frac{LBM}{DF}$. This ratio, indicating coefficient of slenderness, decreased with increasing amounts of fat. It is in negative correlation to cholesterol serum levels at rest (r=−0.45) and after effort (r=−0.39). We can say that slender boys have lower serum cholesterol levels at rest and after effort. The same correlation is after effort in serum cholesterol levels and in amounts of depot fat (r=0.42).

RICCI [5] stated that obese persons produce greater effort during functional examinations because of their lower efficiency. In our two groups there were slender and muscular types only. Even in girls inspite of higher amounts of their depot fat we did not find this correlation. In our examinations this correlation is valid for boys only.

Increased cholesterol levels after effort were studied particularly by ROCHELLE [6], who supposed mobilisation of fat to compensate energetical output. He stated that there is a higher increase in active and trained adult persons. When we compared actual endurance efficiency of our boys and girls in a 300 m run, we did not see any substantial differences between both groups (girls 59,9 sec, boys 57,4 sec).

We have in mind the last difference between the both groups: girls at the age of twelve have already high oestrogen activity. It is proved that oestrogens reduce cholesterol serum levels. May be this increased oestrogen activity in girls produces only a small increase in serum cholesterol after effort in contrast to boys.

Conclusions

1. Serum cholesterol levels at rest are higher in twelve-year-old girls than in boys of the same age.

2. After spiroergometric examinations serum cholesterol increases. This increase is substantially greater in boys than in girls although at rest it was higher in girls.

3. In both groups there are differences in body constitution: girls are heavier, taller, have greater amounts of depot fat, but the same amounts of depot fat, but the same amounts of lean body mass.

4. Serum cholesterol level changes are not in correlation to haematocrit, maximal working capacity, working capacity at the pulse rate of 170 and maximal oxygen consumption. These functional indicators as well as the actual efficiency in 300 m run are in fact the same in both groups.

5. In boys with greater amounts of fat increase of serum cholesterol levels after effort is greater. This was not stated in girls.

6. There is a question whether the smaller increase in serum cholesterol in girls after effort is not due to increased oestrogen activity.

References

1. BIRKE, G. and CARLSON, L. A.: Lipid metabolism and trauma. III. Plasma lipids and proteins in burns. Acta med. scand. *178:* 337–350 (1965).
2. HORÁK, M.; JÍCHA, J. and VOTRUBA, M.: Stanovení cholesterolu a jeho esteru ultramikrometodou. Prakt. Lék. *46:* 710–712 (1966).
3. NAUGHTON, J. and BALKE, B.: Physical working capacity in medical personnel and the response of serum cholesterol to acute exercise and to training. Amer. J. med. Sci. *247:* 286–292 (1964).
4. RATH, R.; VAVŘÍNKOVÁ, H.; PETRÁSEK, R. and MAŠEK, J.: Relationship be-

tween the ratio of body fat and plasma levels of cholesterol, esterified fatty acids, triglycerides and blood pressure values in men and women with different body weights. Rev. Czech. Med. *13:* 106–120 (1967).
5. RICCI, B.: Arbeitsphysiol. *20:* 173 (1963); cit. CAMPBELL, D. E. and LUMSDEN, T. B.: Amer. J. med. Sci. *253:* 155–159 (1967).
6. ROCHELLE, R. H.: Blood plasma cholesterol changes during a physical training program. J. Sports Med. *1:* 63–70 (1961).
7. STOKER, D. J.: Effect of posture on the plamsa cholesterol level. Brit. med. J. Vol. *1/5483:* 336–338 (1966).

Author's address: MUDr. ZD. JIRKA, I. P. Pavlova 6, *Olomouc* (Czechoslovakia).

Repeated Determination of Glucose Concentration in the Synovial Fluid in Haemorrhages into the Knee Joint

J. MOSKWA

Hospital of Traumatic Surgery, Warsaw

Most of the knee injuries in athletes are accompanied by intra-articular haemorrhage due either to the trauma itself or to the surgery.

Among 152 cases of sports injuries treated in 1966 and 1967 in this Department there were 103 cases of knee injury. In 96 cases of that number intra-articular haemorrhages were encountered related directly or indirectly to the trauma.

The present study concerns the synovial glucose in the course of treatment for intra-articular haemorrhage of the knee.

The material of the study considers 22 patients in whom 3–8 examinations of the intra-articular fluid were carried out. The number of examinations in every patient depended upon the duration of the articular exudation. The particular examinations were made at intervals of 3–4 days.

The causes of haemorrhage were as follows:

Surgery (meniscectomy)	11 cases
Posttraumatic haemorrhage	7 cases
Haemorrhage due to arthrosis	2 cases
Haemorrhage due to dissecant osteochondritis	2 cases
Total	22 cases

Parallel to the synovial glucose determination, serum glucose, synovial and plasma osmolarity, the synovial precipitation test and the cellular count of the synovial fluid were determined.

Method

The synovial fluid and venous blood was sampled as usual from patients fasting for 12 hours. Glucose was determined according to NELSON and SOMOGYI.

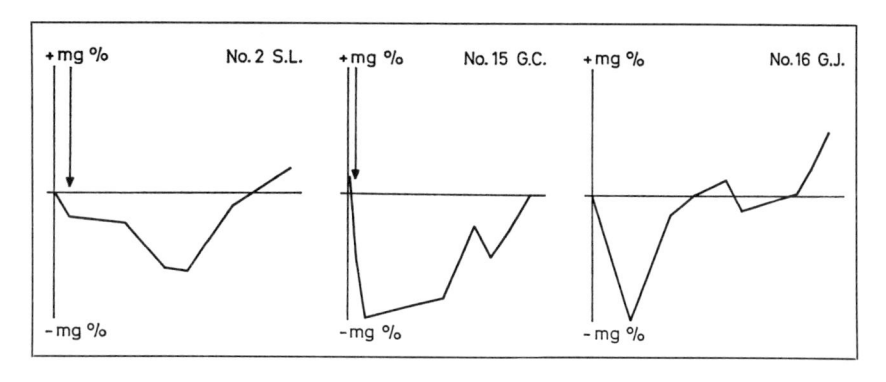

Figure 1   Figure 2   Figure 3

Results and Discussion

According to W. BAUER and M. W. ROPES, the glucose concentration in the synovial fluid is lower by 10 mg percent or equal to the serum glucose. This suggests that the glucose supply is adequate to the glucose uptake by the synovial tissues. In the intra-articular haemorrhage synovial glucose is low due to the increased activity of glycolytic enzymes.

In our observations the synovial glucose in intra-articular haemorrhages was lower by 20 mg percent than that of the serum.

Immediately following the trauma or surgery the difference ranged 40–70 mg percent. In the course of treatment synovial glucose rose and then equalled or almost equalled the serum glucose.

Figure 1 presents a diagram of the differences between the synovial and serum glucose in a patient with protracted haemarthros after meniscectomy.

When the haemarthros subsided, the synovial glucose equalled the serum glucose. In some cases it rose even over the serum level for a short period of time.

In the knee joints previously normal the equalization of the synovial to serum glucose occurred sooner (figure 2) than in the arthrotic joints (figure 3). The same was seen in patients with dissecant osteochondritis with protracted post-surgical exudation.

No distinct correlation was found between the synovial glucose and synovial cellular elements.

The precipitation test was normal in all cases studied.

The osmolarity of the synovial fluid and of the plasma did not show particular differences. On average it was 297 mOsm in plasma and 303 in the synovial fluid.

Conclusions

1. Haemorrhage into the knee joint resulted in a fall of synovial glucose; the difference rose between the synovial and serum glucose.
2. In the course of healing the posttraumatic or postoperative haemarthros synovial and serum glucose equalized.
3. In cases of trauma of a previously healthy joint the equalization of synovial and serum glucose occurred sooner than in joints previously arthrotic.

Author's address: J. MOSKWA, Hospital of Traumatic Surgery, *Warsaw* (Poland).

Variation in Total Body Water with Muscle Glycogen Changes in Man[1]

K. E. OLSSON and B. SALTIN

Department of Physiology, Gymnastik- och idrottshögskolan, Stockholm

It is generally agreed that glycogen is bound with water in the cells [5, 8] and during physical exercise when the glycogen is gradually utilized [1], some water is liberated [7], but different figures are given for this amount, which is especially true in man. Muscle glycogen content can be determined on biopsy samples and previous studies have demonstrated marked variations in muscle glycogen content with prolonged exercise and different diet regimes [1].

In this study we have compared two situations, one when the muscle glycogen stores are almost depleted after hard physical work and the other when the stores are filled above the normal level. In this way it was possible to see whether the total body water was changed between the two situations, and if so, also its relationship to the glycogen content of the muscle.

Material and Methods

Ten young male students were studied. All of them were healthy and had normal kidney function as measured by endogenous creatinine clearance. On the first day all subjects were engaged in hard physical work including leg and arm exercise in order to deplete their glycogen stores.

The next 5 days the subjects had a special diet (3,000 Cal) consisting of only fat and protein during the first two days and then of carbohydrates (2,300 Cal) and protein for the remainder of the time. Water was given in excess every day. Only limited physical effort was permitted during 'the carbohydrate days'.

Total body water (TBW), plasma volume (PV) and glycogen determinations were made three times, first before the hard physical work to get control values, secondly when the glycogen values were expected to be lowest and thirdly after the diet period when the values were expected to be highest. The second determination was performed the morning after the

[1] Supported from project No. K67-14X-2202-01, Swedish Medical Research Council.

hard physical work. The subjects received an excess of water but no carbohydrates after the termination of the exercise.

Glycogen was determined in muscle tissue from thigh and shoulder. Needle biopsies were taken and glycogen analyzed according to the methods described by HULTMAN [4]. Total body water was determined with isotope dilution technique with tritium labeled water as a tracer substance [6, and OLSSON, to be published]. Plasma volume was determined with I^{131} labeled albumin as the tracer substance. Body weight, urine volume, serum and urine electrolytes were measured daily. The specific activity of tritium in plasma water was measured daily to calculate turnover rate of tritium which was used as a measure of water metabolism [2].

Results and Discussion

In figure 1 the results in one of the subjects are given. At the top of the figure is the variation in body weight. The lowest point was reached after the hard physical work, then there was a slight increase, followed by a constancy in weight during the protein and fat diet. During the three days of mainly carbohydrates in the diet body weight increased gradually. The glycogen values were close to zero after the work and up to 3 g/100 g wet muscle after the carbohydrate diet.

The difference between the volume of water intake and urine volume was increasing parallelly to body weight. This has been interpreted to mean an accumulation of water in the body since there was no reason to suspect more than normal loss of water from the skin or the breathing organs during the diet period. The turnover rate of water was 4.4 l/day which is a higher value than in a control material. This was probably due to the fact that water was given in excess.

In the subject presented in figure 1 the total body water increased from 40.3 l during the carbohydrate diet to 43.3 l. The mean increase in body weight for the ten subjects was 2.3 kg, and total body water increased 2.9 liters. This means that there was a definite increase in total body water after the glycogen stores were filled compared to when the stores were depleted. Since the error of the total body water method is around 3.5% [OLSSON, to be published], the mean total body water increase is a more uncertain figure than the mean body weight increase.

An estimation of the increase in the total glycogen stores in the body based on the assumption that the total muscle mass is 40% of the body

Variation in Total Body Water with Muscle Glycogen Changes in Man

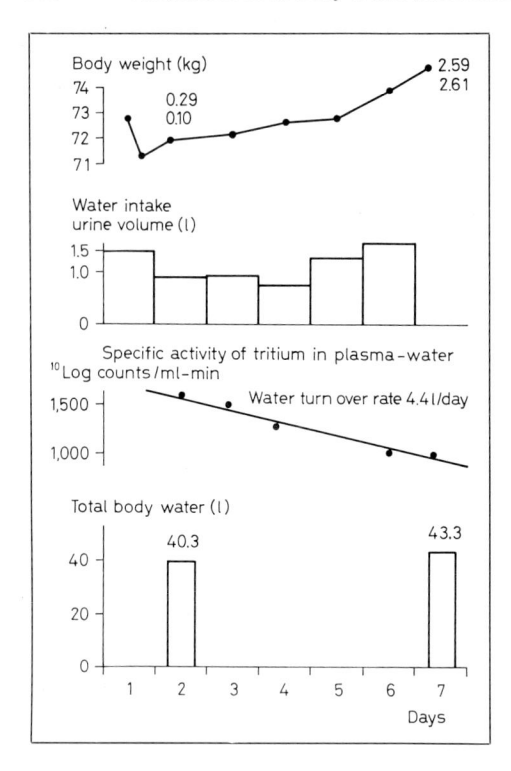

Figure 1. Results on one representative subject during the course of an experiment lasting for seven days. In the top panel is the body weight, and the two figures for the second and the seventh days denote glycogen content (g/100 g wt muscle) in the thigh (lower figure) and the shoulder (upper figure) muscle. The next panel gives the volume of water that the subject drank minus the volume of the urine excreted during the same 24-hours period. The third panel gives the tritium activity in plasma.

The lowest panel indicates the magnitude of the total body water on the second and the seventh day.

weight gave a change in the glycogen store of 0.5 kg in the present study. The error in the determination of the total body water is rather large and it makes it even more difficult to give an exact figure for the amount of water that is bound to the glycogen in the cells. A figure in the order of 4–5 ml/g glycogen seems reasonable from above presented data. How this water is bound or attached to glycogen is impossible to say from this study.

One of the main problems in this study is to be sure that the persons are not hyper- or hypohydrated when studied. There were no statistically significant differences between mean values of plasma volume and serum-electrolytes before and after the diet periods compared to the values taken the first day of study before the hard work. Furthermore the potassium and sodium ratio in urine never exceeded 1, which means that there was no elevated aldesteron activity.

The water released when glycogen is utilized, is probably used when the perspiration is increased during physical work or metabolic efforts. The observed dehydration based on body weight measurements is then probably only partly a true dehydration.

Earlier it has often been stated that thirst is not enough to bring the total body water to normal value after physical work. It has been called the delayed involuntary dehydration [3]. Body weight has been used as a measure of changes in total body water in those works. Perhaps this delayed weight increase is depending on the delayed rebuilding of glycogen and its accompanying water, whereas the extra- and intracellular volumes are immediately restored by thirst.

References

1. BERGSTRÖM, J.; HERMANSEN, L.; HULTMAN, E. and SALTIN, B.: Diet, muscle glycogen and physical performance. Acta physiol. scand. *71:* 140–150 (1967).
2. GAEBLER, O.H. and CHOITZ, H.C.: Studies of body water and water turnover determined with deuterium oxide added to food. Clin. Chem. *10:* 13 (1964).
3. GREENLEAF, J.E.: Involuntary hypohydration in men and animals, a review. National aeronautics and space administration (Washington D.C. 1966).
4. HULTMAN, E.: Muscle glycogen in man determined in needle biopsy specimens. Scand. J. clin. Lab. Invest. *19:* 209–217 (1967).
5. KAPLAN, A. and CHAIKOFF, J.L.: The relation of glycogen, fat and protein to water storage in the liver. K. biol. Chem. *116:* 663 (1936).
6. LANGHAM, W.H.; EVERSOLE, W.J.; HAYES, F.N. and TRUJILLO, T.T.: Assay of tritium activity in body fluids with use of a liquid scintillation system. J. lab. clin. Med. *47:* 819 (1959).
7. SALTIN, B.: Aerobic work capacity and circulation at exercise in man. Acta physiol. scand. *62:* Suppl. 230 (1964).
8. ZUNTZ, N.; LOEWY, A.; MÜLLER, F. und CASPARI, W.: Höhenklima und Bergwanderungen, Berlin, 114 (1906).

Author's address: Dr. K. E. OLSSON, Department of Physiology, GIH, Lidingövagen 1, *S-11433 Stockholm* (Sweden).

Biochemistry of Exercise.
Medicine and Sport, Vol. 3; pp. 163–168 (Karger, Basel/New York 1969)

Inhibition of the Depletion of Diaphragmatic and Cardiac Glycogen by one β-adrenolytic Drug in Mus Musculus Subjected to Swimming Stress

E. MARMO and A. MATERA

Inst. of Pharmacology and Toxicology, Univ. of Naples (Director: Prof. L. DONATELLI)

The possibility of using β-adrenolytic drugs in Sport Medicine induced us to study the effects of these drugs on one of the metabolic modifications induced by prolonged swimming, that is the depletion of diaphragmatic and cardiac glycogen. The β-adrenolytic examined was the CIBA 39089-Ba [dl-1-isopropylamine-2-hydroxy-3(o-allyl-oxyphenoxy)-propane.HCl] (figure 1), that has competitive β-adrenolytic activity with an intensity almost equivalent to that of Propranolol, but associated with lesser inotropic negative effects on the heart. The CIBA 39089-Ba has also an intrinsic β-adrenergic activity.

Material and Methods

The researches were made on 80 *Mus musculus* (Morini breed, ♂, 28–30 g). Some of them were subjected to a swimming experiment in a basin full of *aqua fontis* (24° C). 7 experimental groups were formed. The animals were fasting 12 hours before the experiments, leaving free the access of the water.

A = control animals
B = animals treated with 5 mg/kg i.m. of CIBA 39089-Ba

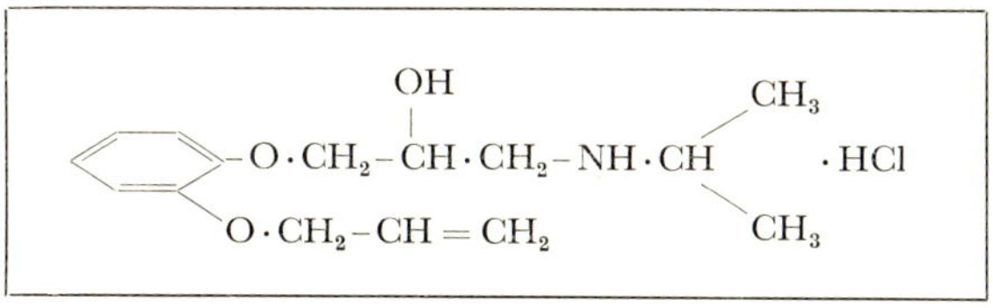

Figure 1. CIBA 39089-Ba [1-isopropylamine-2-hydroxy-3(o-allyl-oxyphenoxy)-propane.-HCl].

C = animals treated with 20 mg/kg i.m. of CIBA 39089-Ba
D = animals subjected to the swimming experiment
E = animals treated with 5 mg/kg i.m. of CIBA 39089-Ba, 20 min before the swimming experiment
F = animals treated with 10 mg/kg i.m. of CIBA 39089-Ba, 20 min before the swimming experiment
G = animals treated with 20 mg/kg i.m. of CIBA 39089-Ba, 20 min before the swimming experiment

The dosage of the glycogen (method of KEMP, A. and KITS VAN HEIYNINGEN, A. J. M.: A colorimetric micro-method for the determination of glycogen in tissues. Biochem. J. 56: 646–648, 1954) at the level of the diaphragm and of the heart's left ventricle was executed at time 0 in the group A,

Table I.

Group	An.	Glycogen g% ± s.e. Diaphragm	Left ventricle
A	20	0.268 ± 0.008	0.080 ± 0.007
B	10	0.256 ± 0.009	0.071 ± 0.005
C	10	0.245 ± 0.010	0.075 ± 0.009
D	10	0.132 ± 0.009 (°) (−50.8%)	0.023 ± 0.004 (°) (−71.3%)
E	10	0.270 ± 0.012 (+0.1%)	0.079 ± 0.007 (−1.3%)
F	10	0.259 ± 0.007 (−3.4%)	0.081 ± 0.006 (+1.2%)
G	10	0.264 ± 0.011 (−1.6%)	0.078 ± 0.005 (−2.5%)

A = control animals; B and C = an. treated respectively with 5 and 20 mg/kg i.m. of CIBA 39089-Ba; D, E, F, and G = an. subjected to the swimming experiment; E, F and G = an. treated 20 min before the swimming experiment with CIBA 39089-Ba [5 (E) – 10 (F) – 20 (G) mg/kg i.m.]; between the brackets the percentage variation in relation to group A; s.e. = standard error; significant values (P<0,05) in relation to group A.

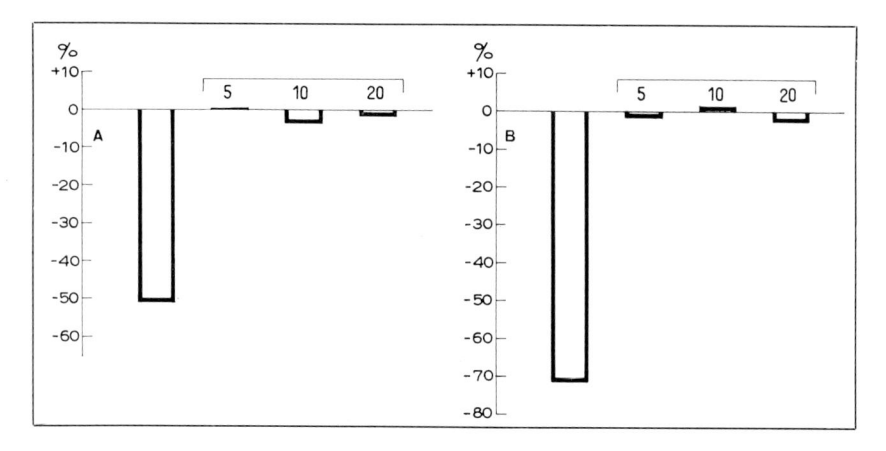

Figure 2. Percentage variations of the glycogen at the level of the diaphragm (graph A) and at the level of the heart (graph B) in relation to value of control animals which were not subjected to the swimming experiment. First column = animals subjected to swimming experiment only; second, third and fourth column = animals treated respectively with 5, 10, 20 mg/kg i.m. 20 min before the swimming experiment.

45 min from the administration of CIBA 39089-Ba, in the groups B, C, E, F, and G, 5 min from the end of the swimming experiment in group D.

Results and Conclusions

Our researches demonstrate (see table I and figure 2) that the depletion of the diaphragmatic and cardiac glycogen in *Mus musculus* caused by prolonged swimming for 20 min can be prevented by the administration of the β-adrenolytic drug, already with a dose of 5 mg/kg i.m.

This preventive action can be explained probably by the lack of the effect of the endogenous catecholamines on the glycogenolysis of the muscles at the cardiac level and at the diaphragmatic level, considering that the muscular glycogenolysis is under the control of the β-adrenergic receptors.

Moreover we documented that the β-adrenolytic used, CIBA 39089-Ba, at the dosages of 5–10–20 mg/kg i.m. administered 20 min before the swimming experiment does not prevent the diminution of the *tigroid substance* (tigrolysis) of the motor cells of the anterior horns. We refer some examples on figure 3 and 4.

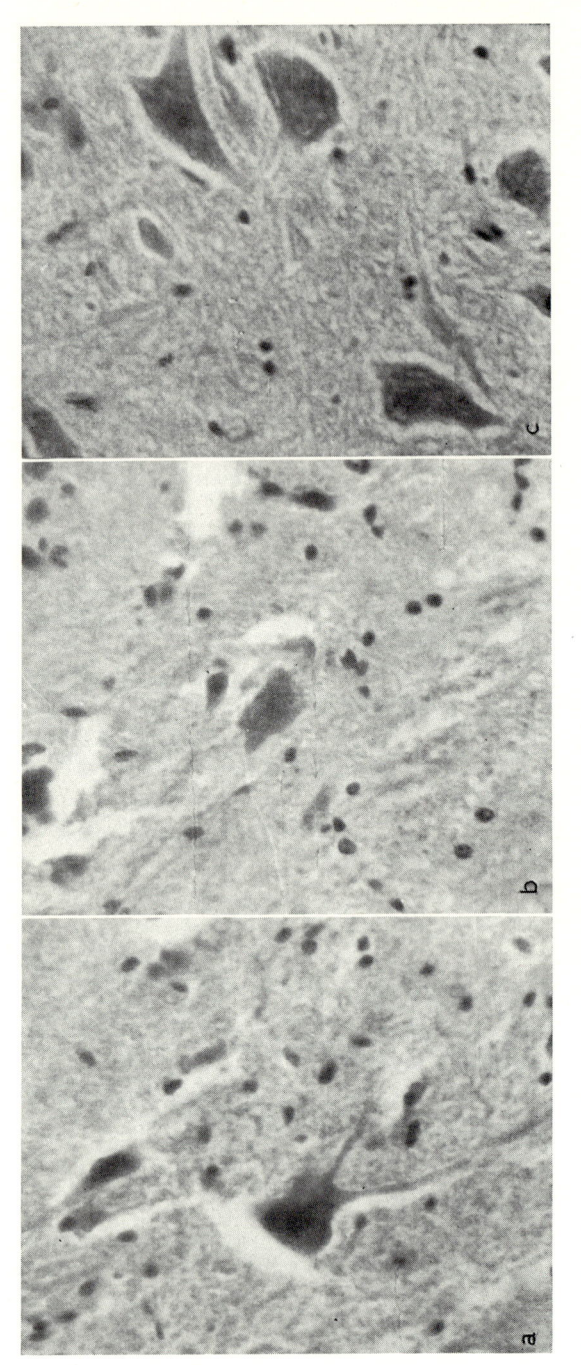

Figure 3. Motor cells of a control animal (a), of an animal subjected to the swimming experiment (b) and of an animal treated with 5 mg/kg i.m. of CIBA 39089-Ba, 20 min before the swimming experiment (c). Method of Nissl (x–400). The animals were killed at time 0 in (a), 5 min from the end of the swimming in (b) and 45 min from the administration of CIBA 39089-Ba in (c).

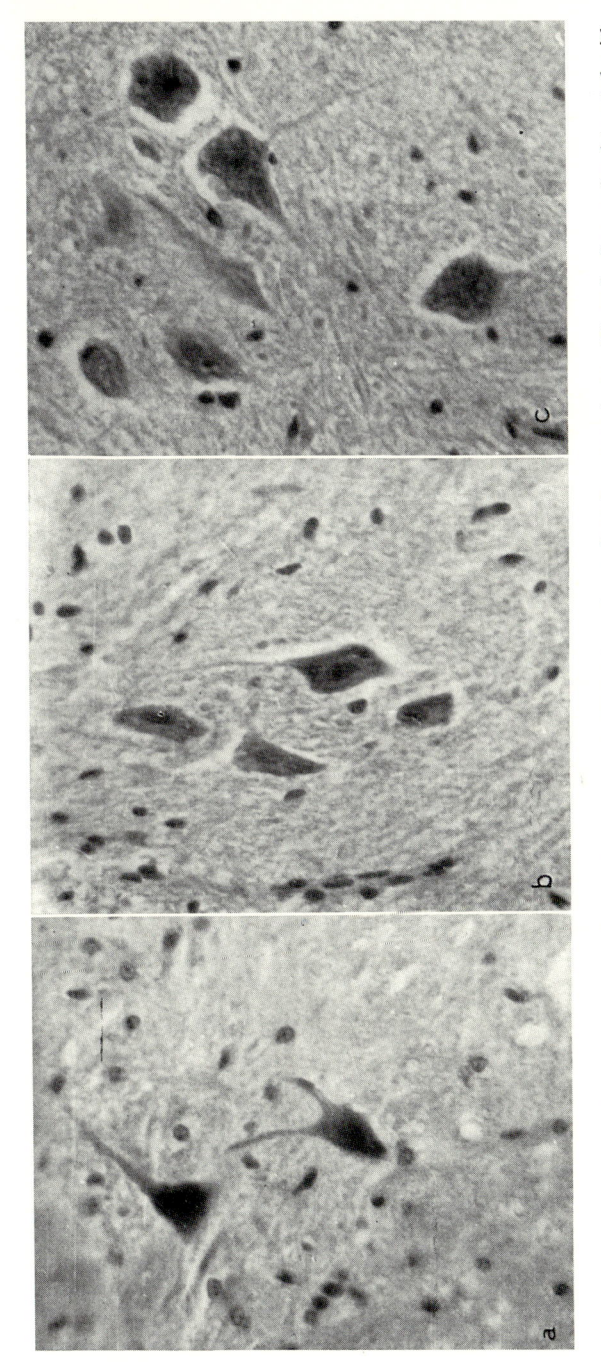

Figure 4. Motor cells of a control animal (a), of an animal subjected to the swimming experiment (b) and of an animal treated with 20 mg/kg i.m. of CIBA 39089-Ba, 20 min before the swimming experiment (c). Method of Nissl (x-400). The animals were killed at time 0 in (a), 5 min from the end of the swimming experiment in (b) and 45 min from the administration of CIBA 39089-Ba in (c).

Summary

The Authors investigated the behaviour of the diaphragmatic and cardiac glycogen and histological aspects of the motor cells of the anterior horns on the *Mus musculus* subjected to a swimming experiment and treated or not with a known β-adrenolytic, the CIBA 39089-Ba.

Authors' address: Prof. E. MARMO and Dr. A. MATERA, Via Cimarosa, 37 – *80127 Naples* (Italy).

III. Hormones

Sympatho-Adrenal Activity and Physical Exercise

U. S. von Euler

Department of Physiology, Karolinska Institute, Stockholm

Physical exercise represents a kind of stress on the organism in which hemodynamic as well as biochemical factors are extensively involved, particularly in exhaustive muscular work. It appears therefore likely that regulative forces in the hormonal and vasomotor area should be brought into play.

While some parameters such as oxygen consumption, ventilation rate and volume, circulatory data and plasma chemistry may be quantitatively related to the work-load, these data give no direct information on the degree of effort of stress which a given physical work imposes upon the subject. It would therefore be desirable to find an indicator of what may be called the effort index, relating the degree of effort to a given work-load, in other words, to obtain a quantitative evaluation of the stresses imposed upon the organism by physical work. It is common experience that a large amount of work output in one individual may require less effort than a smaller physical achievement by another; consequently one should expect mobilization of certain compensatory or regulatory forces to a greater extent in the latter case.

Among the possible regulating factors which might be called into play by the organism to meet the special conditions connected with muscular work, the adreno-medullary hormones and the sympathetic nervous system should be considered in the first place. Not only do these chemical regulators exert a profound influence on the cardiovascular system, but have also far-reaching effects on metabolism, particularly on the mobilization of combustive material.

1. Physical Exercise and Cardiovascular Homeostasis

It is well established that muscular work causes only relatively small alterations in the mean blood pressure. TANGL and ZUNTZ [1898] observed in the dog an average rise of 6 mm during light work and 23 mm during heavy work. LILJESTRAND and ZANDER [1928] found an increase of mean blood pressure of 6–7% at an increase of metabolism of 100%. HOLMGREN [1956] observed a mean pressure rise of 3 mm Hg per 300 kpm/min, i.e. 20 mm Hg for a work-load of 2,000 kpm/min. Considering the large alterations in blood distribution and cardiac output occurring during physical activity the homeostatic mechanisms presumably must involve some important regulatory influence from the vasomotor system.

By various means aiming at removing the influence of the sympathetic system, it has become possible to demonstrate its importance. Such measures are the use of ganglionic blockers, adrenolytic drugs, neuronal blockers, sympathectomy and exclusion of the homeostatic blood pressure reflexes in the sinus and aorta regions. All of these interventions cause a profound change in the normal cardiovascular pattern of response to muscular work. While motor nerve stimuli leading to muscular work in the anaesthetized animal normally are not accompanied by any marked change in blood pressure, the same degree of motor activity after section of the buffer nerves causes a strong fall in blood pressure further accentuated by treatment with an a-blocker, such as ergotamine [EULER and LILJESTRAND, 1946] (fig. 1).

After administration of a ganglionic blocker, such as hexamethonium even moderate muscular work may provoke a substantial fall in blood

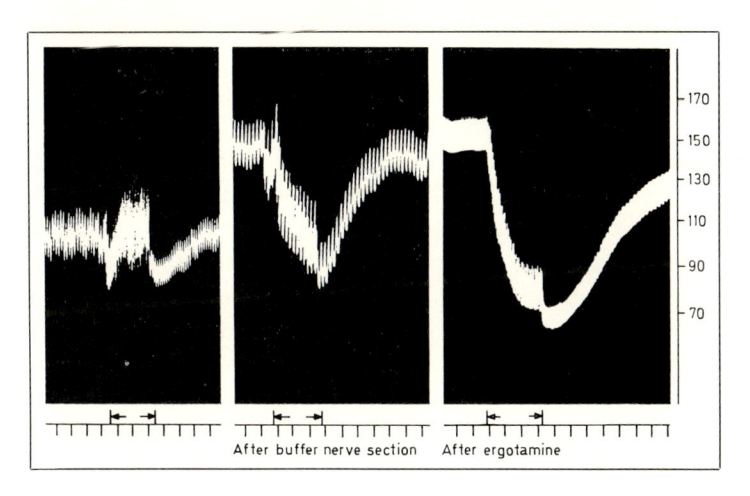

Figure 1. Cat, blood pressure. Motor nerve stimulation in the intact cat, after section of the buffer nerves and both vagi and after administration of ergotamine tartrate 0.2 mg/kg. [After EULER and LILJESTRAND, 1946].

pressure, which in some subjects can lead to dizziness and threatening collapse [RØNNOV-JESSEN, 1953].

From these and numerous other data it seems clear that counter-regulatory mechanisms are evoked during muscular work, consisting in increased activity of vasoconstrictor nerves, presumably to some extent also enhanced adreno-medullary secretion. These reactions are chiefly elicited from the reflexogenic zones of the sinus and aorta receptors.

Earlier experiments by Japanese workers have demonstrated a hypersection from the adrenal medulla of the dog as a result of muscular work. In these cases [WADA, SEO and ABE, 1935] adrenal blood samples were collected from the unanaesthetized dog and evaluated by biological methods. These studies have shown that only in exhaustive work – consisting in runs – did the medullary secretion increase, while moderate work, even over a prolonged period, did not increase the medullary hormone level in the adrenal venous plasma.

HOLTZ, CREDNER and KRONEBERG [1947] were able to demonstrate the appearance in urine of a sympathomimetic substance (urosympathin) having the properties of noradrenaline. They also showed that urine samples taken during or after muscular work in man had a stronger pressor action when tested on the cat's blood pressure than samples from resting periods.

2. Effect of Muscular Work on Urinary Excretion of Catecholamines

The development of methods for estimating the output of catecholamines, adrenaline and noradrenaline in urine, has effectively contributed to the knowledge of secretion of the sympathetic transmitter and of the adrenal medullary hormones. The basis for the use of this method is the finding that different degrees of activity known to influence either the sympathetic nervous activity or the adrenal medullary secretion are reflected in the amount of excreted catecholamines in urine. Even if the amounts of free catecholamines excreted in urine only represent a small portion, some 1–3% of the total amounts of catecholamines released in the blood stream, the analytical findings of catecholamines in urine still give a good idea of the degree of secretion. In addition this technique is simple and accurate and does not to any appreciable extent inconvenience the subjects. In the quantitative study by EULER and HELLNER [1952] urine was collected from subjects who had been engaged in physical exercise of different kinds for various lengths of time. One group of subjects performed work on the ergo-

Table I. Urinary excretion of noradrenaline and adrenaline during physical exercise (ergometer bicycle)

Subject	Exercise min	Work load kpm/min	Excretion ng/min NA	A	Plasma lactic acid mg %	O_2 cons. l/min
G. H.	6	1,950	280	90	114	4.3
v. D.	5.5	1,440	290	60	127	3.1
E. B. ♀	5	1,350	135	15	105	2.6
L. K. (mean of 6 runs)	60	900	110	11	–	2.2

[Euler and Hellner, 1952]

meter bicycle, while other groups were practising general athletics and 1,500 meter runs, or were engaged in a 10 km ski-run competition. The urinary bladder was emptied voluntarily shortly before the onset of the work and then after the work was ended. Urine collecting periods were usually extended to not less than 1 hour in order to obtain sufficient quantities of urine and in order to reduce the error due to incomplete emptying of the bladder. Since the period of work in some cases was much briefer than the total collection time, the secretion rate during the actual work was computed by subtracting the excretion rate during the resting period from the total excretion. The resting excretion rate was set at 50 ng/min of noradrenaline + adrenaline, but since this figure is somewhat high, the figures for the actual excretion during work will be minimum values.

From a large series of estimations the resting values have been determined to about 20 ng/min of noradrenaline and 5 ng/min of adrenaline. During night, resting values are about half as high. As seen in table I, work on the ergometer at a work-load of 900–1,950 kpm/min, during which the oxygen consumption varied between 2.2 and 4.3 l/min, caused a considerable increase in the catecholamine excretion in all cases, both for noradrenaline and for adrenaline in this series. In one subject it was found that in 6 identical runs at 900 kpm/min during 60 min, the output of noradrenaline in urine was on an average 110 ng/min at an oxygen consumption of 2.2 l/min. The adrenaline values were less markedly increased in this subject, and were on an average 11 ng/min.

The members of one group were engaged in a ski-run competition of 10 km length with running times between 39 and 54 min. From figure 2 it

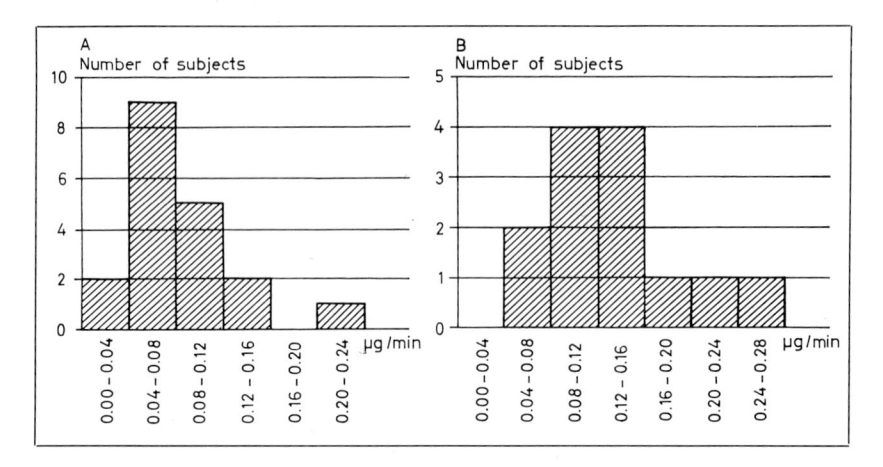

Figure 2. Noradrenaline excretion in μg/min in groups of male students during moderate muscular work in A and during 10 km ski-run competition in B. Ordinate: number of subjects. [After EULER and HELLNER, 1952].

can be seen that the noradrenaline output during the actual ski run was in several cases greatly increased and considerably greater than those observed during moderate work (figure 2A). However, even here the values showed relatively large differences. In 2 of the competitors the excretion was low, between 40 and 80 ng/min. On the other hand there were no less than 7 runners in which the excretion exceeded 120 ng/min and in one even exceeded 240 ng/min. On the whole the most successful competitors showed the highest excretion figures, presumably indicating a strong effort on their side.

In another study on a well trained subject the catecholamine output increased from 30 ng/min during room rest up to values of about 400 ng of noradrenaline and 100 ng of adrenaline per min. Exercise time was from 16 to 60 min. It is of interest to note that even at an oxygen consumption of 2.4 l/min the noradrenaline and adrenaline output was still very moderate. Only at the higher degrees of muscular work with an oxygen consumption of the order of 3.8 l/min there was a definite increase in the output of noradrenaline and adrenaline in urine. The highest figures were not unexpectedly observed at an oxygen consumption of 4–4.1 l/min. In this case both the adrenaline and noradrenaline output values were greatly increased as seen in table II [EULER and HELLNER, 1952].

From the catecholamine excretion in urine certain conclusions may be drawn as regards the amount of catecholamines released into the circula-

Table II. Excretion of noradrenaline (NA) and adrenaline (A) in urine during muscular work in a trained subject

O₂ cons. l/min	Noradr. mμg/min	Adr. mμg/min	% Adr.	Maximal lactic acid mg%
Rest	25	5	17	
1.85	22	8	28	
2.10	24	6	21	
2.40	38	18	32	
3.80	150	29	16	
4.00	350	78	18	47
4.10	390	110	22	47

[EULER and HELLNER, 1952]

tion. By comparison with the figures obtained in urine after infusion of noradrenaline in the experiments of EULER and LUFT [1951], the maximal amount of noradrenaline which would be released into the circulation during heavy work should be of the order of 20 μg/min, assuming an excretion of 2% of the amount released. Amounts of this order, when infused intravenously in man, are known to elicit definite cardiovascular effects as seen by a rise of mean blood pressure of some 30 mm Hg or more [BARNETT et al., 1950]. This again would further substantiate the conclusion obtained with regard to the nature of the homeostatic reactions during muscular work.

HOLMGREN [1956] measured the urinary excretion of noradrenaline and adrenaline in 16 subjects before and during a period of about 1½–2 hours which included up to 20 minutes of muscular work of increasing intensity, followed by 20–35 minutes of work and again a period of ½–3½ hours of rest. The work load was in 8 cases 1,200 kpm/min and in 8 cases 1,500 kpm/min. From resting values of 8.5 ng/min of adrenaline and 27 ng/min of noradrenaline the mean figures increased to 19 ng/min of adrenaline and 63 ng/min of noradrenaline if the total period of work and rest was included. However, if the excretion was calculated for the working period only, by subtraction of the resting output from the non-working period, the figures were 40 ng/min adrenaline and 142 ng/min noradrenaline. These figures are consistent with the values found in other studies for similar work load and working time.

ELMADJIAN, HOPE and LAMSON [1958] measured the catecholamine excretion in ice-hockey players and found large increases, which may be estimated at about 150 ng/min for noradrenaline. Somewhat unexpectedly the adrenaline figures were not higher than 10 ng/min if computed in the same way.

In the study by GARLIND et al. [1960], where the subjects were exposed to 2 minute runs with 2 minute intervals for 1 hour, a moderate increase both in adrenaline and noradrenaline excretion was also observed. In this case ergometer bicycle work was performed causing a heart frequency of 160–170 beats per minute.

A careful, systematic study of the effect of muscular activity of different intensity on the excretion on noradrenaline and adrenaline in man has been made by KÄRKI [1956]. A group of 3 subjects was practising runs and performed various types of gymnastics and athletic activities over periods of 45–70 min. Exhausting competition of long duration was studied in 10 marathon runners and in 10 long distance skiers. In another group 5 subjects took part in a national competition of wood cutters. In the first group, in which the work may be characterized as moderate, the noradrenaline excretion increased from the resting rate of 19 ng/min on an average about 5 times to 99 ng/min. In the following 2–2 ½ hours the average excretion was about 30 ng/min which is still above the resting value. There is reason to believe that the excretion gradually diminished over a period of about 2 hours after the end of the work.

In the marathon run competition the length of the course was the normal one, or 42.2 km, and the ski run 40 km. In these studies the bladders were emptied some 20–30 min before the actual race and again some 15–20 min after the end of the race which lasted for about 2 ½–3 hours. The urine volume during this period was relatively small, from 40–180 ml.

As seen in table III, the noradrenaline excretion in the marathon runners varied from 73 to 191 ng/min with a mean of 131 ng/min while the excretion in the skiers had the same mean value but varied from 49 to 310 ng/min. Since the normal excretion of noradrenaline in adults is about 20 ng/min during rest, it can be seen that the noradrenaline excretion was up to 17 times the normal. The excretion figures in these groups are close to the highest values observed in our previous studies with relatively brief exhaustive work. It is remarkable, however, that this excretion can be kept up during periods of hours.

It is of interest to observe the relative increase in the amount of adrenaline secreted and to compare that with the increase in secretion of noradrenaline. As seen in the table the relative increase in the amount of adrenaline was much larger than that of noradrenaline. However, since the

Table III. Urinary excretion of NA and A in 10 marathon runners and 10 long-distance skiers during competition (2 ½–3 h) ng/min

	Marathon race 42.2 km		40 km ski race	
	NA	A	NA	A
	131	59	131	40
	(73–191)	(37–115)	(49–310)	(11–66)

[KÄRKI, 1956]

adrenaline figure is normally quite low, any increase would be more impressive than for noradrenaline on a percentual basis. The adrenaline excretion was on an average in the marathon runners 59 ng/min, but was markedly lower on an average in the skiers, 40 ng/min. Whereas the normal excretion of adrenaline is about 5 ng/min during rest, the excretion for the competitors varied from 11 to 115 ng/min and was thus increased up to 20–25 times. KÄRKI also noted that the concentration of noradrenaline and adrenaline in urine could be quite high, and values as high as 0.75 μg/ml of urine were observed. In these cases it was even possible to observe direct actions of biological test preparations.

Catecholamine analyses were also performed on urine collected during a national contest in Finland for wood cutters, involving cutting of firewood for a 6½–7 hour period. The 5 participants represented a group of selected skilful woodsmen. Urine samples were collected during the previous night, during the actual contest and also in the evening after the contest and the following night, making 4 estimations in total. During the night preceding the contest the excretion of noradrenaline and adrenaline was normal (table IV). During the competition the excretion per minute for the whole 7 hour period was greatly increased and amounted to 434 ng/min in one of the contestants who was a very big and robust man. Of interest is that the participant who won the competition showed exceptionally low values or 66 ng/min of noradrenaline and 8.1 ng/min of adrenaline. He was a man of slight build but very agile. His resting secretion of noradrenaline was also very low, 4.4 ng/min. During the following period the average figures had fallen considerably although not to the resting levels but in the night following the contest the figures were back to normal.

From these studies it can be seen that during muscular work the excretion of noradrenaline as well as adrenaline tends to increase. The

Table IV. Urinary excretion of NA and A before, during and after a wood cutting competition (5 participants). Mean values, ng/min

| Night before 23–7 | | Work period 7–14 | | Evening after 14–23 | | Night after 23–7 | |
NA	A	NA	A	NA	A	NA	A
17	5.2	239	31	24	6.9	15	5.6
(11–18)	(2.5–6.7)	(66–434)	(8.1–51)	(6.5–52)	(2.2–10)	(4.4–19)	(2.5–10)

[Kärki, 1956]

increase is also clearly dependent on the intensity of work rather than on the amount of work done and presumably also depends on the degree on effort exerted in the special case. It can also be seen that not only noradrenaline, released from the sympathetic nerves and in all likelyhood chiefly from the vasoconstrictor nerves, is increased, but also the adrenaline excretion. From other experiments there are good reasons to assume that the adrenaline is mainly excreted from the adrenal medulla. Thus it seems that physical exercise causes an increased secretion both from the adrenergic nervous system and from the adrenal medulla.

In the studies by Euler and Hellner [1952] there was some evidence that the catecholamine excretion during a given work load depended on the training of the subject tested. Thus in trained subjects the output was only moderately increased even at an oxygen consumption of the order of 2 l/min. In other subjects, however, who were not in the same state of physical fitness, even a work load corresponding to 2 l/min produced a marked increase in the catecholamine excretion. It is interesting to note that in one of the subjects the adrenaline excretion was rather small during exercise, consisting of 900 kpm/min, while the noradrenaline excretion was markedly increased.

Kärki also studied whether the amount of adrenaline excreted would diminish as the organism became accustomed to this kind of stress. However, no decrease in the amount excreted was noted over a month's time when the subjects performed the same work.

The increase in noradrenaline excretion during muscular work is in agreement with the previously reached conclusion that the sympathetic nervous system plays an important part in the maintenance of blood pressure during work. It has been observed by Freeman and Rosenblueth [1931],

LORD and HINTON [1945] and HOLMGREN [1956] that after sympathectomy the blood pressure diminishes during muscular work, as it does after hexamethonium [RØNNOV JESSEN, 1953].

It may be assumed that both noradrenaline and adrenaline are secreted during heavy muscular work as a response of the organism to a stress situation. Since mental stress does not need to be associated with increased excretion of noradrenaline, even if adrenaline excretion is increased, while the reverse is true during postural stress, it seems that the two catecholamines are released in response to different kinds of stress.

The noradrenaline release seems to be reflexogenic in nature and to be elicited by an action of the blood pressure homeostatic mechanisms, while the output of adrenaline appears to indicate another kind of regulatory force. It might be assumed that the increase in adrenaline excretion is at least partly elicited by some metabolic alteration, in which case it could be classified as a metabolic or biochemical reflex. Although little is known about the receptor areas stimulated under these conditions, it should be noted that hypoglycemia, for instance after insulin administration in man, causes a strong increase in the adrenaline secretion from the adrenal medulla [DUNÉR, 1954] and excretion in urine [EULER and LUFT, 1952]. It has been observed that in marathon runners the blood sugar level may fall to 45 mg/100 ml as observed by LEVINE et al. [1924]. This might be one factor, but the presence of other biochemical reflexes cannot be excluded.

Some other questions also present themselves in connection with these observations. Firstly it might be of interest to study more systematically what the noradrenaline and adrenaline excretion would be in a number of subjects who differ in condition, training and physical capacity, when exposed to the same work load. In this way it might be possible to test the hypothesis whether the degree of subjective effort involved in a certain work is correlated to the excretion of noradrenaline or adrenaline or both. It might also be possible to evaluate an individual's capacity for physical work not only by mechanical and physical parameters but also by estimating the degree of strain acting on the organism. By introducing standard tests it should be possible to relate a given work load to the catecholamine excretion and construct an index on this basis.

A second question, perhaps of more theoretical interest, is the capacity of the adrenergic nervous system to release noradrenaline. During recent years it has been repeatedly claimed that a large percentage, up to 90% of the catecholamines released from the nerve endings, should be recaptured [cf. FOLKOW, HÄGGENDAL and LISANDER, 1967]. The excretion of 400 ng/min of noradrenaline in urine, assuming an excretion percentage of 2% of the amount released into the blood stream from the nerve endings [cf. EULER and LUFT, 1951; ELMADJIAN, HOPE and LAMSON, 1958] would correspond to 20 µg/min. If the noradrenaline stores in the human organism outside the suprarenals are estimated at some 3 mg, the net release per min would be about 0.7% of the stores per min. Should 90% of the total amount released be recaptured one arrives at the figure of 7% release of the stores per min. This would require that half of all adrenergic nerve endings are releasing transmitter at maximal rate or 15% per minute [EULER and LISHAJKO, 1967], which appears unlikely. Some of the noradrenaline excreted in urine may be derived from the adrenal medulla, although the relatively small excretion of adrenaline, which constitutes more than 80% of the total amount of catecholamines in the adrenal medulla in man, does not speak in favour of a considerable excretion of noradrenaline from this source.

References

BARNETT, A. J.; BLACKET, R. B.; DEPOORTER, A. E.; SANDERSON, P. H. and WILSON, G.: The action of noradrenaline in man and its relation to phaeochromocytoma and hypertension. Clin. Sci. 9: 151–179 (1950).
DUNÉR, H.: The effect of insulin hypoglycemia on the secretion of adrenaline and noradrenaline from the suprarenal of cat. Acta physiol. scand. 32: 63–68 (1954).
ELMADJIAN, F.; HOPE, J. M. and LAMSON, E. T.: Excretion of epinephrine and norepinephrine under stress. Recent Progr. Hormone Res. 14: 513–553 (1958).
EULER, U. S. v. and HELLNER, S.: Excretion of noradrenaline and adrenaline in muscular work. Acta physiol. scand. 26: 183–191 (1952).
EULER, U. S. v. and LILJESTRAND, G.: The regulation of the blood pressure with special reference to muscular work. Acta physiol. scand. 12: 279–300 (1946).
EULER, U. S. v. and LISHAJKO, F.: Re-uptake and net uptake of noradrenaline in adrenergic nerve granules with a note on the affinity for l- and d-isomers. Acta physiol. scand. 71: 151–162 (1967).
EULER, U. S. v. and LUFT, R.: Noradrenaline output in urine after infusion in man. Brit. J. Pharmacol. 6: 286–288 (1951).
EULER, U. S. v. and LUFT, R.: Effect of insulin on urinary excretion of adrenalin and noradrenalin. Metabolism 1: 528–532 (1952).
FOLKOW, B.; HÄGGENDAL, J. and LISANDER, B.: Extent of release and elimination of noradrenaline at peripheral adrenergic nerve terminals. Acta physiol. scand. Suppl. 307 (1967).
FREEMAN, N. E. and ROSENBLUETH, A.: Reflex stimulation and inhibition of vasodilators in sympathectomized animals. Amer. J. Physiol. 98: 454–462 (1931).
GARLIND, T.; GOLDBERG, L.; GRAF, K.; PERMAN, E. S.; STRANDELL, T. and STRÖM, G.: Effect of ethanol on circulatory, metabolic, and neurohormonal function during muscular work in men. Acta pharmacol. 17: 106–114 (1960).
HOLMGREN, A.: Circulatory changes during muscular work in man. Scand. J. clin. Lab. Invest. 8: Suppl. 24 (1956).

Holtz, P.; Credner, K. and Kroneberg, G.: Über das sympathicomimetische pressorische Prinzip des Harns ('Urosympathin'). Arch. exp. Path. Pharmakol. *204:* 228–243 (1947).

Kärki, N. T.: The urinary excretion of noradrenaline and adrenaline in different age groups, its diurnal variation and the effect of muscular work on it. Acta physiol. scand. *39:* Suppl. 132 (1956).

Levine, S. A.; Gordon, B. and Derick, C. L.: Some changes in the chemical constituents of the blood following a marathon race. J. amer. med. Ass. *82:* 1778 (1924).

Liljestrand, G. and Zander, E.: Vergleichende Bestimmungen des Minutenvolumens des Herzens beim Menschen mittels der Stickoxidulmethode und durch Blutdruckmessungen. Z. ges. exp. Med. *59:* 105 (1928).

Lord, J. W. and Hinton, J. W.: Effect of exercise on blood pressure of patients with advanced hypertension. J. amer. med. Ass. *129:* 1156–1158 (1945).

Rønnov-Jessen, V.: Blodtryks- og pulsvariationer hos hexamethoniumbehandlede hypertensions-patienter under arbejde. Nord. Med. *50:* 1356–1360 (1953).

Tangl, F. and Zuntz, N.: Über die Einwirkung der Muskelarbeit auf den Blutdruck. Arch. ges. Physiol. *70:* 544 (1898).

Wada, M.; Seo, M. and Abe, K.: Effect of muscular exercise upon the epinephrine secretion from the suprarenal gland. Tohoku J. exp. Med. *27:* 65–86 (1935).

Author's address: Dr. U. S. von Euler, Department of Physiology, Karolinska Institute, *Stockholm 60* (Sweden).

Influence of Exercise on Serum Free Thyroxine and Binding Proteins

Ph. de Nayer[1], M. Ostyn[2] and M. de Visscher

Laboratoire de Pathologie Générale, University of Louvain

Only the free-thyroxine (T_4-f), a small fraction of the total circulating thyroxine is likely to enter the tissue cells and to exert the hormonal effect. In serum, the T_4-f is in equilibrium with thyroxine (T_4) bound to specific proteins: 'the Thyroxine-binding Globulin' (TBG), the 'Thyroxine-binding Prealbumin' (TBPA) and to albumin (TBA) [14]. Lashof et al. reported that in human subjects muscular exercise does not affect the peripheral utilization of the thyroid hormone, as measured by the concentration of circulating hormone and by the turnover rate of radiothyroxine [5]. No information, however, is available on the T_4-f level during muscular exercise. The present study was undertaken to assess the evolution of the T_4-f level after strenuous physical exercise.

Method

The T_4-f was measured using the dialysis method described by Oppenheimer et al. [10]. Diluted serum labelled with ^{125}I-T_4 (1 μg/100 ml) was dialyzed for 20 hours against phosphate buffer pH 7.4, ionic strength 0.15. The fraction of unbound T_4 (DF or dialysable fraction) was computed from the ratio of the radioactivity in the outer to the inner compartment. The T_4-f was obtained by multiplying the DF times the total T_4 in the system, i.e. the PBI and the added radiothyroxine.

The distribution of the radiothyroxine on the binding proteins; and the binding capacity of TBG and TBPA were determined by paper electrophoresis in tris-maleate buffer pH 8.6, 0.075 M [15]. In some experiments other electrophoretic systems, the reverse flow technique [13] and the glycine acetate method [9] were also tested.

[1] Aspirant FNRS, Belgium.
[2] Hoger Inst. Lich. Opl., Univ. of Louvain (Dir. Prof. P. P. de Nayer).

The 'Harvard step-test' was performed at a rhythm of 30 steps p. minute during 5 minutes, by 7 male athletes (age ranging from 20 to 24 years).

Blood was drawn from each subject before the test, 30 min and 150 min after completion of the exercise. Each subject served as his own control.

Statistical evaluation of the data is based on the 'paired t test' [16].

Results

The data pertinent to the concentration of thyroid hormone in the serum are summarized in table I. The level of T_4-f is significantly decreased in the blood samples obtained 30 min after the end of the test. This value had returned to normal levels in the samples collected 150 min after the exercise.

The characteristics of the binding-proteins remained unmodified (table II). Neither the application of the 'Reverse-flow' technique for assessing the TBG binding-capacity, nor the use of Glycine-acetate buffer at pH 9.0 for measuring the TBPA binding-capacity revealed any change in the binding-proteins.

No difference was found in the hematocrit, nor in the hemoglobin and protein concentration before and after exercise. The electrophoretic distribution of the serum proteins was identical in the three samples.

The serum chloride concentration measured 30 min and 150 min after exercising was similar to the pre-exercise value.

Discussion

A short-period of strenuous exercise induced a temporary decrease in T_4-f. Under this condition there is no noticeable change in the binding proteins.

Exercise affects the distribution of the body fluids. After this type of exercise, however, the hemoconcentration is transient: 30 min after the end of the test the blood volume is normalized [6]. Alterations of the interstitial space are less documented, and conflicting results have been reported [1, 17]. In our experiments no changes were observed in the serum chloride concentration. Although this parameter represents only a rough estimation

Table I. Dialysis data (mean ± S.E.M.) n = 7

	A[1]	B[2]	C[3]	paired 't' test A–B	B–C
PBI (μg/100 ml)	5.48 ± 0.435	5.04 ± 0.344	5.60 ± 0.394	N.S.	$0.005 > p > 0.001$
DF (fraction)	0.0378 ± 0.00231	0.0354 ± 0.00182	0.0384 ± 0.00194	N.S.	N.S.
T$_4$f × 10^{11} mole/l	2.693 ± 0.234	2.323 ± 0.147	2.827 ± 0.236	$0.05 > p > 0.025$	$0.01 > p > 0.005$

A[1] = Before exercising
B[2] = 30 min after exercising
C[3] = 150 min after exercising

Table II. Electrophoretic data (mean ± S.E.M.)

– Binding capacity (µg/100 ml)	Before exercise	30 min after exercise	150 min after exercise
n = 8			
TBG	20.1± 1.45	20.3± 1.66	23.2± 1.87
TBA	176.3±16.15	186.5±13.8	187.6±13.6
– Distribution (in % of total radioactivity)			
n = 4			
TBG	42.6± 3.34	44.9± 3.48	44.3± 3.98
TBA	17.3± 0.65	17.9± 1.05	19.9± 0.96
TBPA	37.8± 3.53	35.7± 4.47	34.4± 3.55

of the evolution of the extracellular space, a variation of 15%, i.e. the variation of T_4-f, would have been detected by this method. Since there is no change in the blood volume persisting after 30 min, we may conclude that at the time of blood sampling, the interstitial space was also restored.

Considering that in our experimental conditions the distribution of the body fluids would not interfere, we may assume that the decrease of serum T_4-f is due to a shift of T_4 to the cellular compartment. Increased cellular metabolism during exercise may involve an increased T_4 utilization. In this connection it is interesting to mention that training results in an increased T_4 metabolism [3]. Evidence has also been presented that in rats muscular activity increased T_4 utilization [2, 12].

The interference of pH, body temperature and free fatty acids with the binding of T_4 to the binding proteins has been discussed elsewhere [7]. It may be added that an increase in the perfusion rate, may result in an increased degradation of T_4 [11].

The mechanism of action of epinephrine on the metabolism of T_4 is not clearly understood, but it is admitted that it increases the rate of degradation of the thyroid hormone [4].

The return of T_4-f to normal level, i.e. to the former equilibrium, may be favoured by the mobilization of T_4 from extrathyroidal exchangeable tissue stores [8]. Such a mechanism, indeed, is more likely to occur than an increased secretion of hormone by the thyroid gland itself.

In conclusion, muscular exercise is associated to a temporary decrease in the circulating T_4-f level. Increased cellular utilization of T_4 is a possible mechanism for explaining this observation.

Summary

A short period muscular exercise induced a transient decrease in serum free tyroxine level. Indirect evidence is presented for an increased cellular utilization of thyroxine as a possible interpretation for this observation.

Acknowledgement

These studies have been supported in part by the Fonds de la Recherche Scientifique Médicale, Belgium.

References

1. CULLUMBINE, H. and KOCH, A. C. E.: The changes in plasma and tissue fluids volume following exercise. Quart. J. exp. Physiol. *35:* 39–46 (1949).
2. ESCOBAR DEL REY, F. and MORREALE DE ESCOBAR, G.: Studies on the peripheral disappearance of thyroid hormone (III). Acta Endocrin., Kbh. *23:* 400–406 (1956).
3. IRVINE, C. H. G.: Thyroxine secretion rate in the horse in various physiological states. J. Endocrin. *39:* 313–320 (1967).
4. KALLMAN, B. and STARR, P.: The effects of epinephrine on thyroxine metabolism: iodine excretion after various thyroid derivates. Endocrinology *64:* 703–706 (1959).
5. LASHOF, J. C.; BONDY, P. K.; STERLING, K. and MAN, E. B.: Effect of muscular exercise on circulating thyroid hormone. Proc. Soc. exp. Biol., N.Y. *86:* 233–235 (1954).
6. MOORE, R. and BUSKIRK, E. R.: Exercise and body fluids: in JOHNSON, W. R. (ed.): Science and Medicine of Exercise and Sports, pp. 207–235 (Harper, New York 1960).
7. DE NAYER, PH.; MALVAUX, P.; OSTYN, M.; VAN DEN SCHRIECK, H. G.; BECKERS, C. and DE VISSCHER, M.: Serum free thyroxine and binding proteins after muscular exercise. J. clin. Endocrin *28:* 714–716 (1968).
8. OPPENHEIMER, J. H.; BERNSTEIN, G. and HASEN, J.: Estimation of rapidly exchangeable cellular thyroxine from the plasma disappearance curves and simultaneously administered thyroxine-^{131}I and albumin-^{125}I. J. clin. Invest. *46:* 762–777 (1967).
9. OPPENHEIMER, J. H.; MARTINEZ, M. and BERNSTEIN, G.: Determination of the maximal binding capacity and protein concentration of thyroxine-binding prealbumin in human serum. J. lab. clin. Med. *67:* 500–509 (1966).
10. OPPENHEIMER, J. H.; SQUEF, R.; SURKS, M. I. and HAUER, H.: Binding of thyroxine by serum proteins evaluated by equilibrium dialysis and electrophoretic techniques. Alterations in non-thyroidal illness. J. clin. Invest. *42:* 1769–1782 (1963).
11. RALL, J. E.: Mechanisms for the control of the distribution of thyroid hormones. Gunma Symposia on Endocrinology *3:* 137–152 (1966), (Maebashi, Japan 1966).
12. RHODES, B. A.: Effect of exercise on the thyroid gland. Nature *216:* 917–918 (1967).

13. Robbins, J.: Reverse flow zone electrophoresis. A method for determining the thyroxine-binding capacity of serum protein. Arch. Biochem. *63:* 461–469 (1956).
14. Robbins, J. and Rall, J. E.: The iodine containing hormones; in Gray, C. H. and Bacharach, A. L. (eds.): Hormones in blood, vol. I pp. 382–490 (Academic Press, London, New York 1967).
15. van den Schrieck, H. G.; De Nayer, Ph.; Beckers, C. and De Visscher, M.: Endemic goiter in the Ueles: A study of thyroxine-binding proteins. J. clin. Endocrin. *25* :1643–1648 (1965).
16. Snedecor, G. W.: Statistical methods; 5th ed. (The Iowa State University Press, Ames, Iowa, USA 1956).
17. Welt, L. G.; Orloff, J.; Kydd, D. M. and Oltman, J. E.: An example of cellular hyperosmolarity. J. clin. Invest. *29:* 935–939 (1950).

Authors' address: Ph. de Nayer, M.Ostyn and M. de Visscher, Laboratoire de Pathologie Générale, University of Louvain, 69, Brusselsestraat, *Louvain* (Belgium).

Sympathoadrenal Response to Hypoxia

E. J. BECKER and F. KREUZER

Dept. of Physiology, Faculty of Medicine, University of Nijmegen, *Nijmegen,* The Netherlands

Stress in general evokes a systemic response from the organism through two main mechanisms: the pituitary-adrenocortical axis and the sympathoadrenal medullary system. The corresponding chemical mediators are steroid hormones and catecholamines and the advent of modern methods for the accurate determination of these chemical agents has contributed much to the better understanding of the reactions of the human body to a variety of stress conditions. It is clear that in most situations both systems are at work but their relative activity will depend on the type of stress factors operating at that particular set of conditions. It is practically impossible to isolate for study one single stress factor; in all studies on the conscious human usually several physical and also emotional stress factors are mixed and are acting at the same time. For this reason evaluation of experiments designed to quantitate the effects of stress conditions by measuring the concentrations of the chemical mediators is frequently a difficult problem.

The well known diurnal rhythm of the excretion of adrenocortical hormones and catecholamines must be taken into consideration especially in studies of shorter duration. Direct comparison of analytical results obtained on samples collected at different times of the day will lead to erroneous conclusions.

Even in well designed experiments one usually finds considerable variations not only between different subjects but also large day-to-day variations for the same individual. Therefore, a large number of subjects or experimental runs is essential in order to make statistical evaluation possible.

We would like to present some experimental results from our laboratory to illustrate the points mentioned above.

In table I results are shown from an experiment in which the effect of moderate work on the catecholamine excretion was studied.

The results are in accord with the long recognized association [VON EULER, 1952] between moderately hard physical exercise and the pattern of catecholamine release: there is a significant increase in noradrenaline

Table I. Effect of moderate work on catecholamine excretion

	NE ng	E ng	HMMA μg
		per milligram creatinine	
Before work	18.8 ± 8.0	0.9 ± 0.8	2.20 ± 0.72
After work	34.8 ± 10.0	2.4 ± 2.3	3.84 ± 1.16
	$P<0.01$	$P>0.1$	$P<0.01$

Figures are averages ± standard deviation of 20 runs on the same subject.

excretion while the increase in adrenaline excretion remains statistically insignificant. The great increase in the excretion of the major metabolite confirms the increased release of the active amines.

The subject of this experiment was a well trained young man who had, in connection with other projects, a long experience in treadmill exercise. From previous analyses it was known that his normal adrenaline excretion was always exceptionally low which, in our subjective evaluation, seems to be in accord with his personality. It appears that on the treadmill he was primarily under the physical stress of the actual work with very little, if any, emotional stress.

In our laboratory we are interested in the various effects of hypoxia. In 1963 we have organized an expedition to the Monte Rosa (4,560 m) and in one of the projects [CUNNINGHAM et al., 1965] of this expedition it was found that at high altitude urinary catecholamine excretion was about twice as much as at sea level. The increased catecholamine excretion was almost entirely due to norepinephrine; the epinephrine excretion remained essentially unchanged. Since most of the norepinephrine in the human originates from adrenergic nerve endings, it would appear that, under the conditions to which the members of the Monte Rosa expedition were exposed, low oxygen tension affected the sympathetic nerves more than the adrenal medulla.

In another series of experiments low oxygen tension of high altitude was simulated in a low pressure chamber. Again, the subjects excreted more catecholamines at reduced oxygen tension but now it was the epinephrine excretion that increased; the small increase in norepinephrine excretion was statistically insignificant.

The results of these experiments are summarized in table II.

The most important or, perhaps, the only important common parameter of the two sets of experiments was reduced oxygen tension and at

Table II. Average excretion of free norepinephrine, epinephrine and hydroxymethoxy mandelic acid at sea level and at high altitude

		NE nanogram	E nanogram	HMMA microgram
		per milligram creatinine		
Monte Rosa Expedition (3,000–4,560 m)	sea level (29)	17.2 ± 6.1	4.6 ± 2.4	Lower[1]
	altitude (62)	35.6 ± 12.5	4.8 ± 2.7	Higher[1]
		p<0.01	p>0.1	
Simulated high altitude (3,000–4,000) m	sea level (40)	11.2 ± 5.4	2.0 ± 1.2	3.2 ± 1.5
	altitude (40)	12.8 ± 6.3	4.4 ± 2.3	5.5 ± 2.5
		p>0.1	p<0.01	p<0.001

Values are means ± standard deviation of the number of samples given in parantheses. All figures are uncorrected for recovery. With the methods used average recoveries for NE and E were about 70–75%, for HMMA about 80–85%.

[1] The method used for HMMA in this series was not quantitative enough, it merely indicated that excretion was higher at altitude than at sea level.

first glance it is difficult to understand why hypoxia in itself, produced by actual high altitude on the one hand and by simulated high altitude on the other hand, should result in different patterns of catecholamine excretion.

As pointed out earlier, in experiments with conscious human subjects there are usually several stress factors at work besides the one which is being studied and various combinations of such additional stresses can influence the outcome of the experiment. In comparing the two sets of experiments discussed here other possible stress factors than hypoxia should be taken into consideration.

The members of the Monte Rosa expedition performed a great deal of physical work and participated in a number of exacting experiments during their 3 week sojourn at real high altitude. In contrast, the subjects of the low pressure chamber experiments performed no physical work at all and were exposed to low oxygen pressure only for 90 min. It is well demonstrated that muscular exercise is accompanied primarily by an increase in norepinephrine excretion and it is highly probable that physical activity was an important contributing stress factor in the Monte Rosa study, explaining at least partly the increase in norepinephrine excretion.

Undoubtedly, emotional stress factors were also involved in the two series of experiments and, because of the difference in the conditions of the two series, the emotional stress factors were certainly also of different types. In the Monte Rosa study the participants looked forward with exhilaration to the experience of climbing a high mountain; they were in an active, aggressive mood anticipating all the expected rigors of the expedition. These types of mental state, according to current opinion, influence primarily the sympathetic nerves and, therefore, are associated with increased norepinephrine secretion. In the low pressure chamber series the mental state of the subjects could be characterized by passivity, anxiety and the unpleasant feeling of being confined to a small, potentially hazardous container. These kinds of mental states correspond to emotional stress factors which are believed to affect primarily the adrenal medulla and, therefore, will be accompanied by an increased epinephrine production. Interestingly, in a series of 'mock runs' where the subjects did not know that they were not exposed to reduced pressure, we have found a noticeable increase in the epinephrine excretion of some of our subjects.

In another series of experiments in the low pressure chamber we have found that consumption of moderate amounts of coffee or tea (1–2 cups) as well as moderate smoking had no measurable effect on the epinephrine excretion.

In conclusion it may be stated that hypoxia in general activates the sympathoadrenal system in man as evidenced by the increased catecholamine excretion. The ratio in which the medullary and nervous portions of the sympathoadrenal system respond to hypoxia will depend on the nature of the other stress factors, mainly emotional, which in man will always be present. The overall effect will be reflected in the relative concentrations of excreted norepinephrine and epinephrine but quantitative separation of the effect of individual stress factors from urinary catecholamine analysis in such complex situations does not seem to be possible at present.

References

Cunningham, W. L.; Becker, E. J. and Kreuzer, F.: Catecholamines in plasma and urine at high altitude. J. appl. Physiol. *20:* 607–610 (1965).
Von Euler, U. S. and Hellner, S.: Excretion of noradrenaline and adrenaline in muscular work. Acta physiol. scand. *26:* 183–191 (1952).

Authors' address: E. J. Becker and F. Kreuzer, Dept. of Physiology, Faculty of Medicine, University of Nijmegen, Kapittelweg 40, *Nijmegen* (The Netherlands).

Influence of Anterior Pituitary Hormones and Physical Activity Levels on Intact and Repaired Knee Ligaments of Hypophysectomized Rats[1]

C. M. Tipton, D. S. Sandage and W. Mergner

Exercise Physiology Laboratory and the Department of Pathology, University of Iowa, Iowa City, Iowa

Considerable evidence is available that demonstrates that the level of physical activity will influence the strength of intact ligaments in normal rats [Adams, 1966; Tipton et al., 1967b]. We also have unpublished data that show a six week training program will improve the "strength" of repaired ligaments in normal mongrel dogs. It has repeatedly been demonstrated that various hormones will significantly alter the tensile strength of connective tissue; therefore, studies were undertaken with male hypophysectomized rats to determine the relationship between activity levels, exogenously administered hormones, and the strength of repaired ligaments.

Methods

Male Sprague-Dawley hypophysectomized rats of similar ages were used that weighed between 210–250 g at the time of surgery. A 30-day recovery period was permitted after which the animals were assigned to a given experimental group. The experimental period was 6 weeks for most groups. The exceptions were the animals in the trained (10 weeks), the repaired plus trained group (16 weeks), and their controls. Animals that failed to exhibit anatomical and physiological evidence for the removal of the hypophysis were not included in the statistical analysis. When surgery was performed, ether anesthesia was used and the right medial collateral ligament was exposed and sectioned over the intercondyular space. The ligament was repaired with two strands of 6–0 ophthalmic thread. The wound was then closed and the animal returned to its cage. Problems associated with infections were minimized by application of a sulfa powder and several intramuscular injections of 10,000 units of Strep-Distyrillin. The details concerning the

---

[1] Supported by funds provided by PHS Grant Number AM-08893-04.

insertion of bone pins and the method of immobilization have been published elsewhere [TIPTON et al., 1967b].

We previously showed that there were no significant differences between right and left legs in measures of ligamentous strength and that ligamentous strength can best be expressed on a strength/body weight ratio. The details concerning the techniques used to measure ligamentous strength have been already published [TIPTON et al., 1967a]. The animals were trained as before [TIPTON et al., 1967b]. In essence the animals were capable of running an hour/day at a speed of 1 mile/hour at the completion of their experimental period. The animals were housed in quarters that were temperature and light controlled. Purina rat chow and water were provided *ad libitum*.

Exogenous hormones were injected daily in the following dosages: ACTH: 25 μg per 100 grams BW., ICSH: 25 μg/100 grams BW., STH/mg/rat, TSH: 7 μg/100 grams BW., testosterone: 25 μg/100 grams BW., and thyroxine 7.5 μg/100 grams BW. Measurements of organ weights and resting oxygen consumptions indicated that these dosages had a significant anatomical and physiological effect.

Results

To facilitate interpretation, results are presented under the four headings listed in table I. When the strength of intact ligaments from hypophysectomized rats maintained for 6 weeks were compared to those maintained for 10 weeks, no significant differences occurred; therefore, these results were combined in a single value. Animals maintained for more than 10 weeks were significantly different than the 6 week groups and were treated separately. It can be seen in table I under heading A and B that the activity level of the animals will influence the separation force ratio; namely, training is associated with higher values whereas immobilization is associated with lower values. Since the sham procedures involved the insertion of pins, it appears that the presence of these pins reduced the use of that limb. The lighter gastrocnemius muscle weights from legs with bone pins reinforces this statement. It can also be seen in table I that the combination of TSH and training will markedly alter the separation force ratio obtained from intact ligaments. Under headings C and D the measures obtained from repaired ligaments can be observed. The influence of activity levels is again present because the immobilized legs have the lowest values and the animals that

Table I. The influence of exogenous hormones and physical activity on ligamentous strength

Sub groups	No. of animals	Body wt. in kg	Rt. leg. separation force in kg	Rt. leg separation force ratio
A. Intact Ligaments				
Hypophysectomy	28	0.230±0.004	1.90±0.08	8.309±0.336
Hypophysectomy + Sham Procedures	11	0.203±0.003	1.52±0.10	7.324±0.525
Hypophysectomy + Immobilization	10	0.182±0.002	1.42±0.13	7.854±0.315
Hypophysectomy + Training	13	0.218±0.005	2.11±0.12	9.732±0.568*
B. Intact Ligaments + Exogenous Hormones				
Hypophysectomy + STH	13	0.300±0.005	1.86±0.11	6.212±0.391
Hypophysectomy + STH + Training	9	0.288±0.007	1.73±0.09	6.009±0.372*
Hypophysectomy + TSH	15	0.222±0.004	2.09±0.08	9.369±0.488
Hypophysectomy + TSH + Training	10	0.220±0.004	2.73±0.11	12.488±0.694*
C. Repaired Ligaments				
Hypophysectomy + Repair + Immobilization	12	0.189±0.003	0.89±0.11	4.784±0.584*
Hypophysectomy + Repair	22	0.239±0.004	1.85±0.12	7.719±0.478
Hypophysectomy + Repair (16 weeks)	9	0.220±0.007	2.36±0.13	10.729±0.598*
Hypophysectomy + Repair + Training (16 weeks)	10	0.183±0.003	2.13±0.11	11.604±0.566*
Hypophysectomy (16 weeks)	8	0.186±0.003	2.09±0.04	11.227±0.371*
D. Repaired Ligaments + Exogenous Hormones				
Hypophysectomy + Repair + ACTH	9	0.201±0.004	1.25±0.16	6.160±0.742*
Hypophysectomy + Repair + ICSH	15	0.205±0.002	1.73±0.10	8.396±0.471
Hypophysectomy + Repair + STH	13	0.291±0.006	1.59±0.08	5.454±0.363*
Hypophysectomy + Repair + TSH	11	0.205±0.004	1.19±0.11	5.809±0.536*
Hypophysectomy + Repair + Testosterone	16	0.199±0.002	2.16±0.10	10.889±0.539*
Hypophysectomy + Repair + Thyroxine	9	0.172±0.004	1.05±0.12	6.066±0.650*

* Values are means and standard errors of the mean. The asterisk denotes a separation force ratio that is significantly different ($p=0.05$) from the ratio obtained from the hypophysectomized rats with intact ligaments.

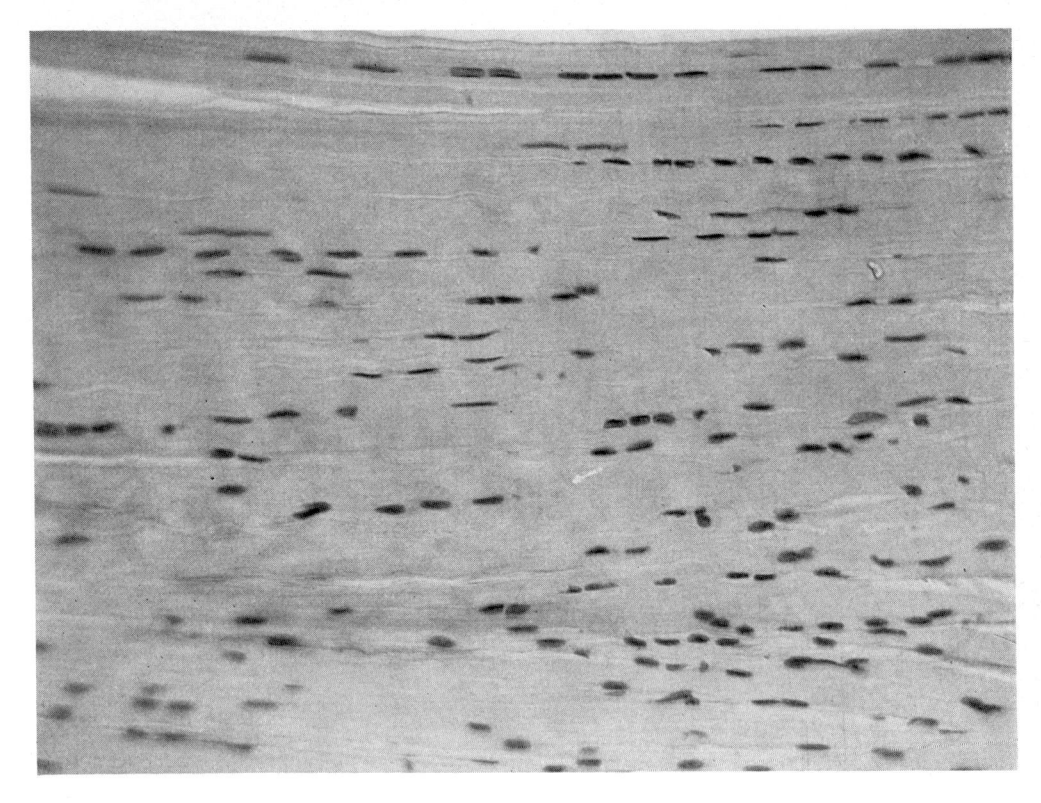

Figure 1. An intact medial collateral ligament from a hypophysectomized rat. Hematoxylin and Eosin stain, 300×.

were trained have the highest values. When the effects of exogenous hormones are examined, it is apparent that ICSH and testosterone will enhance the strength of repaired ligaments.

The histological results in figures 1 and 2 show longitudinal sections through an intact and a repaired ligament taken five weeks after surgery. It appears that after this time the collagen fiber bundles and the long axis of the fibroblasts are well oriented. The thickness of the collagen fiber bundles between rows of fibroblasts is much less compared to normal ligaments. Increased cellularity and vascularity can be noted.

Discussion

The results in table I reinforce the concept that the level of physical activity will markedly influence the strength of intact or repaired ligaments.

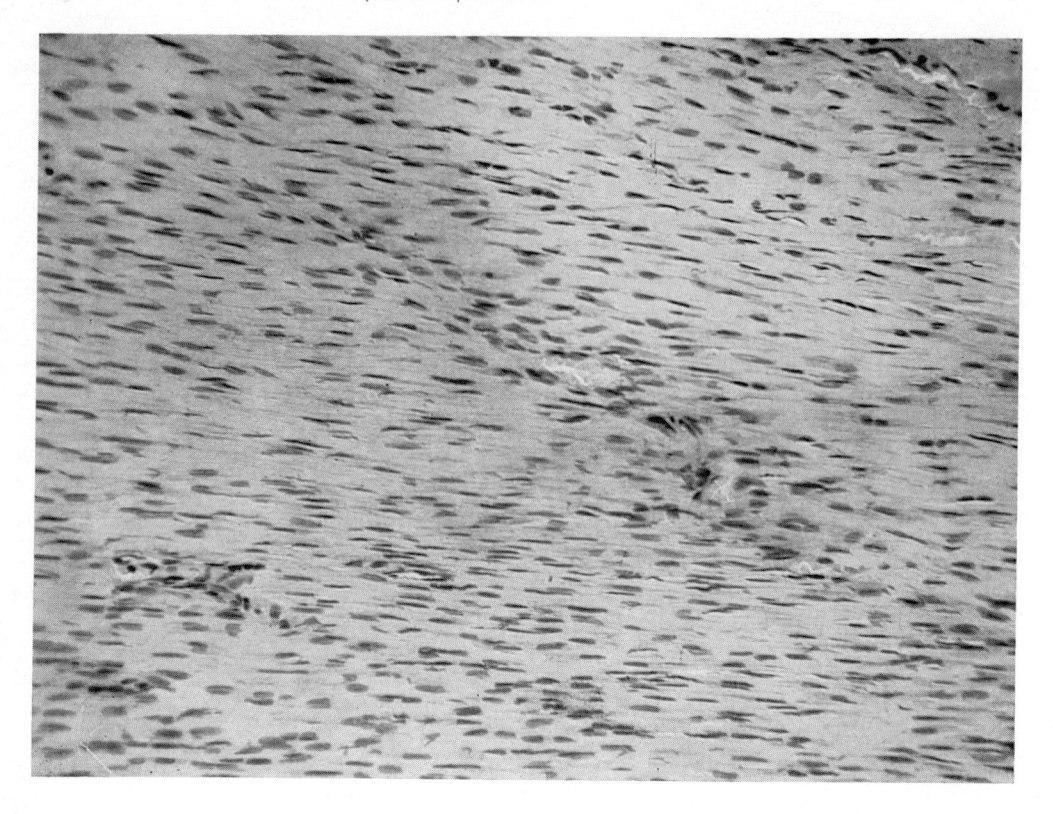

Figure 2. A repaired medial collateral ligament from a hypophysectomized rat five weeks after knee surgery. Stain and magnification are the same as in Figure 1.

As intact ligaments invariably separate from their osseous attachments, the chronic effect of activity is causing a change somewhere in the transition from ligament – nonmineralized fibrocartilage – mineralized fibrocartilage – bone [TIPTON *et al.*, 1967b]. The histological and biochemical data are insufficient at this time to delineate the sites involved.

It has been reported that the tension exerted upon a wound will influence the rate of the repair process [MASON and ALLEN, 1941; BRUNIUS, 1967; CHVAPIL, 1967]. According to CHVAPIL, when tensile strength is used to evaluate the healing of wounds, two phases are involved. The first occurs during the first two weeks and the second occurs from the second to the sixth week or longer. Our animals were measured during the second phase and during the histological period known as the collagenous phase. [CHVAPIL, 1967].

To explain the effects of activity on repaired ligaments, we have postulated an increase in the amount of collagen present. Our light and electron microscope data from trained and nontrained hypophysectomized rats indicate that repaired ligaments from trained animals have a greater collagen fiber density and a larger fiber diameter than repaired ligaments from nontrained animals. Unpublished hydroxyproline results from dog ligaments show a higher concentration in trained than in nontrained animals. CHVAPIL also reports that trained rats have higher bone hydroxyproline levels than nontrained rats. Included within this explanation is the point that activity improves the blood supply to the repaired ligament. Blood flow and metabolic measurements are in progress to test this hypothesis.

Table I also shows that the strength of intact ligaments is enhanced when TSH is injected, particularly when injected into animals that are in the process of training. It has been reported that TSH will increase the level of mucopolysaccharides in tissue, [ZACHARIAE and THORSOE, 1966]. Whether this explanation is appropriate for our findings is unknown.

Of the hormones injected into animals with repaired ligaments, only ICSH and testosterone had any appreciable effect. Although there is not complete agreement as the precise effect of testosterone on repaired tissue, several reports are available that demonstrate that collagen formation is increased when this hormone is injected [JØRGENSEN and SCHMIDT, 1962; ASBOE-HANSEN, 1963; LAITINEN, 1967]. The lower strength values with ACTH [CHVAPIL, 1966; LAITINEN, 1967; PRIEST, 1967], and thyroxine [MOELKE, 1966] were not surprising but we did anticipate that STH would cause an increase in the strength measure. It is possible that we failed to inject high enough dosages [PRUDEEN et al., 1958].

Our intent was to investigate the interrelationships between physical activity, exogenous hormones and ligamentous strength and to gain an insight into the responsible mechanisms. The results indicate that the level of physical activity, and the amounts of TSH, ICSH and testosterone present are an important consideration when interpreting strength results.

Acknowledgement

Gratitude is extended to the Committee on Hormone Distribution of the National Institutes of Health for the generous supply of TSH, ICSH, and STH used within this study.

References

Adams, A.: Effect of exercise upon ligament strength. Res. Quart. *37:* 163–167 (1966).
Asboe-Hansen, G.: The hormonal control of connective tissue. In: International Review of Connective Tissue Research, edited by D. A. Hall. New York: Academic Press (1963), vol. 1, p. 29–61.
Brunius, U.; Zederfeldt, B. and Åhrén, Chr.: Healing of skin incisions closed by non-suture technique. Acta chir. scand. *133:* 509–516 (1967).
Chvapil, M.: Physiology of Connective Tissue. London: Butterworth (1967), p. 258–305.
Jørgensen, O. and Schmidt, A.: Influence of sex hormones on granulation tissue formation and on healing of linear wound. Acta chir. scand. *124:* 1–10 (1962).
Laitinen, O.: The metabolism of collagen and its hormonal control in the rat. Acta Endo. Suppl. *120:* 8–86 (1967).
Mason, M. L. and Allen, H. S.: Rate of healing of tendons: Experimental study of tensile strength. Ann. Surg. *113:* 424–459 (1941).
Moltke, E.: Influence of thyroid hormones on wound healing. In: Hormones and Connective Tissue, edited by G. Asboe-Hansen. Munksgaard: Williams and Wilkins (1966), p. 167–179.
Priest, R. E.: Endocrine control of connective tissue metabolism. In: The Connective Tissue. Baltimore: edited by B. M. Wagner and D. E. Smith. Williams and Wilkins, (1967) p. 50–60.
Prudden, J. F.; Nishihara, G. and Ocampo, L.: Studies on growth hormone. III. The effect of wound tensile strength on marked postoperative anabolism induced with growth hormone. Surg. Gynec. Obstet. *107:* 481–482 (1958).
Tipton, C. M.; Schild, R. J. and Flatt, A. E.: Measurement of ligamentous strength in rat knees. J. Bone Joint Surg. *49A:* 63–72 (1967a).
Tipton, C. M.; Schild, R. J. and Tomanek, R. J.: Influence of physical activity on the strength of knee ligaments in rats. Amer. J. Physiol. *212:* 783–787 (1967b).
Zachariae, F. and Thorsøe, H.: Hormonal control of acid mucopoly saccharides in the female genital tract. In: Hormones and Connective Tissue, edited by G. Asboe-Hansen. Munksgaard, Williams and Wilkins (1966), p. 257–281.

Authors' address: C. M. Tipton, Ph. D., D. S. Sandage, B. S., and W. Mergner, M. D., Exercise Physiology Laboratory and the Dept. of Pathology, University of Iowa, *Iowa City*, Iowa (USA).

Inhibition of Insulin Secretion During Exercise

P. H. WRIGHT and W. J. MALAISSE

Department of Pharmacology, Indiana University, Indianapolis,
and Laboratory of Experimental Medicine, Brussels University, Brussels

Muscular exercise performed by normal subjects produces a marked and immediate augmentation in the rate of glucose utilization by the tissues. The role of insulin in this phenomenon has been questioned. The level of circulating insulin is either unchanged, or decreased, during or after muscular exercise in healthy patients [1, 3, 4, 5]; but no attempt to measure the actual rate of insulin secretion during exercise has yet been undertaken. In the present study, reported in greater detail elsewhere [7], insulin secretion was estimated after intravenous injection of guinea-pig anti-insulin serum (GPAIS) into normal rats, and induction of insulin deficiency.

Fully fed male albino rats were injected intravenously with GPAIS and labeled human albumin. 45 min after this injection and for the ensuing 30 min, the animals were either (i) maintained under control conditions in their cages; (ii) injected subcutaneously with epinephrine (0.2 mg, each 10 min); (iii) submitted to electrical impulses (2 shocks per min); or, (iv) placed in tanks of deep, tepid water. Blood was obtained either from the severed end of the tail (0, 2, and 45 min after the injection of GPAIS), or, at sacrifice, from the neck (75 min after the injection of GPAIS). The rate of endogenous insulin secretion was estimated from the progressive neutralization of the insulin-antibodies, and their redistribution in the body fluids [8].

As shown in the figure, administration of GPAIS resulted within 45 min in hyperglycemia and high rates of insulin secretion. During the ensuing 30 min, further increases in plasma sugar concentration and insulin secretion rate were noticed in the control rats. Despite comparable or even more marked hyperglycemia, the rate of insulin secretion was markedly reduced in the rats injected with epinephrine, submitted to electrical shocks, or compelled to swim. None of these animals showed evidence of systemic ill-effects, or any sign of exhaustion or distress.

The findings in rats receiving exogenous epinephrine confirm that this hormone, as well as other alpha-adrenergic agents, abolishes the stimulant effect of glucose upon insulin secretion [2]. Furthermore, the present results suggest that sufficient endogenous catecholamine may be secreted

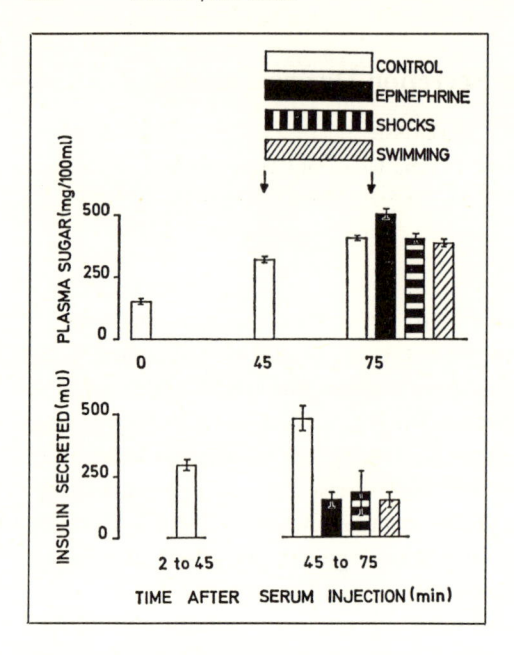

Figure 1. Effects of epinephrine, stress, and exercise upon insulin secretion by the rat. Mean values (±SEM) for plasma sugar concentration and insulin secretion rate.

during stress and exercise to cause a comparable obliteration of insulin secretion.

The dramatic reduction in the rate of insulin secretion observed here contrasts with the minor changes in the level of circulating insulin found during exercise in healthy subjects. This difference is thought to be technical in origin, rather than to be a matter of species. Induction of insulin deficiency represents, indeed, an optimal condition to detect inhibition of insulin secretion, whereas this may be difficult or impossible in normoglycemic subjects, since the level of circulating insulin under resting condition is usually at the lower limit of sensitivity for most methods of plasma-insulin assay [6].

As previously suggested [2], the catecholamines, by inhibiting insulin secretion during stress and exercise, might be better able to mobilize glucose from the liver and fatty acids from adipose tissue, and thus, maintain an adequate supply of nutrients for peripheral and brain metabolism under such conditions. The present observations also demonstrate that insulin is not necessary for the performance of work.

References

1. COCHRAN, B.; MARBACH, E. P.; POUCHER, R.; STEINBERG, T. and GWINUP, G.: Effect of acute muscular exercise on serum immunoreactive insulin concentration. Diabetes *15:* 838–841 (1966).
2. MALAISSE, W.; MALAISSE-LAGAE, F.; WRIGHT, P. H. and ASHMORE, J.: Effects of adrenergic and cholinergic agents upon insulin secretion *in vitro*. Endocrinology *80:* 975–978 (1967).
3. NIKKILA, E. A.; TASKINEN, M. R.; MIETTINEN, T. A.; PELKONEN, R. and POPPIUS, H.: Effect of muscular exercise on insulin secretion. Diabetes *17:* 209–218 (1968).
4. RASIO, E.; MALAISSE, W.; FRANCKSON, J. R. M. and CONARD, V.: Serum insulin during acute muscular exercise in normal man. Arch. int. Pharmacodyn. *160:* 485–491 (1966).
5. SCHALCH, D. S.: The influence of physical stress and exercise on growth hormone and insulin secretion in man. J. lab. clin. Med. *69:* 256–269 (1967).
6. WRIGHT, P. H.: The measurement of insulin secretion: a review of current methods. Diabetes *17:* 641–645 (1968).
7. WRIGHT, P. H. and MALAISSE, W. J.: Effects of epinephrine, stress and exercise upon insulin secretion by the rat. Amer. J. Physiol. *214:* 1031–1034 (1968).
8. WRIGHT, P. H.; RIVERA-CALIMLIM, L. and MALAISSE, W. J.: Endogenous insulin secretion in the rat following injection of anti-insulin serum. Amer. J. Physiol. *211:* 1089–1094 (1966).

Author's address: Dr. W. J. MALAISSE, Laboratoire de Médecine Expérimentale, Université Libre de Bruxelles, 115, boulevard de Waterloo, *Bruxelles 1* (Belgium).

Ergometric Exercise and Urinary Excretion of Noradrenaline, Adrenaline, Dopamine, Homovanillic and Vanilmandelic Acid

A. DE SCHAEPDRYVER and M. HEBBELINCK

Department of Pharmacology, University of Ghent, Ghent, and
Laboratoire de l'Effort, University of Brussels, Brussels

Several investigators have shown that muscular work affects the urinary excretion of noradrenaline (NA) and adrenaline (A) [4, 8, 7, 9, 3, 15, 11, 1], whereas but few data on dopamine (DA), homovanillic acid (HVA) and vanilmandelic acid (VMA) have been reported.

In the present paper we report the results of two types of ergometric work on the urinary output of NA, A, DA, HVA and VMA.

The subjects were three healthy male students and one female student, all of whom were accustomed to physical training and ergometric experiments.

Two types of workload were imposed by means of a Lannooy bicycle ergometer:

1. Aerobic capacity (type A): stepwise increase by 50 W (men) and by 25 W (woman) every 6 minutes, starting at 100 W until a heart rate of over 180 is attained. Pedalling rate remained ± 60 RPM. Mean duration of workload for this type of ergometric work amounted to 15 min.

2. Anaerobic capacity (type B): a constant load of 3,5–4 W/kg B.W. (men) and 3–3.5 W/kg B.W. (woman), cycling until exhaustion at a rate of 100–120 RPM. Mean duration of workload for this type of ergometric work did not exceed 3 minutes.

Cardiorespiratory parameters were continuously registered on a Dargatz Magnotest Spirograph and blood lactic acid determinations were made just before the start of the experiment, immediately after stopping exercise, and finally 30 min after the end of work. Changes in blood lactic acid most clearly discriminated between aerobic and anaerobic work.

In each experiment urine was collected in the two hours interval before the ergometric work (sample a), and subsequently in intervals of two hours three more times (samples b, c, d) after the start of the exercise.

Analyses for NA and A were made according to the trihydroxyindole method [13], DA, HVA and VMA determinations were made according

Table I

Subject	Experiment		NA	A	DA	HVA	VMA
MJ	A1	b	+48	*+116*	+107	−65	+572
		c	*+121*	+60	*+117*	−20	*+977*
		d	+83	+67	+65	−9	
	B2	b	*+297*	*+128*	+12	*+2*	+108
		c	+288	−29	−25	−40	*+155*
		d	+45	0	−51	−13	−29

b, c, d: 2, 4 and 6 h after the start of the exercise respectively.

to the methods of CARLSSON and WALDECK [2], SATO [12] and GEORGES [5], respectively.

In this paper we are mainly concerned with the urinary excretion of the catecholamines (i.e. NA, A and DA) and their major catabolites VMA and HVA under work stress.

The data have been expressed in percentage changes of NA, A, DA, HVA and VMA compared to the resting values.

Table I is typical for the results obtained.

In the 14 experiments performed very variable increases were registered in the urinary excretion of NA, A, DA and their metabolites. The stimulating effect of muscular work on the sympatho-adrenomedullary system tended to be enhanced in the anaerobic type of work, where NA and A reached maximal values sooner than in the aerobic type of exercise. Although lacticacidemia showed a pronounced difference between the aerobic and anaerobic work, the determination of catecholamines and their metabolites failed to differentiate between these 2 types of work.

References

1. BANISTER, E.W.: Urinary catecholamine secretion. *XVI*. Weltkongr. Sportmed., Hannover (1966). Kongressbericht, Hannover (1967), p. 649–657.
2. CARLSSON, A. and WALDECK, B.: A fluorimetric method for the determination of dopamine (3-hydroxytyramine). Acta physiol. scand. *44:* 293–298 (1958).
3. ELMADJIAN, F.; HOPE, J.M. and LAMSON, E.T.: Excretion of epinephrine and norepinephrine under stress. Recent Progr. Hormone Res. *14:* 513–553 (1958).
4. EULER, U.S. VON, and HELLNER, S.: Excretion of noradrenaline and adrenaline in muscular work. Acta physiol. scand. *26:* 183–191 (1952).

5. GEORGES, R.J.: A colorimetric modification of the Pisano method for the estimation of 3-methoxy-4-hydroxymandelic acid in urine. Clin. chim. Acta *10:* 583–585 (1964).
6. HÄGGENDAL, J. and WERDENIUS, B.: Dopamine in human urine during muscular work. Acta physiol. scand. *66:* 223–225 (1966).
7. HASSELMAN, M.; SCHAFF, G. et METZ, B.: Influences respectives du travail, de la température ambiante et de la privation de sommeil sur l'excrétion urinaire des catécholamines chez l'homme normal. C.R. Soc. Biol. *154:* 197–201 (1960).
8. HOLMGREN, A.: Circulatory changes during muscular work in man. Scand. J. clin. Lab. Invest. *8:* Suppl. 24 (1956).
9. KÄRKI, N.T.: The urinary excretion of noradrenaline and adrenaline in different age groups, its diurnal variation and the effect of muscular work on it. Acta physiol. scand. *36:* Suppl. 132 (1956).
10. KLEPPING, J.; TRUCHOT, R.; DIDIER, J.-P.; ESCOUSSE, A. et EYGONNET, J.-P.: Etude de l'élimination urinaire de l'acide vanillyl-mandélique (VMA) pendant l'effort comme critère de la capacité d'adaptation à l'exercice musculaire. C.R. Soc. Biol. *158:* 2007–2009 (1964).
11. KLEPPING, J.; DIDIER, J.-P. et ESCOUSSE, A.: Essai d'évaluation de la capacité d'adaptation à l'effort par détermination de l'élimination urinaire des catécholamines et de l'acide vanillyl-mandélique. Rev. suisse Méd. Sport. *14:* 266–278 (1966).
12. SATO, T.L.: The quantitative determination of 3-methoxy-4-hydroxyphenylacetic acid (HVA) in urine. J. lab. clin. Med. *66:* 517–525 (1965).
13. SCHAEPDRYVER, A.F. DE: Differential fluorimetric estimation of adrenaline and noradrenaline in urine. Arch. int. Pharmacodyn. *115:* 233–245 (1958).
14. SCHMID, E. VON und SCHMERWITZ, K.: Untersuchungen über die Aktivierung des sympathiko-adrenalen Systems bei Baskettballsportlern an Hand der Vanillinmandelsäurebestimmung im Harn. Sportarzt *12:* 399–415 (1964).
15. TAKAHASHI, A.: Muscle exercise and the hypothalamo sympathico-adrenomedullary system. Nagoya J. Med. Sci. *24:* 37–71 (1661).

Authors' addresses: A. DE SCHAEPDRYVER, Department of Pharmacology, University of Ghent, *Ghent,* and M. HEBBELINCK, Laboratoire de l'Effort, University of Brussels, *Brussels* (Belgium).

The Turnover of Sympathico-Adrenal Hormones of Sportsmen in Training, Anticipation and During Competition, Judged by Measurements of the Urinary Excretion of 3-methoxy-4-hydroxy-mandelic Acid

P. NOWACKI, E. SCHMID and F. WEIST

1st Dept. of Medicine, Medical Academy, Lübeck

Estimations of adrenal medullary hormones during physical exercise have been done by several authors, for instance by VON EULER [4], KÄRKI [5], and others. In competitive sport, it was shown by ELMADJIAN *et al.* [3] that various emotional states figure largely in the raise of noradrenaline and/or adrenaline of ice-hockey players and boxers. Recently this has been confirmed by EHRINGER and SPREITZER [2] for speed skaters.

The urinary excretion of 3-methoxy-4-hydroxy-mandelic acid (MHMA, vanilmandelic acid) is supposed to represent the major part of catecholamines metabolized within the human body. Thus our group has studied for several years the effect of bodily and mental stress upon this metabolite (SCHMID [6]; ADAM *et al.* [1]).

We would like to report on 450 MHMA-determinations from 54 sportsmen done in urine collected for periods ranging between 2 and 12 hours. The subjects came from clubs in higher or national leagues and even

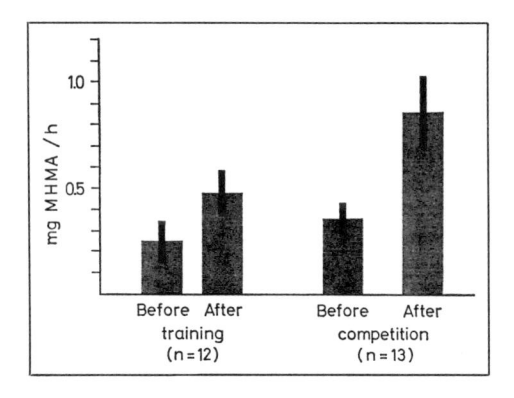

Figure 1. Rise of urinary MHMA in basketball players during training (at left, n=13) and during competition (at right, n=12). The brackets in this and the following figures correspond to the standard deviation.

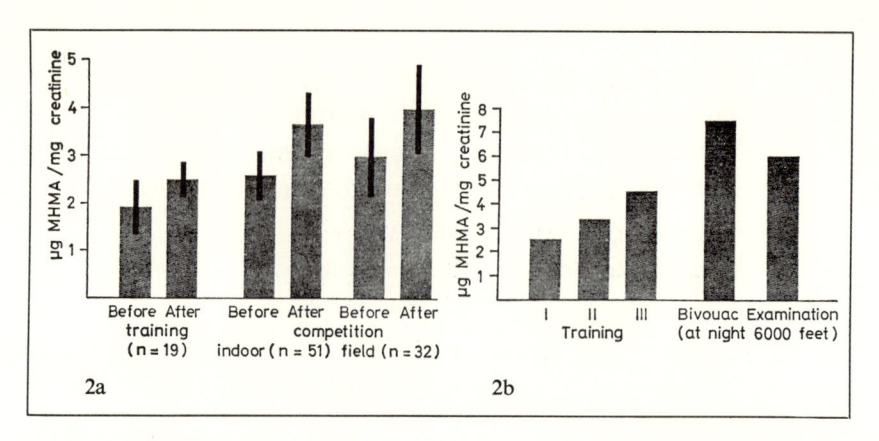

Figure 2a. Effect of playing handball upon the urinary excretion of MHMA. At left: before and after training (n=19); at right: before and after competition either indoor (n=51) or on the field (n=32).

Figure 2b. Rise of MHMA caused by bodily and emotional stress in trainees for skiing instructorship (n=9).

from an olympic rowing crew which won the European championship and the olympic gold medal in the rowing-eights competition 1967 and 1968 respectively.

MHMA was determined photometrically after separation of acid urinary metabolites by thin layer chromatography (TAUTZ et al. [7]).

In basketball players the urinary excretion of MHMA rose during training periods significantly (figure 1). The values before competition were slightly elevated compared with pre-training levels. However the means of MHMA after competition were approximately twice as high as after training sessions. The maxima were found in three field players during a decisive game. Quite similar results were obtained in handball players (figure 2a). In these series and the following ones we preferred to refer the MHMA-values obtained to creatinine levels as timed urine specimens could not be always obtained. A significant rise of vanilmandelic acid could be demonstrated again in training and during competitions. The comparison of the means with Student's t-Test showed significant differences at the 1% level between the values after competitions and after training. Interestingly enough anticipation values before competitions either indoor or on the field were significantly higher than MHMA before training, too.

When a comparison was made between the various games, anticipation values before decisive events which were won were significantly higher than in games which were lost or in nondecisive plays which were

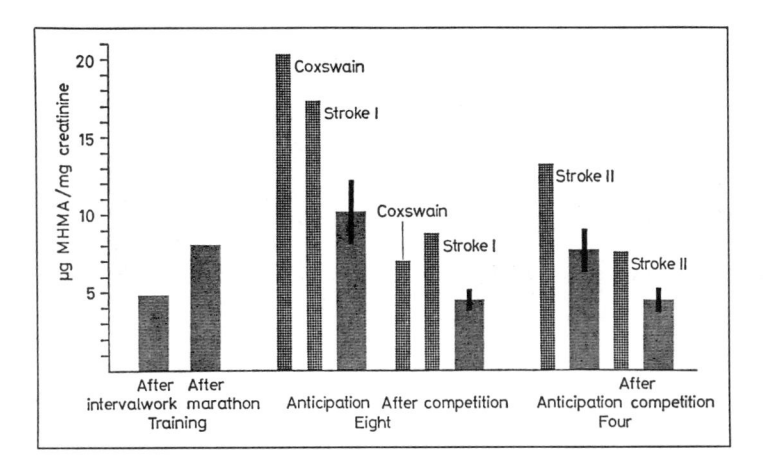

Figure 3. Means and individual values of MHMA in an olympic rowing crew.

won easily (field 3.28±0.78 and 2.42±0.60, indoor 3.11±0.65 and 2.45± 0.47; p<0.005 and <0.005 respectively).

In a group of 9 skiers which were training for instructorship (figure 2b) a rise of MHMA was observed with increasing bodily stress. However, the highest values were found in these persons during a bivouac at 6,000 feet at night done to test their ability to survive together with their pupils in critical situations such as blizzards, and during final verbal examination. The trend of a rising MHMA-excretion was confirmed with the non-parametrical tests of FRIEDMAN and DE JONGHE ($2a<0.01$ and <0.001 respectively).

Finally, serial determinations of vanilmandelic acid were done in the rowing eights from Ratzeburg in training and in competition. Generally the values in these sportsmen, well-trained by ADAM, were higher than in ball players. During interval training (500–600 m, 5 to 7 times) an adaptation was seen characterized by a continuous decline of MHMA in successive training periods, which was not found in marathon training for distances of 15–30 km. The highest values were observed in 2-hour anticipation periods before 2 important races (Gilette Cup and National championship, figure 3). The urine samples collected after the races contained significantly lower quantities of vanilmandelic acid, which were, however, still higher than at rest. As to individual boat members, it was interesting to note that the maximum MHMA-levels in anticipation were found in the coxswain – subject only to mental stress – and in two strokes of the eight and the four.

This result again emphasizes the importance of emotional influences upon the sympatho-adrenal activity in sportsmen. We believe that emotional stress is a necessary element enabling sportsmen to perform at their best.

Acknowledgement

This work was supported by the Deutsche Forschungsgemeinschaft, Bad Godesberg.

References

1. ADAM, K.; NOWACKI, P. und SCHMID, E.: Untersuchungen über die sympathikoadrenale Reaktion bei Hochleistungssportlern im Training und im Wettkampf. Sportarzt und Sportmedizin *9:* 389 (1968).
2. EHRINGER, H. und SPREITZER, G.: Die Ausscheidung von Adrenalin und Noradrenalin im Harn bei Eisschnelläufern während des Wettkampfes und vor dem Start. Wien. klin. Wschr. *79:* 832 (1967).
3. ELMADJIAN, F.; HOPE, J. M. and LAMSON, E. T.: Excretion of epinephrine and norepinephrine in various emotional states. J. clin. Endocr. *17:* 608 (1957).
4. VON EULER, U. S. and HELLNER, S.: Noradrenaline excretion in muscular work. Acta physiol. scand. *26:* 183 (1952).
5. KÄRKI, N. T.: The urinary excretion of noradrenaline and adrenaline in different age groups, its diurnal variations and the of effect muscular work on it. Acta physiol. scand. *39:* 132 (1956).
6. SCHMID, E.: Untersuchungen über Physiologie und Pathophysiologie des sympathikoadrenalen Systems durch Bestimmung der Vanillin-Mandelsäure-Ausscheidung im Harn mit dünnschichtchromatographischer Technik. Arch. KreislForsch. *49:* 83 (1966).
7. TAUTZ, N. A.; VOLTMER, G. und SCHMID, E.: Methode zur quantitativen Bestimmung von Homovanillinsäure, Vanillinmandelsäure und Vanillinsäure im Urin mit dünnschichtchromatographischer Trennung. Klin. Wschr. *43:* 233 (1965).

Authors' address: Dr. P. NOWACKI, Priv.-Doz., Dr. E. SCHMID, Dr. F. WEIST, I. Medizinische Klinik der Medizinischen Akademie Lübeck, *24 Lübeck*, Kronsforder Allee 71/73 (Germany).

Adrenosympathetic Activation and NEFA Metabolism

A. Gerola, R. Dringoli, P. Ravaioli and P. L. Orsucci

Istituto di Patologia Medica, Univ. of Siena Medical School, Siena

It has long been demonstrated that a neurohumoral adrenosympathetic activation accompanies and precedes muscular effort. Among the effects of this adrenosympathetic activation, the cardiovascular ones have been studied particularly. Rushmer first recorded many cardiovascular parameters in the dog, and their variations during runs on the treadmill; in some dogs however, the same changes can take place before any muscular effort and they appear to be quite similar to the effects of either electrical hypothalamic stimulation or catecholamine infusions [5].

On the other hand, it is well known that adrenosympathetic activation, besides cardiovascular effects, brings about some metabolic changes, as far as carbohydrates are concerned; moreover, adrenergic amines are known to give rise to some 'pharmacological' effects concerning both carbohydrate and lipid metabolism [2]. Conversely, the relationships between central nervous system and lipid metabolism are not yet equally well clarified [1, 2]. The present study is aimed to verify whether the adrenosympathetic activation, besides the well known cardiovascular 'hyperkinetic' effects and the hyperglycemic effect, by means of a hypothalamic stimulation, can actually interfere in some way with lipid metabolism.

Material and Methods

Eleven cats were studied under general anesthesia induced with chloralose (40 mg/kg) and urethane (100 mg/kg). In all the animals the left femoral artery was cannulated for continuous blood pressure recording. A polyvinyl catheter also was driven through the left femoral vein up to the right atrium for collecting mixed venous blood.

Finally the animals were placed in a stereotaxic apparatus (Horsley Clarke). Thus a couple of silver electrodes, insulated except for the tips (1 mm apart) could be implanted in the posterior and lateral part of the right hypothalamus. Electrical stimulations (Tectronix square wave stimulator

160A, 161, 162) were given in six runs (100 Hz, 1 msec, 2–4 V) of 5 sec duration with a 5-sec interval between one run and the following. Thus the entire stimulation period lasted 1 min.

Stimulations were considered effective when followed by a marked, immediate rise of blood (systolic, diastolic and pulse) pressure, which reverted at the end of the first run and repeated with the beginning of the following one. We have never made any trial stimulation. Two animals were discarded because the first stimulation had no cardiovascular effect. In eight animals a second stimulation was repeated after 30 min or after 60 min. In six cats only the second electrical stimulation could evoke the same cardiovascular effect previously observed.

Before and directly after the stimulation, mixed venous blood samples were drawn for glucose and NEFA estimations (Folin-Wu and Itaya methods, respectively).

Results

Our data are summarized in the following order: initial values, effects of the first stimulation, interval between the first and the second stimulation, effects of the second stimulation when we observed a cardiovascular response.

Initial values

Blood sugar data are quite dispersed and ranging from 150 to 315 mg%. NEFA also are widely ranging from 112.3 to 531.2 μEq/l.

Effect of the first electrical stimulation

In spite of great dispersion of initial values, both glucose and NEFA levels rise directly after the stimulation. Figure 1 clearly shows that blood sugar went up in 6 out of 7 cats while NEFA did so in all cases.

Interval between the first and the second stimulation

In just a few animals blood sugar and NEFA concentrations went down to the initial values; in other cats the decrement was only partial;

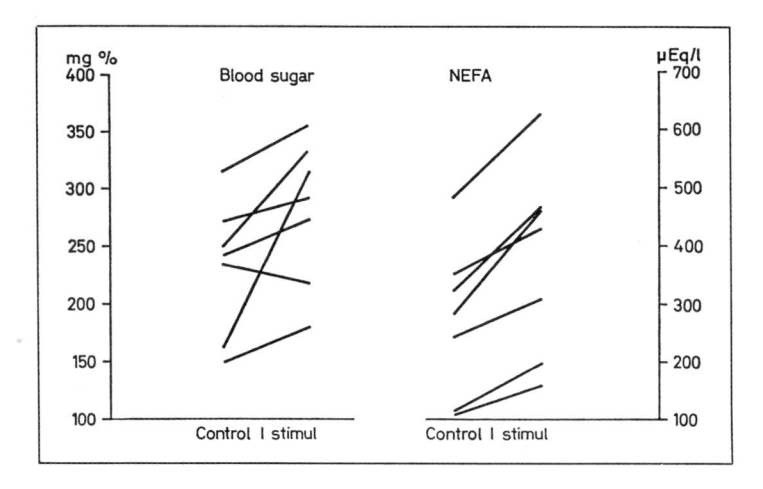

Figure 1. Blood sugar and NEFA values before and immediately after an electrical stimulation of the cat hypothalamus.

in some others, sugar and NEFA levels kept rising after 30 min and even after 60 min.

Effects of the second stimulation

In 6 out of 8 cats the electrical hypothalamic stimulation gave rise to a cardiovascular effect exactly similar to the first stimulation. In these 6 animals, however, we have not observed similar changes as far as blood sugar and NEFA are concerned.

Figure 2 clearly shows that the hypothalamic stimulation repeated after 30 min could no longer evoke the expected increments of blood sugar and NEFA except in 1 case out of 3. After 60 min the second stimulation raises blood sugar and NEFA in 1 out of 3 cases. In one experiment (68.05.07) one stimulation repeated after 30 min brought about a decrement of both glucose and NEFA which rose only with a third stimulation after 30 min interval.

Discussion

Undoubtedly, our experimental preparation suffers from serious limitations: general anesthesia, acute surgical procedure and the strength of

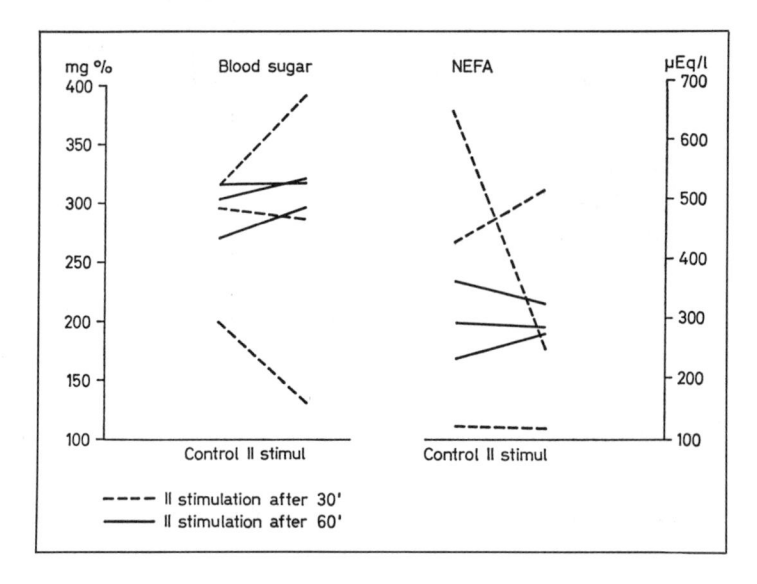

Figure 2. Blood sugar and NEFA values before and immediately after the second electrical stimulation of the cat hypothalamus.

electrical hypothalamic stimulation, all create unphysiological conditions which are at least responsible for a great dispersion of initial blood values. On the other hand it is hard to figure out another way of separating an adrenosympathetic activation, central nervous in origin, which anticipates muscular effort (conditioning, training) from the activation which follows the effort, and appears to be its effect.

On this ground our results seem to suggest two quite reliable conclusions. First of all we believe we have demonstrated that the electrical stimulation of the posterior and lateral part of the hypothalamus in the cat, evoking a cardiovascular 'hyperkinetic' effect and a hyperglycemic effect, can also bring about a NEFA increment in the blood. These increments of rapidly utilized metabolites can be reasonably interpreted as the result of a regulation integrated at high level in order to assure and even anticipate both a cardiovascular and metabolic support of muscular effort.

Furthermore, we have observed that the two aspects (cardiovascular and metabolic) studied here, do not get exhausted simultaneously and proportionally; on the contrary, the metabolic exhaustion appears before the cardiovascular one. It is fair to remember the observed discrepancy between metabolic and cardiovascular effects of noradrenaline [4].

These conclusions appear to have quite a few relevant implications. First, the metabolic consequences of recurrent stressing situations which are supposed to prepare for, but are not actually followed by, a neuromuscular effort. Another important implication, which deserves further study, concerns the damage which might be brought about by recurrent adrenosympathetic activations (artificially, as in our experimental model, or pharmacologically induced) when such an activation becomes metabolically ineffective although capable to involve the cardiovascular system; involvment which might be deceiving and dangerous as well.

References

1. ANDREOTTI, L.; GUARNIERI, E.; NUZZACI, G.; GIARDINA, A. and BIANUCCI, G.: La regolazione nervosa della mobilizzazione dei lipidi. Rass. Neurol. Veg. *18:* 438 (1964).
2. CORREL, J. W.: quoted by 1.
3. HAVEL, R. I.: in *Lipid pharmacology*. PAOLETTI, R. ed. (Academic Press, New York 1964).
4. NESTEL, P. J.: Plasma triglyceride concentration and plasma FFA change in responses to noreprinephrine in man. J. clin. Invest. *43:* 77 (1964).
5. SMITH, O. A.; JABUR, S. J. and RUSHMER, E. P.: in *Symposium on central nervous system and control of circulation*. EICHAN, L. W. and MCQUARRY, D. C., ed. Physiol. Rev. *40:* suppl. 4 (1960).

Authors' address: A. GEROLA, R. DRINGOLI, P. RAVAIOLI and P. ORSUCCI, Istituto di Patologia Medica, Univ. of Siena Medical School, *Siena* (Italy).

IV. Enzymes

Enzyme Modifications During Activity

E. Schmidt and F. W. Schmidt

Division of Gastroenterology, Department of Medicine, Medical Academy of Hannover

Physical activity is a complex process. It requires a differentiated regulation by enzyme systems of many organs. A survey on the multiplicity of the variations of enzyme activities is not possible at the present time. Hence, I shall confine myself to a description of the enzymatic changes in skeletal muscle and in serum during exercise.

At first some remarks about the relevance of enzyme determinations: Certainly, we measure enzyme activities *in vitro* under standard conditions, which justifies the comparison of the obtained values. These values, however, are primarily irrelative. They do not reflect the actual turnover rates of substrates *in vivo*. Only the consideration of the relation of groups of enzymes or of characteristic key enzymes establishes a relation between enzyme alterations and alterations of substrate turnover on the basis of comparative analysis.

The homogeneity of the tissues under investigation is of essential importance. Their cellular composition should not change during the experiments, thus bringing about further experimental difficulties. It is well

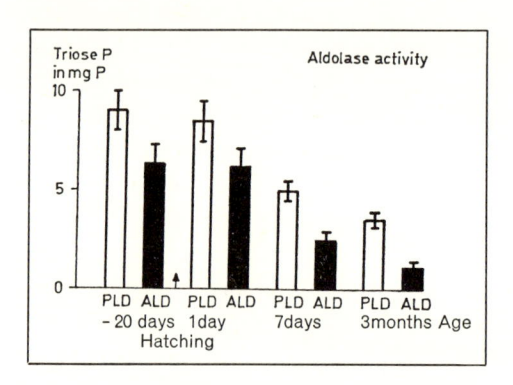

Figure 1. Aldolase activity (triosephosphate in phosphorus lib. 30 min/mg non-collag. protein) in M. posterior latissimus dorsi P.L.D. and M. anterior latissimus dorsi A.L.D. before (20-day embryo), immediately and 7 days and 3 months after hatching. [E. Gutman, 1966]

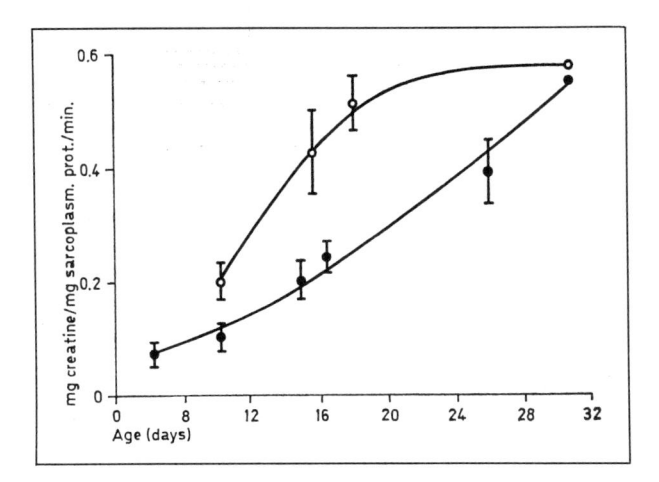

Figure 2. Effect of activity on the creatine phosphokinase activity of the leg muscles of young rabbits. The figure summarises the results obtained with 6 litters. ○ litters disturbed at 5 days post partum. ● undisturbed control litters. [KENDRICK-JONES and PERRY, 1966]

known, that the vertebrate muscle we are dealing with, is by no means homogeneous. On the contrary, it shows a pronounced heterogeneity. That makes generalization or transfer of information hazardous. A very exact topical and temporal characterization of the muscle specimens is therefore required for comparative study, in order to exclude the influence of different or varying proportions of phasic or tonic muscle fibers.

Let me demonstrate the significance of the definition of age – that is, the definition of the actual developmental stage of the phasic and tonic fibers – with GUTMAN's [29] studies on the activities of aldolase in the tonic *M. anterior latissimus dorsi* and the phasic *M. posterior latissimus dorsi*.

In both muscles the activity of aldolase decreases in the course of maturation, but the decrease is much greater during the differentiation to the red muscle type (figure 1).

The finding, that the velocity of the differentiation of fiber types seems to depend upon exercise, is interesting with respect to our problem, but it also complicates the base of reference further.

The figure 2 of KENDRICK-JONES and PERRY [38] shows the earlier increase of CPK activity in the leg muscle of young rabbits, which were physically exercised.

The enzymatic and metabolic differentiation in fully developed muscles is shown on the following figure 3 from PETTE [53].

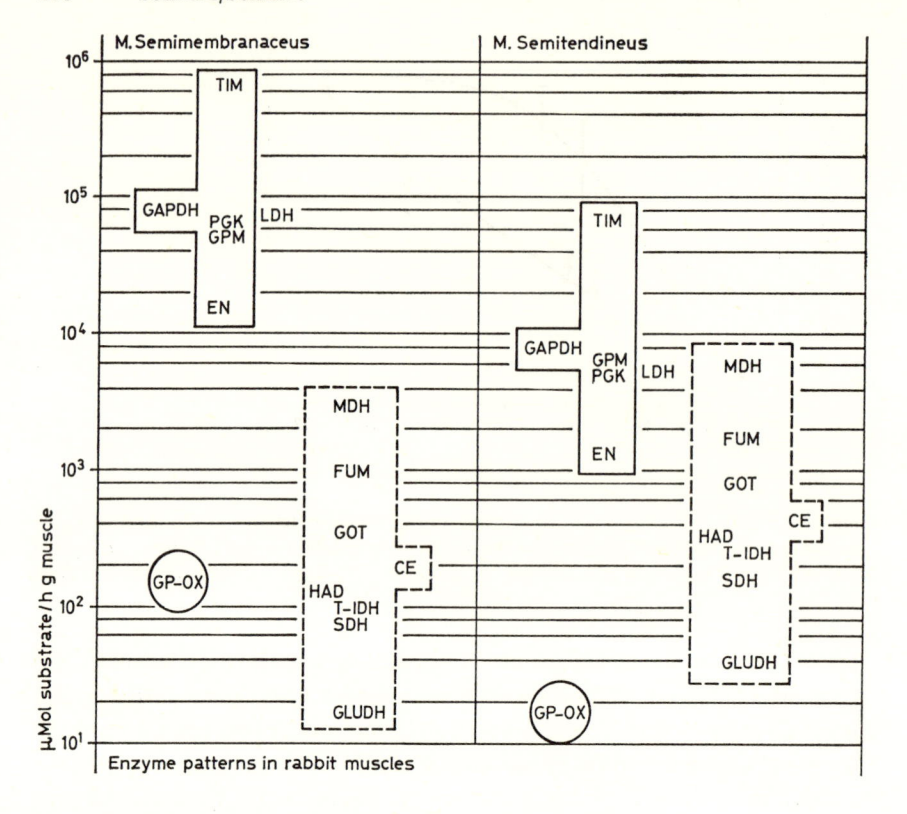

Figure 3. Enzyme patterns in rabbit muscles. [D. PETTE, 1966]

Here, the constant proportion groups of glycolytic enzymes – within the single line –, of the enzymes of citrate cycle and fatty acid oxidation – within the broken line –, and the enzymes of glycerophosphate cycle are plotted. The glycolytic enzymes appear in the phasic *M. semimembranaceus* in tenfold higher activity than in the tonic *M. semitendineus*. On the other hand, the enzymes of the mitochondrial metabolism are two- to fourfold higher in the tonic muscle. This correlates well with its greater supply with mitochondria. Thus, the systems glycolysis /citrate cycle and glycolysis/ fatty acid oxidation respectively, are differing from each other by a factor of twenty to thirty in both muscles. This represents lastly the different proportions of aerobic and anaerobic metabolism in both tissues. It becomes particularly apparent, if the capacity of anaerobic lactate formation is compared to the capacity of aerobic glucose oxidation, that means, the oxidation of pyruvate via the Krebs-cycle, as it was done by PETTE (table I).

Table I.

	LDH	Enzyme activity μMol/h gm muscle Cond. Enzyme	Ratio LDH/CE
M. semimembranaceus (phasic)	80,500	180	450
M. semitendineus (tonic)	6,100	420	15

[D. PETTE, 1966]

These relations permit the statement, that the continuous tonic function is largely maintained by the oxidative metabolism, whereas the discontinous phasic function is primarily supported by glycolysis. The stress is on 'primarily', as the glycolytic capacity of tonic muscle is still very high in comparison to other organs, which are specialized in oxidative glucose metabolism as, for instance, the cerebral cortex of the rat. We may conclude, thus, that glycolysis possesses an appreciable importance in tonic muscle, especially to meet the peak requirements of action metabolism. This is further evidenced by the considerable increase of lactate under exhaustive exercise conditions.

These considerations are in line with the results of KEUL [39] and other authors, who found that during sub-maximal exertion oxidative metabolism prevails and only under exhaustive work about one third of the glucose extracted from the blood, reappears as pyruvate and lactate.

The possibility to assess the relative capacity of metabolic pathways from enzyme activities also indicates to what extent the energy-linked carbohydrate metabolism of the different muscle types involves glycogenolysis or direct glucose breakdown.

Table II compares the activities of phosphorylase, hexokinase and condensing enzyme as representatives for glycogenolysis, glucose uptake and pyruvate oxidation respectively, in phasic, tonic and as an extreme variant in heart muscle.

The correlation of the systems indicates that glycogenolysis is of greater importance in the phasic muscle than in the tonic or heart muscle, while in all types of muscles the ability for direct uptake of glucose is paralleled by the respiratory capacity. The latter features are more marked in

Table II.

		M. adduct. magn. (rabbit)	M. soleus (rabbit)	heart muscle (rat)
Metabolic System	Key Enzyme	Activity (μMol/h gm muscle)		
Glykogenolysis	Phosphorylase	2,800	135	340
Glucose phosphorylation	Hexokinase	12	93	460
Citrate-Cycle	Cond. Enzyme	86	340	3,900
	System Correlations			
Glykogenolysis / Citrate-Cycle	Phosph./CE	32	0.4	0.09
Glucose phosphorylation / Citrate-Cycle	HK/CE	0.14	0.26	0.12

[D. Pette]

tonic muscle and especially in heart muscle, as evidenced by the absolute activities.

In the human the selection of muscles with a distinct type of fibers is usually not possible for technical reasons. Therefore the enzyme patterns at hand are not so sharply distinct from each other. One may, however, conclude from the investigations of Laudahn, that the muscles of the trunk have higher glycolytic activities than the muscles of the limb, which in contrast are better supplied with oxidative enzymes (figure 4). The enzyme patterns of different human muscles – predominantly of the tonic type – are plotted in reference to GAPDH = 1.

The question, whether changes of the innervation lead to metabolic changes and consequently to variations of the enzyme pattern, is also interesting with regard to our subject. It is well known, that cross-innervation of tonic muscles with nerves from phasic muscles results in a considerable acceleration of contraction. On the other hand, the innervation of *M. flexor digitorum longus* with the *N. soleus* produces nothing more than the preservation of the muscle in the slow state that was caused by denervation before re-innervation [17]. These facts correspond well to the respective changes of the enzyme patterns: cross-innervation of a red muscle leads to a significant increase of glycolytic enzymes and a decrease of the enzymes of citrate cycle

Enzyme Modifications During Activity

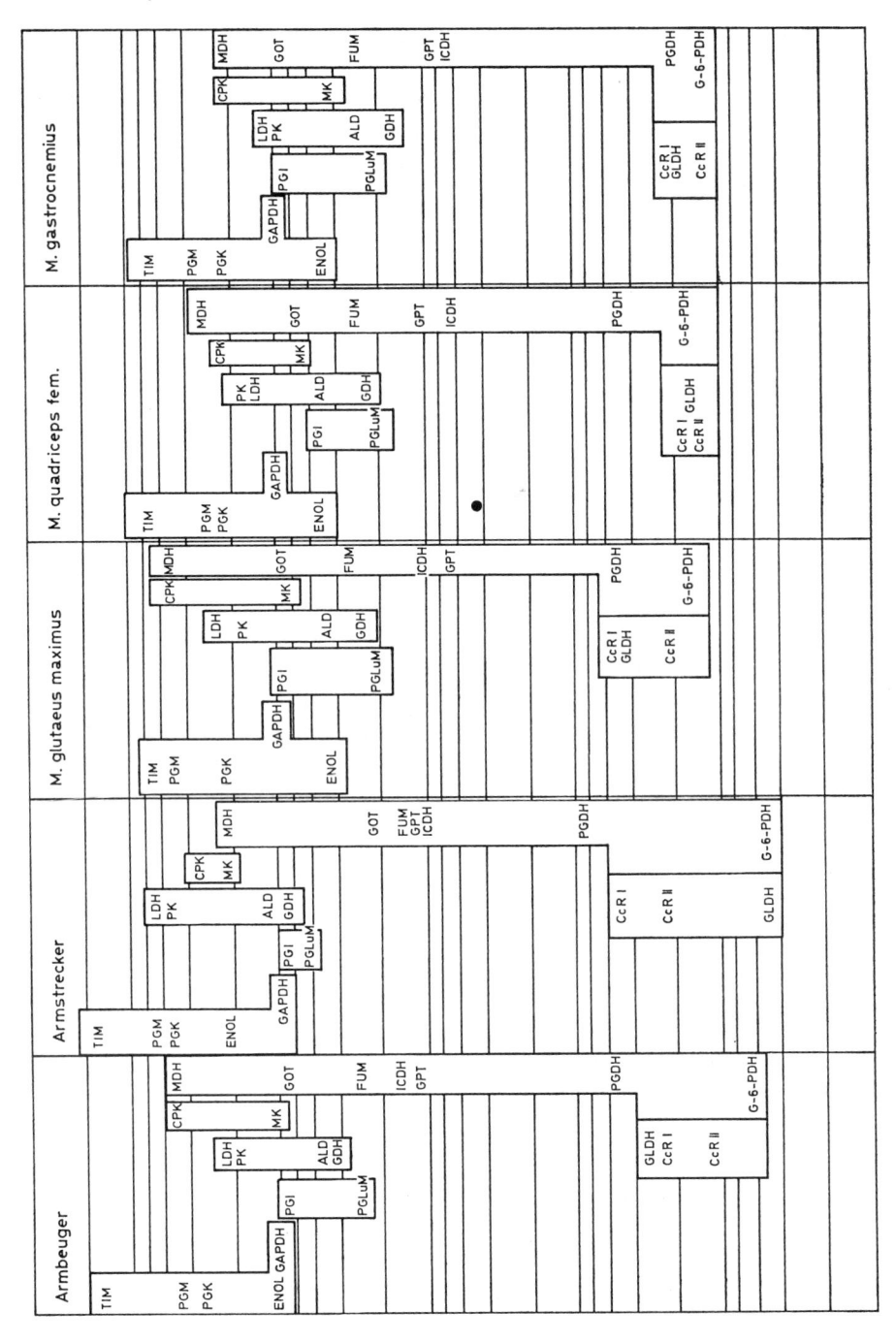

Figure 4. Enzyme patterns in human muscles. [G. LAUDAHN, 1967]

and fatty acid oxidation. In the inverse case, the variation is of minor extent: with the activities of glycolytic enzymes unchanged, the activities of mitochondrial enzymes are diminished [24]. After all we find a picture of dedifferentiation to a more primitive type of metabolism.

Compared to the progress of fundamental knowledge in recent years, our informations about the variation of enzyme activities in tissues under exercise conditions are still relatively poor.

In principle we must discriminate the changes in acute exercise from those under long-term exertion, that is, after training. Enzyme activities as measured *in vitro* would permit a multifold higher turnover rate than exists *in vivo*; only in the tetanized muscle the rate of glycogen breakdown is of the same order of magnitude as the phosphorylase activity under optimal conditions of substrate concentration and pH [11]. Thus true augmentation of enzyme protein by induction, which takes some time, is not to be expected early. At the moment the interest is focussed – speaking in the terms of CORI and HELMREICH [34] – to 'the on- and off-effect of enzymatic activation related to the contraction-relaxation cycle of the muscle'. The key enzymes in this respect are phosphorylase and PFK. The activities of both enzymes rise synchronously and proportionally under stimulation (figure 5).

The activation of phosphorylase is accomplished according to CORI and HELMREICH [34] by the conversion of phosphorylase B, which is inactive in the absence of cyclic 5-AMP, to phosphorylase A with phosphorylase-kinase. Phosphorylase-kinase can be activated by calcium ions,

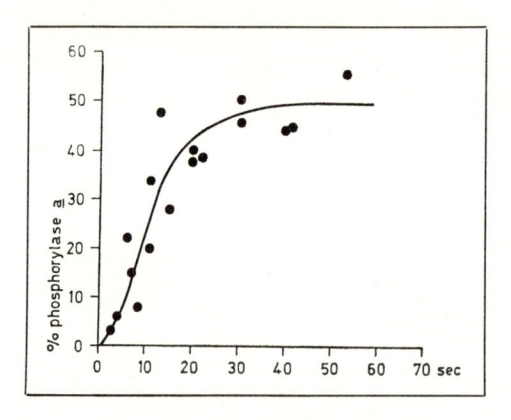

Figure 5. Appearance of phosphorylase A in stimulated muscle. The muscles were stimulated at 20° at 6 shocks per sec. [E. HELMREICH and C. F. CORI, 1964]

PFK by ADP. A linkage of glycolysis and the respiratory chain seems to be given with the powerful inhibition of PFK by citrate.

The data reported on the variations of enzyme activities during long-term exercise – under training conditions – are not only very different, but indeed contradictory. The reasons for the discrepancies are probably to a lesser extent due to differences in the methods of enzyme determinations, than to the great differences in experimentally applied exertion. Obviously, the latter often did not surpass the critical value. Furthermore, differences in response to various types of exercise are to be expected, because of the fact, that other substrates constitute the source of energy under conditions of repeated maximal exertion of short duration than under conditions of long-term training.

HULTMAN [26] has demonstrated unequivocally the close relationship of muscle glycogen content and working capacity under exhaustive exercise, and he had thus shown, that in this case glycogen breakdown and glucose oxidation are the main factors (figure 6). Prolonged, sub-maximal exertion however can be continued even with a largely diminished glycogen reserve. In that case glucose phosphorylation and fatty acid oxidation become more

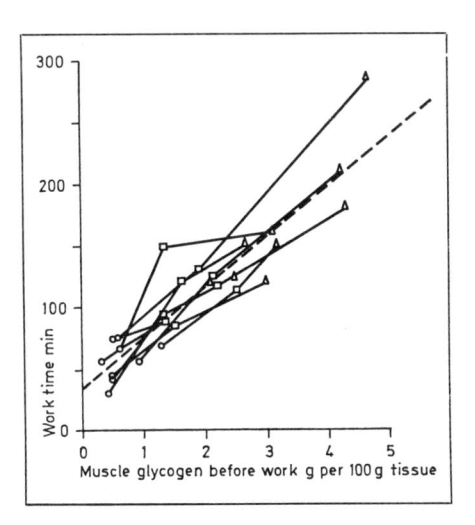

Figure 6. Relation between initial glycogen content of quadriceps femoris muscle and work time. 9 subjects worked on a bicycle ergometer with a load corresponding to 75% of their max O_2 uptake to complete exhaustion. Each subject worked three times, and the experiments were preceded by 3 days or more of dietary regime. □ = after mixed diet; ○ = after fat+protein diet; △ = after carbohydrate diet. [E. HULTMAN, 1967]

prominent. The energy production for prolonged work shifts from glycolysis to the more efficient and economical oxidative pathway.

Hence we may postulate for the long-term training an increase in the oxidative capacity. The enzyme pattern of skeletal muscle would become more similar to that of heart muscle. Moreover, because of the constant proportion between the surface of mitochondrial membranes and the content of oxidative enzymes, we may postulate an augmentation or multiplication of mitochondria. This is exactly what was found by LAGUENS et al. [41, 42] in the heart muscle of rats after a relatively short period of exercise.

Earlier comparative studies showed a fair correlation between the capacity for endurance work of various muscles and their content of respiratory enzymes. The breast muscles of non-flying chicken have low O_2-values and are poor in mitochondria. In the breast muscles of mellards and pigeons, which spend long periods in active flight, these values are ten times higher [51]. LAWRIE [44] has reported that the levels of cytochrome oxidase, succinate oxidase and succinate dehydrogenase in the *psoas muscle* of sedentary laboratory rabbits are approximately one third to one half as high as those found in the wild hare, and only one forth to one sixth as high as values obtained in horse *psoas*.

Variations of enzyme activities after training were first reported by YAKOVLEV et al. [73]. Later experiments however with an intensified exercise program failed. HEARN and WAINIO [32], who trained their rats by daily swimming of thirty minutes duration for 5 to 8 weeks, found no increase of

Table III. Enzyme activities in muscles of rats in exercising and sedentary groups

Group	Cytochrome oxidase	Succinate oxidase	NADH-dehydrogenase	NADH-Cytochrome reductase
	μl O_2/min/g		μmol/min/Mito g muscle	
M. gastrocnemius				
Sedentary	305 ± 15	73 ± 5	5.6 ± 0.6	0.25 ± 0.05
Exercising	551 ± 31	117 ± 8	11.8 ± 1.5	0.60 ± 0.09
M. Soleus			Mitochondrial protein mg/g muscle	
Sedentary	427 ± 16	95 ± 10		
Exercising	691 ± 52	160 ± 8		
			Sedentary	2.97 ± 0.20
J. O. HOLLOSZY, 1967			Exercising	4.67 ± 0.30

succinate dehydrogenase activity in the skeletal muscles. Under similar conditions neither ALD, LDH, MDH, CPK nor phosporylase activities increased [25, 26, 27, 33]. Only a considerable increase of the exertion by treadmill running made HOLLOSZY [36] succeed in producing enzyme elevations (table III).

Expressed per gram of muscle the activities of succinate dehydrogenase, NADH dehydrogenase, NADH cytochrom C reductase, succinate oxidase and cytochrom C oxidase increased by an average factor of 2 in response to the training. The cytochrom C levels increased to the same extent. Unfortunately the author did not measure glycolytic enzymes. PETER *et al.* [52] reported an increase of hexokinase, KENDRICK-JONES and PERRY [37] one of CPK and ALD. I hope that the papers of this symposion will provide the missing informations.

In response to muscular exercise the liver metabolism is also enhanced. BERGSTRÖM and HULTMAN [6] found the glucose production considerably increased under work in man with a tendency towards further rise during exercise. This increase of substrate turnover under work corresponds with the higher oxygen uptake in liver mitochondria of rats in the night [21, 22], when the animals display maximal physical activity, and with the higher oxidation rates of citrate cycle intermediates after experimental work [23].

Data on the variations of enzyme activities in the liver under exertion are scarce: CRITZ [13] found an increase of GOT activity, SANGSTER and BEATON [57] one of the MDH levels.

In contrast to the predictable alterations of the enzyme activities in tissues, the causal connection of exercise with the release of enzymes of cell metabolism and the elevation of their activities in the serum was surprising. Beyond its fundamental significance, this phenomenon has attracted widespread attention for its implications upon the basis of enzyme diagnostics: namely, the assumption, that merely damaged cells release intracellular enzymes into the serum.

Figure 7 shows the results of some of our own studies [50]. In response to 50-W-exertion on ergometer with a duration up to 5 h several enzyme activities become more or less elevated in serum. Most other authors report similar results [1, 3, 4, 5, 8, 9, 12, 14, 18, 20, 28, 35, 40, 45, 50, 55, 56, 58, 62, 67, 69].

The discrepancies of the extent of the enzyme elevations can be attributed in part to the different extent of the work executed, but are mostly due to the heterogeneity of the test-groups (table IV).

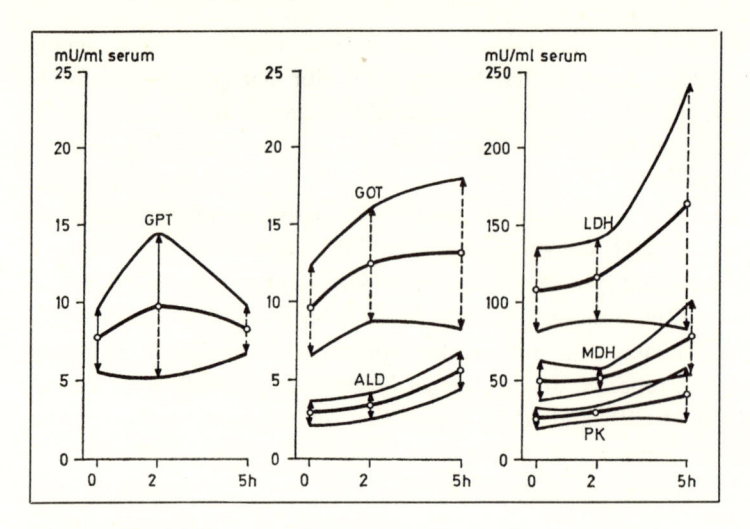

Figure 7. Enzyme activities in the serum before and after exercise.

HOLLMANN [35] is right to point out that the terms 'trained' and 'untrained' are insufficient as a description of physical properties. A good weight-lifter is well trained with respect to the strength of his skeletal muscles, while his cardio-vascular system may be untrained and in conformity with that of any other person of the same age. On the other hand, a long-distance runner has a well trained cardio-vascular system, whereas the strength of his skeletal muscles may be virtually untrained.

The impressive experiments of GARBUS *et al.* [20] demonstrate, that the state of training is a decisive factor.

Table V shows, that under equal working conditions the untrained rats displayed three- to fivefold higher elevations of enzyme activities in the serum.

In spite of some discrepancies between the results of the numerous investigations, we may come to three conclusions:

1. The elevation of enzyme activities in the serum depends upon the duration and the degree of exertion.
2. Preceding training lowers the enzyme elevations after exercise.
3. The individual enzymes show different modifications.

Most of the authors assume that the increase of enzyme activities in serum is due to an enhanced efflux of enzymes from the active muscles. Other possibilities should be discussed at least: The higher enzyme activities

Table IV. Serum enzyme changes following exercise (Enzyme activities in % of the initial values)

Author	exercise	duration	degree	GOT	GPT	LDH	ALD	MDH	CPK	remarks
RICHTER [55]	Ergometer	15 min	180–200 W	–	–	–	∽100	–	–	untrained, increase under exercise
RICHTER [55]	Ergometer	15 min	200 W	–	–	–	∽100	–	–	trained, decrease under exercise
BAUMANN [5]	Ergometer	15 min	100 W	–	–	95	–	–	?	trained
BAUMANN [5]	Ergometer	15 min	200 W	–	–	118	–	–	332	moderately trained
HOLLMANN [35]	Ergometer	∽20 min	30 W – exhaustion	125	160	110	154	–	166	sports students
KÜSTNER [40]	Ergometer	15 min	100 W	–	–	–	–	–	240	female untrained
KÜSTNER [40]	Ergometer	15 min	150 W	–	–	–	–	–	100	male untrained
KÜSTNER [40]	Ergometer	3 × 15 min intervals	100 W	–	–	–	–	–	230	female untrained
KÜSTNER [40]	Ergometer	3 × 15 min intervals 4 and 8 hours	150 W	–	–	–	200	–	–	male untrained
CANTONE [9]	treadmill	30 min	8 km/hour	–	–	–	200	–	–	untrained
VETTER [69]	Ergometer	20 min	200 W	83	72	74	75	84	–	untrained
MASSARRAT [45]	staircase-mounting		1200–1600 steps	112	102	111	–	–	–	untrained
CRITZ [14]	Harvard step test			53	–	–	–	–	–	trained
CRITZ [14]	Harvard step test			90	–	–	–	–	–	untrained

Table IV (continued)

Author	exercise	duration	degree	GOT	GPT	LDH	ALD	MDH	CPK	remarks
SCHNEIDER [62]	Ergometer	5 min 5 min 5 min	50 W 100 W 150 W	131	–	–	–	–	8,560	?
FOWLER [18]	treadmill	15 min	8 km/hour 3°–5°	110	130	105	108	130	–	untrained
FOWLER [18]	treadmill	15 min	8 km/hour 5°–8°–11°	150	156	120	125	150	–	trained
FOWLER [18]	running		8 miles	220	200	166	145	200	–	trained
OTTO [50]	Ergometer	25 min	10 min 25 W 10 min 50 W 5 min 150 W	80	104	97	–	104	–	moderately trained
BAUMANN [5]	boxing	30 min		79	76	77	101	–	92	trained
SCHMIDT [58]	gymnastics (ground work)	2 hours		200	125	180	350	155	–	trained
OTTO [50]	Ergometer	2 hours	50 W	119	114	111	110	112	–	moderately trained
AHLBORG [1]	Ergometer	2 hours	up to exhaustion	125	127	130	–	–	140	untrained
BAUMANN [5]	running	2 hours		–	–	91	–	–	390	trained
BAUMANN [5]	running	2 hours		–	–	83	–	–	96	untrained
OTTO [50]	gymnastics (ground work)	2 hours		111	–	121	–	131	–	trained
OTTO [50]	Ergometer	5 hours	50 W	157	122	147	207	149	–	moderately trained
GRILLITH [28]	walking	53 miles	3,5 miles/h	–	–	–	–	–	240	untrained

Table IV (continued)

Author	exercise	duration	degree	GOT	GPT	LDH	ALD	MDH	CPK	remarks
Cornelius [12]	racetraining			180	–	–	–	–	–	horses
Cornelius [12]	swimming-training	2–25 min		330	–	–	–	–	–	horses
Ullrich [67]	trotting race		3,300 m	137	200	–	–	–	–	trotters
Altland [4]	treadmill	4 hours	6,9 m/min	200	150	160	270	220	–	rats: untrained
Altland [3]	treadmill	16 hours		510	405	253	807	–	–	rats: weight gain 13%; fatty changes of the liver, muscle cell necroses
Garbus [20]	treadmill	6 hours daily/10 h	6,9 m/min	340	350	580	–	–	–	rats: untrained/trained

Long-term exertion

Author	exercise	duration	degree	GOT	GPT	LDH	ALD	MDH	CPK	remarks
Baumann [5]	exercise	1,5 days		108	92	127	137	–	171	moderately trained
Cantone [9]	treadmill	5–7 days daily 30 min	8 km/h	–	–	–	>200	–	–	untrained
Cantone [9]	running	10 days daily 30 min	10 km/h	–	–	–	160	–	–	trained
Richterich [56]	soldiers training			190	120	–	–	–	–	recruits/civilians
Calvy [8]	soldiers training	6 months		–	–	95	–	126	–	ICDH: 51

Table V. Serum enzyme and urea nitrogen values in unexercised controls and changes in trained and untrained rats exercised 16 h

Enzyme	Trained unexercised controls	Exercised 16 h Trained	Exercised 16 h Untrained	Ratio Trained/control	Ratio Untrained/trained
SLDH	730 ± 192	614 ± 104	2,270 ± 162	0.8	3.7
SAld	51 ± 10	74 ± 6	431 ± 28	1.4	5.8
SGOT	346 ± 25	380 ± 24	1,320 ± 65	1.1	3.4
SGPT	62 ± 3	52 ± 4	187 ± 17	0.8	3.6
SUN	23.1 ± 1.3	26.2 ± 0.8	41.4 ± 1.8	1.1	1.6

Values of glutamic oxalacetic transaminase (SGOT), glutamic pyruvic transaminase (SGPT), aldolase (SAld), and lactic dehydrogenase (SLDH) are expressed as units/ml of serum ± SEM. Serum urea nitrogen (SUN) values are expressed as mg/100 ml serum ± SEM. Values are for 8 unexercised, 14 trained, and 18 untrained rats, except for SLDH determinations of 13 unexercised controls [J. Garbus *et al.*, 1964].

in serum after physical work might be due to an activation of the normally present enzymes by the altered composition of serum under exercise, or, possibly, to a delay in their elimination as a consequence of – for instance – the reduced hepatic blood flow. Until now there are no clues for either of the two possibilities. In our studies on the alterations of cellular enzymes after addition of serum, we found inhibitory effects and also short-term activations [61]. However the latter were of minor extent and confined to some enzymes only.

Investigations on the elimination of injected enzymes brought no reliable connections between physical activity an the velocity of elimination.

Conclusions as to the origin of the elevated enzyme activities in serum after exercise can be drawn from the comparison of enzyme proportions.

Figure 8 shows the changes of the enzyme pattern of normal serum under exercise, referred to LDH = 100. For comparison, the serum pattern in acute idiopathic myoglobinuria is also plotted. The left and the right column shows the tissue patterns of liver and skeletal muscle respectively.

In these relative patterns, the isolated increase of the activities of CPK and ALD, which are very prominent in skeletal muscle, demonstrates, that the efflux of enzymes from the muscle alters the serum pattern. It is particularly evident in myoglobinuria and to a somewhat lesser extent under exercise, that the serum pattern approaches that of muscle tissue.

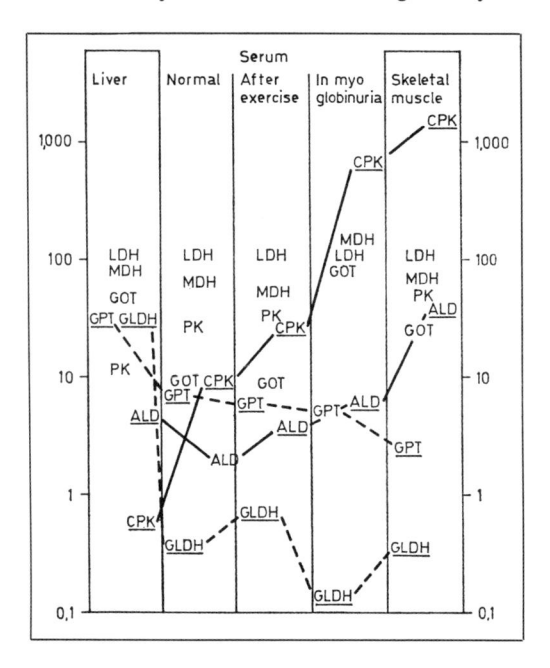

Figure 8.

Beside this dominating effect, the absence of a marked decrease of GPT and the relative elevation of the virtually liver specific GLDH show that under exertion an increased leakage of enzymes from the liver is also to be observed. These findings can be interpreted as an expression of the enhanced functional activity of the liver under exercise.

The cause for the efflux of enzymes under exercise is entirely unknown. Damage of muscle cells was considered to be responsible, especially after exhaustive work, in analogy to the elevation of serum enzyme activities owing to disease. As a morphologic proof for this assumption, ALTLAND [3] could demonstrate necrotic cells in the striated muscle fibers and fatty changes in heart, liver, kidney, and skeletal muscle of his untrained rats. Certainly these changes must be considered an extreme. In later publications, the same authors [20] reported that the necrotic muscle fibers constituted only a minute fraction of the total fibers and were not seen in many animals. The serum elevations were noted within two hours after beginning the exercise, before the appearance of fatty changes, and persisted long after fatty changes in the organs had disappeared. These findings

Table VI. Concentration gradients

	Skeletal muscle/ serum	Liver/serum
ALD	21 800	2 700
PK	6 200	1 400
LDH	1 400	1 400
MDH	2 000	2 600
GOT	5 700	9 000
GPT	750	7 600

Activities/g wet weight: activities/ml serum

suggest, that the enzymes are derived mainly from the cells showing no overt histologic changes, but probably having an altered cellular permeability appearing earlier and persisting longer than the fatty changes [20].

Several authors assume relative hypoxia of the active skeletal muscles to be the cause of the enzyme leakage. This is not probable because of the slight reduction of pO_2 during work [39], and because of the lack of a higher increase of enzyme activities after exertion under hypoxic conditions [35].

The causative effect of the increased release of catecholamines also appears to be unlikely, as shown by the investigations of GARBUS [20].

In view of the extremely high concentration gradients between the intra- and extracellular space and the lack of a static cell membrane, it appears more productive to us to raise the question, which active mechanisms maintain these concentration gradients in preventing the leakage of metabolites and enzymes. The present concept of active transport is mostly based upon observations on the transfer of small ions through red cell membranes. It can hardly be transferred to our problem, which may be defined as 'prevention of leakiness' [ZIERLER, 74, 75, 77] rather than as active transport.

From the morphological point of view, the so-called water-containing pores, the width and the charge of which determinate the membrane permeability, offer themselves as the sites of transfer. Their diameters are estimated to be 3 to 4 Å [19, 63, 66, 74]. Pores of this kind however are not permeable for molecules of the size of enzyme proteins, the smaller diameter of which lies in the range of 50 to 200 Å [10, 31, 49]. On the other hand, ZIERLER [74, 76] showed that the release rates of aldolase and potassium from skeletal muscle behave like their diffusion coefficients. Hence he suggests the same sites of release for both molecules.

ZIERLER [76] in his fundamental work on the release of aldolase postulates an oscillation of the cellular membrane, where smaller and larger gaps with altering localisation open and close alternately. This concept could substantiate that by stimulation of the muscle fibers the movements of the cell membrane become faster and the opening of the gaps more frequent. Metabolic lesions then would cause irregular movements and thus produce larger and longer persisting holes. Both mechanisms could contribute to an enhanced enzyme leakage.

On the other hand nobody has ever seen such holes. On the contrary, some years ago, WOHLFARTH-BOTTERMANN [70] pointed out that he was never able, in spite of greatest efforts, to produce naked protoplasm, because each gap was closed immediately by a demonstrable membrane, even if it was of traumatic origin.

In a modified manner the membrane oscillation with their openings of more than 100 Å postulated by ZIERLER, can be visualized and proven, if we extend our considerations to the micropinocytotic and cytopemptic processes, which begin or end within the interior of the cells during secretion or uptake of substances of higher molecular size [59, 64]. The cell membrane cannot be separated from the inner cellular structures, neither functionally, nor substantially, but is in permanent exchange. Thus we find it hard to stick to the definition of the cell membrane as a sort of skin with particularly reduced permeability.

It seems not reasonable, even not from the morphological point of view, to start the reflections on the leakage of enzymes at the cell membrane, as if the enzyme molecules were permanently assaulting this wall, in order to escape eventually, when it crumbles. It is more likely that the enzymes remain within the cell compartments at their sites of action, as long as sufficient energy is supplied to maintain the structural order. It is well known that disturbances of the cellular metabolic efficiency, which reduce energy output, cause morphological modifications and enzyme release as well [7, 15, 16, 30, 46, 47, 48, 54, 60, 65, 71, 72].

The dependance of enzyme release upon energy yield is only a global and therefore unsatisfactory answer to our initial question, which factors might prevent the leakage of enzymes.

Thus, explanations of the enzyme release during physical activity can be nothing but pure assumptions:

1. Under severe exertion there is a competition for the energy-rich phosphates, which results in a relative deficiency of structure-maintaining energy.

2. The efflux of enzymes is an undesired side-effect of the necessarily increased permeability under exercise, which serves for the accelerated exchange of substrates and products, and due to an incomplete selectivity of the limiting membranes. This possibility has been pointed out particularly by ZIERLER.

3. It can be suggested, though it is not likely, that aged enzymes, which are already impaired in their functional mobility and elasticity are not intracellularly removed, but released into the serum, or that

4. due to disturbances of translocation within the cell, enzymes produced newly and in greater amounts cannot be transferred from the ribosomes to their sites of action, but leak out into the serum in connection with the increased substrate exchange.

Further investigations must show, whether one of these suggestions holds true.

References

1. AHLBORG, B. and BROHULT, J.: Metabolic changes after long-term physical exercise. Särtryck ur Försvars medicin 2: 35 (1966).
2. AHLBORG, B.; BERGSTRÖM, J.; EKELUND, L. and HULTMAN, E.: Muscle glycogen and muscle electrolytes during prolonged physical exercise. Acta physiol. scand. 70: 129 (1967).
3. ALTLAND, P. and HIGHMAN, B.: Effects of exercise in serum enzyme values and tissues of rats. Amer. J. Physiol. 201: 393 (1961).
4. ALTLAND, P.; HIGHMAN, B. and NELSON, B. D.: Serum enzyme and tissue changes in rats exercised repeatedly at altitude: effects of training. Amer. J. Physiol. 214, 28 (1968).
5. BAUMANN, P.; ESCHER, J. und RICHTERICH, R.: Das Verhalten von Serum-Enzymen bei sportlichen Leistungen. Schweiz. Z. Sportmed. 10: 33 (1962).
6. BERGSTRÖM, J. and HULTMAN, E.: A study of the glycogen metabolism during exercise in man. Scand. J. clin. Lab. Invest. 19: 218 (1967).
7. BRUNS, F. H.; BROSSWITZ, E.; DENNEMANN, H.; HORN, H. D. und NOLTMANN, E.: Studien über die Ursachen des Enzym-Verlustes der geschädigten Zelle. Klin. Wschr. 39: 342 (1961).
8. CALVY, G. L.; CADY, L. D.; MUTSON, A.; NIERMAN, J. and GERTLER, M. M.: Serum lipids and enzymes. Their levels after high-caloric, high-fat intake and vigorous exercise regimen in Marine Corps recruit personnel. J. amer. med. Ass. 183: 1 (1963).
9. CANTONE, A. and CERTELLI, P.: The effect of muscle work on serum aldolase activity in trained and untrained men. Int. Z. angew. Physiol. 18: 107 (1960).
10. COLOWICK, S. P. and KAPLAN, N. O.: Methods in Enzymology. Acad. Press N.Y. 1955.

11. Cori, C. F.: Regulation of enzyme activity in muscle during work. in: Enzymes: Units of biological structure and function. Ed. O. H. Gaebler Acad. Press N. Y. 1956, p. 573.
12. Cornelius, C. E.; Burnham, L. G. and Hill, H. E.: Serum transaminase activities of thoroughbred horses in training. J. amer. vet. med. Ass. *142:* 639 (1963).
13. Critz, J. B.: The effect of exercise on tissue and serum glutamic-oxalacetic transaminase. Dissertation Abstr. *22:* 2852 (1962).
14. Critz, J. B. and Merrick, A. W.: Serum glutamic oxalacetic transaminase levels after exercise in men. Proc. Soc. exper. Biol. *109:* 608 (1962).
15. Dawson, D. M.: Efflux of enzymes from chicken muscle. Biochim. Biophys. Acta *113:* 144 (1966).
16. Dinman, B. D.; Hamdi, E. A.; Fox, C. F. and Frajola, W. J.: CCl_4 toxicity. III. Hepato-structural and enzymatic changes. Arch. environm. Hlth *7:* 630 (1963).
17. Eccles, J. C.: The effects of nerve cross union on muscle contraction; in: Exploratory Concepts in Muscular Dystrophy and Related Disorders. Exerpta, Med. Foundation. Internat. Congr., Ser. No. 147, Amsterdam, New York, London 1967, p. 151.
18. Fowler, W. M.; Chowdhury, S. R.; Pearson, C. M.; Gardner, G. and Bratton, R.: Changes in serum enzyme levels after exercise in trained and untrained subjects. J. appl. Physiol. *17:* 943 (1962).
19. Frey-Wyssling, A.: Submikroskopische Zytologie. Nova Acta Leopoldina *22:* 147 (1960).
20. Garbus, J.; Highman, B. and Altland, P.: Serum enzymes and lactic dehydrogenase isoenzymes after exercise and training in rats. Amer. J. Physiol. *207:* 467 (1964).
21. Glick, J. L. and Cohen, W. D.: Nocturnal changes in oxidative activities of rat liver mitochondria. Science *143:* 1184 (1964).
22. Glick, J. L. and Bronk, J.: The effect of exercise on the rate of oxygen uptake by rat liver mitochondria. Biochem. Biophys. Acta *82:* 167 (1964).
23. Glick, J. L.: Effects of exercise on oxidative activities in rat liver mitochondria. Amer. J. Physiol. *210:* 1215 (1966).
24. Golisch, G.; Pette, D. und Pichlmeir, H.: Einflüsse der Innervation auf das Enzymaktivitätsmuster weisser und roter Skelettmuskeln. Z. klin. Chem. *3:* 202 (1965).
25. Gollnick, P. D. and Hearn, G. R.: Lactic dehydrogenase activities of heart and skeletal muscle of exercised rats. Amer. J. Physiol. *201:* 694 (1961).
26. Gollnick, P. D.; Struck, P. J. and Boggo, T. P.: Lactic dehydrogenase activities of rat heart and sceletal muscle after exercise and training. J. appl. Physiol. *22:* 623 (1967).
27. Gould, M. K. and Rawlinson, W. A.: Biochemical adaptation as a response to exercise. 1. Effect of swimming on the levels of lactic-dehydrogenase, malic-dehydrogenase and phosphorylase in muscles of 8-, 11-, and 15-week-old rats. Biochem. J. *73:* 41, 44 (1959).
28. Griffith, P. G.: Serum-levels of ATP: Creatine-Phosphotransferase (Creatine-Kinase). The normal range and effect of muscular activity. Clin. chim. Acta *13:* 413 (1966).
29. Gutman, E.: Basic muscle type differentiation; in: Exploratory Concepts in Muscular Dystrophy and Related Disorders. Exerpta Med. Foundation. Internat. Congr., Ser. No. 147, Amsterdam, New York, London 1967, p. 132.

30. Hanson, H. und Bohley, P.: Enzym-Freisetzung während der Perfusion autolysierender Rattenlebern. Hoppe-Seylers Z. physiol. Chem. *337:* 32 (1964).
31. Haurowitz, F.: Chemistry and biology of proteins. Acad. Press N.Y. (1950).
32. Hearn, G. R. and Wainio, W. W.: Succinic dehydrogenase activity of the heart and skeletal muscle of exercised rats. Amer. J. Physiol. *185:* 348 (1956).
33. Hearn, G. R. and Wainio, W. W.: Aldolase activity of the heart and skeletal muscle of exercised rats. Amer. J. Physiol. *190:* 206 (1957).
34. Helmreich, E. and Cori, C. F.: Regulation of glycolysis in muscle. In: Advances in Enzyme Regulation. Vol. 3 Ed. G. Weber Pergamon Press (1956) p. 91.
35. Hollmann, W.; Schlüssel, H. und Spechtmeyer, H.: Einige Enzym-Spiegel bei dosierter dynamischer und statischer Arbeit unter Atmung variabler O_2-Gemische. Sportarzt und Sportmed. (1965), p. 166.
36. Holloszy, J. O.: Biochem. adaptations in muscle. Effects of exercise on mitochondrial oxygen uptake and respiratory enzyme activity in skeletal muscle. J. Biol. Chem. *242:* 2278 (1967).
37. Kendrick-Jones, J. and Perry, S. V.: Enzymatic adaptation to contractile activity in skeletal muscle. Nature *208:* 1068 (1965).
38. Kendrick-Jones, J. and Perry, S. V.: Biochemical adaption in muscle. In Exploratory Concepts in Muscular Dystrophy and Related Disorders. Exerpta Med. Foundation. Intern. Congr. Ser. No. 147, Amsterdam, New York, London 1967, p. 64.
39. Keul, J.; Doll, E. and Keppler D.: The substrate supply of the human skeletal muscle at rest, during and after work. Experientia *23:* 977 (1967).
40. Küstner, W.; Paetzel, A. und Weinreich, J.: Veränderungen der Kreatin-Phosphokinase-Aktivität im Serum bei körperlicher Belastung. Med. Klin. *47:* 1858 (1966).
41. Laguens, R. P.; Lozada, B. B.; Gómez-Dumm, C. L. and Beramendi, A. R.: Effect of acute and exhaustive exercise upon the fine structure of heart mitochondria. Experientia *22:* 244 (1966).
42. Laguens, R. P. and Gómez-Dumm, C. L. A.: Fine structure of myocardial mitochondria in rats after exercise for one-half to two hours. Circulat. Res. *21:* 271 (1967).
43. Laudahn, G.; Heyck, H. und Feustel, F.: Enzyme im Serum bei Muskelkrankheiten. Symp. über prakt. Enzym-Diagnostik. Ed. F. W. Schmidt, Huber Verlag Bern 1968, p. 249.
44. Lawrie, R. A.: The activity of the cytochrome system in muscle and its relation to myoglobin. Biochem. J. *55:* 298 (1953).
45. Massarrat, S. und Lang, N.: Änderungen der Aktivitäten von SGOT, SGPT und anderen Serumenzymen sowie des Bromsulphthaleintestes unter körperlicher Belastung bei entzündlich aktiven und inaktiven Lebererkrankungen. Gastroenterologia (Basel), Suppl. ad Vol *97:* 231 (1962).
46. Matschinsky, F. und Wieland, O.: Über Serumveränderungen und Störungen der Mitochondrienfunktion bei experimenteller Phalloidin-Vergiftung. Biochem. Z. *333:* 33 (1960).
47. McLean, A. E. M.: Leakage of enzymes from human and rat liver slices. Biochem. J. *89:* 54 (1963).
48. Möhr, J. R.: Untersuchungen über den Austritt von Zellenzymen unter der Einwirkung verschiedener Gifte am Modell der isolierten perfundierten Rattenleber. Diss. Marburg/Lahn 1965.
49. Netter, H.: Theoretische Biochemie. 288 ff. (Springer, Berlin/Göttingen/Heidelberg 1959).

50. OTTO, P.; SCHMIDT, E. und SCHMIDT, F. W.: Enzymspiegel im Serum bei körperlicher Arbeit und ambulanten Patienten. Klin. Wschr. *42:* 75 (1964).
51. PAUL, M. H. and SPERLING, E.: Cyclophorase system. XXIII. Correlation of cyclophorase activity and mitochondrial density in striated muscle. Proc. Soc. exp. Biol. N.Y. *79:* 352 (1952).
52. PETER, J. B.; JEFFRES, R. N. and LAMB, D. R.: Exercise: effects on hexokinase activity in red and white skeletal muscle. Science *160:* 200 (1968).
53. PETTE, D.: Energieliefernder Stoffwechsel des Muskels unter zellphysiologischem Aspekt. In Symp. über progressive Muskeldystrophie, p. 492. Ed. E. Kuhn, Springer Verlag, Berlin/Heidelberg/New York (1966).
54. REES, K. R. and SINHA, K. P.: Blood enzymes in liver injury. J. path. Bact. *80:* 297 (1960).
55. RICHTER, K. und KONITZER, K.: Veränderungen der Aldolase-Aktivität im Blutserum bei Muskelarbeit. Klin. Wschr. *38:* 998 (1960).
56. RICHTERICH, R.; VERREY, R.; GAUTIER, R. und STAMPFLI, K.: Serum-Enzyme bei Blutspendern. I. Oxalacetat- und Pyruvat-Transaminase bei Rekruten mit Gelbsuchtanamnese. Schweiz. Med. Wschr. *91:* 601 (1961).
57. SANGSTER, J. F. and BEATON, J. R.: Alterations in enzyme activities as a consequence of exercise (swimming) in the rat. Proc. Soc. exper. Biol. *122:* 542 (1966).
58. SCHMIDT, E. und SCHMIDT, F. W.: Zur Pathophysiologie von enzymatischen Veränderungen bei Lebererkrankungen. In Fortschritte der Gastroenterologie. Ed. E. WILDHIRT. Urban und Schwarzenberg, München 1960.
59. SCHMIDT, W.: Morphologische Aspekte der Stoffaufnahme und intrazellulären Stoffverarbeitung, Sekretion und Exkretion p. 147, Springer Berlin/Göttingen/Heidelberg 1965.
60. SCHMIDT, E.; SCHMIDT, F. W.; HERFARTH, C.; OPITZ, K. und VOGELL, W.: Analyse des bei Perfusion unter Hypoxie entstehenden intrazellulären Enzym-Musters. III. Mitt. über Studien zum Austritt von Zellenzymen am Modell der isolierten perfundierten Rattenleber. Enzym. biol. clin.*7:* 185 (1966).
61. SCHMIDT, E.; SCHMIDT, F. W. und HERFARTH, C.: Studien zum Austritt von Zell-Enzymen am Modell der isolierten, perfundierten Rattenleber. Enzym. biol. clin. *7:* 53 (1966).
62. SCHNEIDER, K. W. und HEISE, E. R.: Die diagnostische Bedeutung einer erhöhten Kreatin-Phosphokinase-Aktivität im Serum. Dtsch. Med. Wschr. *88:* 520 (1963).
63. SOLOMON, A. K.: Measurement of the equivalent pore radius in cell membranes. Membrane Transport and metabolism. Proc. Symp. Prag 1960, p. 4 Acad. Press N.Y. 1961.
64. STAUBESAND, J.: Cytopempsis, Sekretion und Exkretion p. 162, Springer Berlin/Göttingen/Heidelberg 1965.
65. STREFFER, C. and WILLIAMSON, D. H.: The effect of calcium ions on the leakage of protein and enzymes from rat liver slices. Biochem. J. *95:* 552 (1965).
66. THEORELL, T.: Attempt to formulate quantitative theory of membrane permeability. Proc. Soc. exper. Biol. *33:* 282 (1935).
67. ULLRICH, W.: Über das Verhalten der Serum-Transaminasen bei Trabrennpferden nach Bewegungs-Belastung. Wien. tierärztl. Mschr. *33:* 95 (1966).
68. VOGELL, W.: Phasen der Bildung morphologischer und enzymatischer Muster des Flugmuskels der Wanderheuschrecke. Naturwissenschaften *52:* 465 (1965).
69. VETTER, K.; GRIESCHE, H. und MOCH, K.: Serumfermente und ihr Verhalten unter physiologischen Bedingungen. Z. ges. inn. Med. *17:* 359 (1961).
70. WOHLFARTH-BOTTERMANN, K. E.: Diskussionsbemerkung zum Vortrag von

A. Sievers: Funktion des Golgi-Apparates in pflanzlichen und tierischen Zellen. Sekretion und Exkretion. p. 118, Springer/Berlin/Göttingen/Heidelberg 1965.

71. Wolfson, S. K., Jr.; Spencer, J. A.; Sterkel, R. L. and Williams-Ashman, H. G.: Clinical and experimental studies on serum pyridine nucleotide linked dehydrogenases in liver damage. Ann. N. Y. Acad. Sci. *75:* 260 (1958).

72. Wrogemann, K.: Untersuchungen über den Austritt von Zellenzymen aus der akut oder chronisch vorgeschädigten isolierten perfundierten Rattenleber. Diss. Marburg/Lahn 1966.

73. Yakovlev, N. N.: Sechenov J. Physiol. *36:* 744 (1950); Yampolskaya, L. I. a. Yakovlev, N. N.: Sechenov J. Physiol. *37:* 110 (1951); Yampolskaya, L. I.: Sechenov J. Physiol. *38:* 91 (1952). (cited from Gould, M. K. 1959).

74. Zierler, K. L.: Movement of aldolase from excised rat diaphragm. Amer. J. Physiol. *185:* 1 (1956).

75. Zierler, K. L.: Diffusion of aldolase from rat sceletal muscle. An index of membrane permeability. Amer. J. Physiol. *190:* 20 (1957).

76. Zierler, K. L.: Increased muscle permeability to aldolase produced by depolarization and by metabolic inhibitors. Amer. J. Physiol. *193:* 534 (1958).

77. Zierler, K. L.: Muscle membrane as a dynamic structure and its permeability to aldolase. Ann. N.Y. Acad. Sci. *75:* 227 (1958).

Author's address: Prof. Dr. F. W. Schmidt Medizinische Hochschule Hannover, Medizinische Klinik, Abteilung für Gastroenterologie, *3 Hannover*, Osterfeldstrasse 5 (Germany).

Biochemistry of Exercise.
Medicine and Sport, Vol. 3; pp. 239–244 (Karger, Basel/New York 1969)

The Immediate and Chronic Effect of Exercise on the Number and Structure of Skeletal Muscle Mitochondria

P. D. GOLLNICK and D. W. KING

Exercise Physiology Laboratory, Department of Physical Education for Men and Electron Microscope Laboratory Washington State University, Pullman, Wash.

Adenosine triphosphate (ATP) is generated within the cell primarily in the mitochondria. Oxidation by these organelles produces about 95% of the total energy made available to the cell. The oxidative capacity of a given tissue is therefore dependent upon its mitochondrial concentration. Thus, the red fibers of mammalian muscle that engage in sustained activtiy have high oxidative capacity and many mitochondria, whereas the white fibers that are fast acting with little endurance have low oxidative capacity and few mitochondria. Similarly, the flight muscles of migratory birds have more mitochondria than those in nonmigratory birds, while the nonflying domestic chicken has relatively few mitochondria in these same muscles [7].

Recently it has been shown that the shape and total mass of mitochondria in the myocardium can be changed in rats and dogs by a single swim to exhaustion [5, 6]. A training program of swimming up to 6 h/day also produced an increase in the total mitochondrial mass of rat myocardium [1]. HOLLOSZY [4] has reported that a training program of strenuous running increased the oxidative capacity, total protein and enzymatic activity of the mitochondrial fraction of rat skeletal muscle.

The effects of training and exhaustive exercise on the mitochondria of rat gastrocnemius muscle were investigated in the present study. Comparisons were also made between exhaustion of trained rats by running and untrained rats by swimming.

Materials and Methods

Twenty male rats of the Sprague-Dawley strain with initial body weights ranging from 180–200 g were used in the study. Eight of these rats were trained to exercise in motor-driven work wheels. After 4 weeks all were capable of running continuously for 60 min at 1.0 mph or faster. Each animal ran 40 min at 1.0 mph followed by 20 min at 1.4 mph each day for an additional 6 weeks.

Four of the trained rats were killed immediately after running to exhaustion at speeds between 1.0 and 2.0 mph and the remaining four rats were killed 24 h later. Four of the sedentary rats were sacrificed at rest, while the remaining 8 swam to exhaustion in groups of 4 in 35°C water. Four of these fatigued rats were killed immediately at the point of exhaustion and the remaining four 2 h later.

The animals were sacrificed by decapitation. Samples form the belly of the relaxed gastrocnemius muscle were quickly removed, fixed in cold 1% osmium tetroxide in barbital acetate buffer and embedded in Epon [8]. Longitudinal sections were stained with uranyl acetate and REYNOLDS lead acetate [9, 10] and examined with a Philips 100 B electron microscope. Micrographs were made at 2,600 diameters and enlarged photographically to 25,000 and 60,000 diameters for evaluation of number and size of mitochondria. Mitochondrial counts were made in an area (arbitrary units) and expressed as mitochondria/100 square microns.

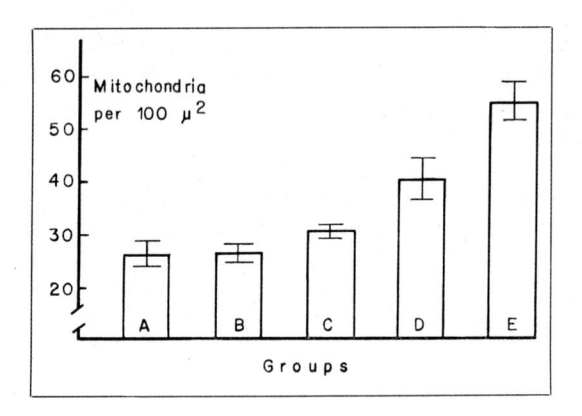

Figure 1. Mitochondrial concentration in rat skeletal muscle after various expermental treatments. Groups are: A. Untrained rats sacrificed at rest; B. Untrained animals killed immediately after being exhausted by swimming; C. Untrained rats killed 2 h after being exhausted by swimming; D. Trained rats killed at the point of exhaustion produced by running; and E. Trained animals sacrificed 24 h after a final exercise bout.

Number and Structure of Skeletal Muscle Mitochondria

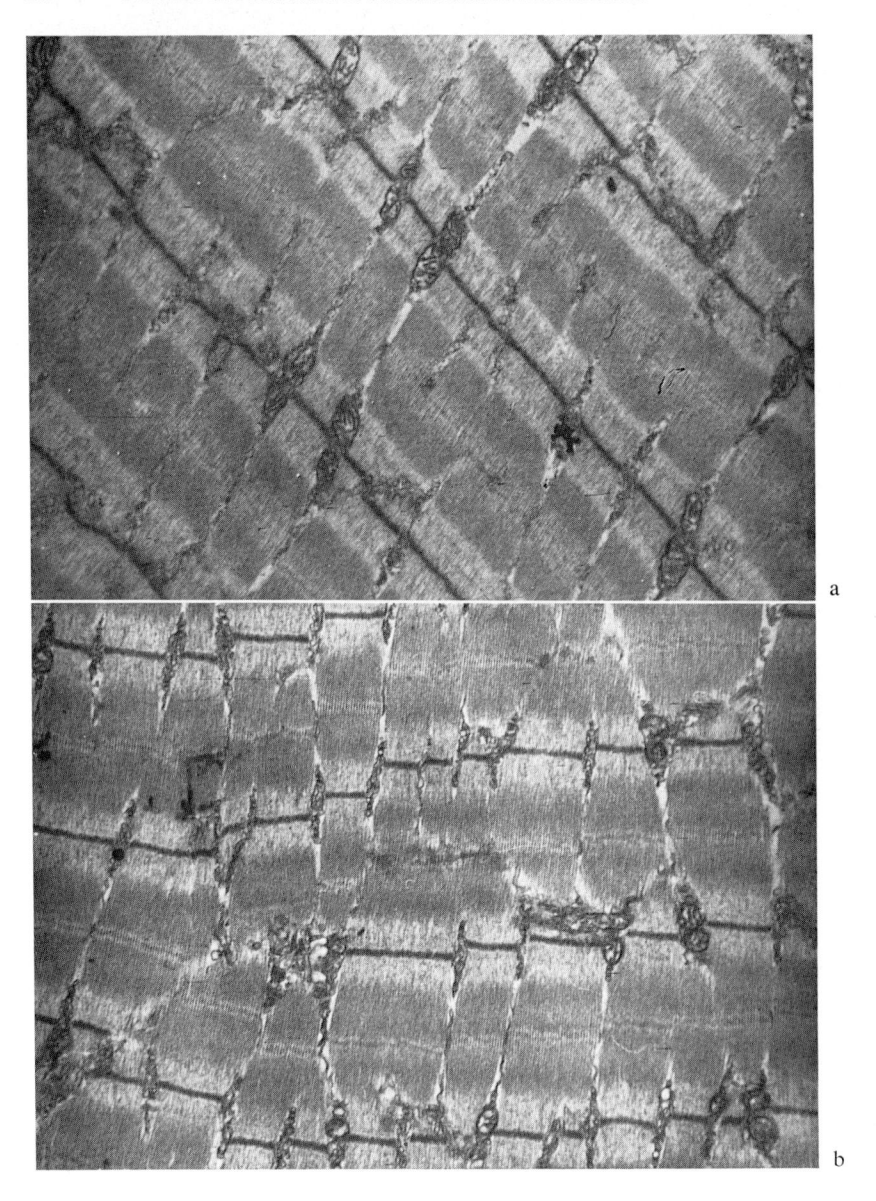

Figure 2. Skeletal muscle from untrained rats. a. Rats killed at rest and b. rats sacrificed immediately after becoming exhausted while swimming (10,050×).

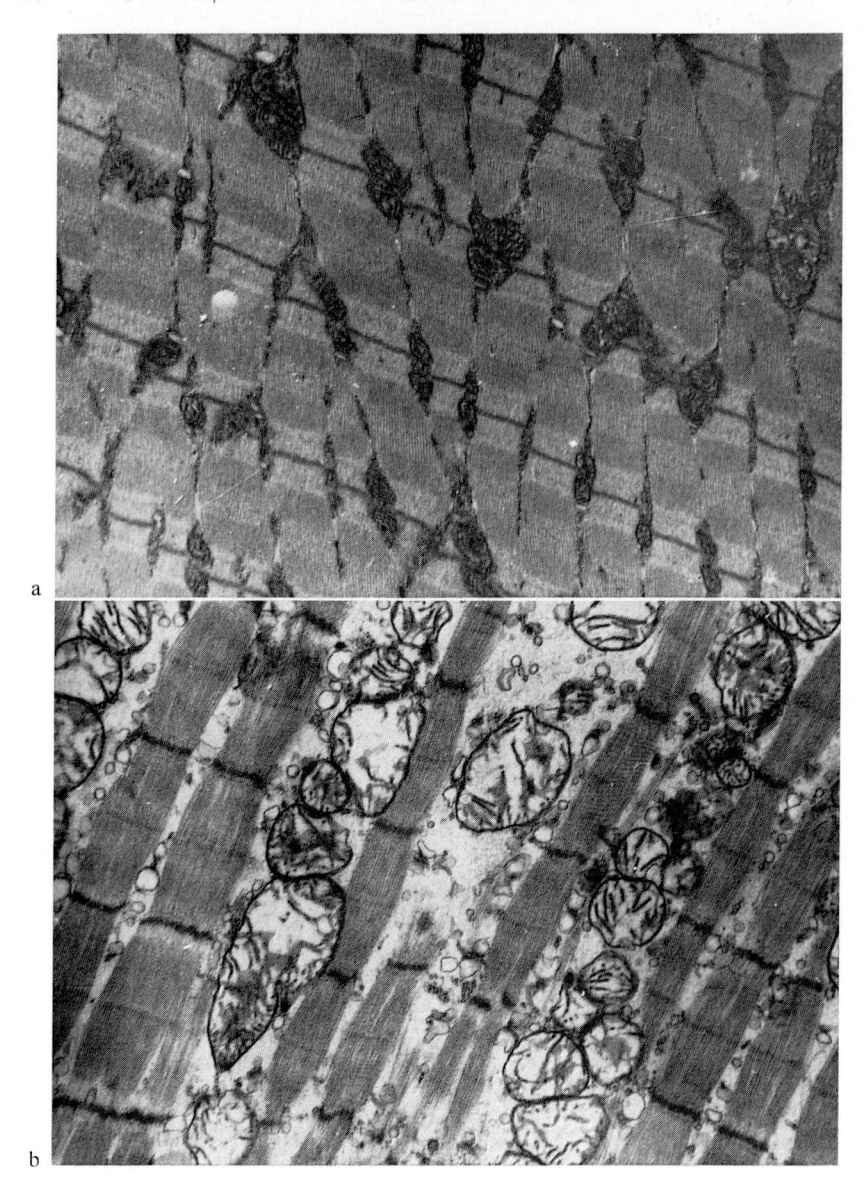

Figure 3. Skeletal muscle from trained rats. a. Animals sacrificed 24 h after a final exercise bout and b. those killed immediately after an exhaustive run (10,050 ×).

Results

The gastrocnemius muscles of the trained rats contained more than twice as many mitochondria per unit area as sedentary controls (figure 1). Swimming to exhaustion did not significantly alter the concentration of mitochondria in the skeletal muscle of the sedentary group. However, a slight reduction in number of mitochondria/100 square microns did occur in the muscles of the animals killed immediately after an exhaustive run.

Mitochondria in the skeletal muscle of trained rats were not only more numerous, but also appeared to be larger with more densely packed cristae (figure 3). After running to exhaustion gross swelling in both the tissue and mitochondria was observed in the skeletal muscle. Similar changes did not occur in the gastrocnemius muscle of the untrained rats killed immediately or 2 h after a swim to exhaustion.

Discussion

The increased mitochondrial concentration in muscle from trained rats of this study is consistant with the report of HOLLOSZY [4] that a similar training program produced an augmented oxidative capacity of skeletal muscle. The enlargement of the mitochondria and increase in cristae concentration in the muscles of the trained animals killed 24 h after exercise is also indicative of an increased metabolic capacity. The severity of the exercise used for training apparently is an important factor in determining whether these metabolic adaptations occur in skeletal muscle because they do not occur in the rat after a program of daily swimming [3, 4].

The swelling in the skeletal muscle of the rats killed after running to exhaustion was probably responsible for reducing the mitochondrial concentration of this group. This reduction, however, was probably more apparent than real and was no doubt caused by a reduction in myofibillar tissue in the counting area due to spreading of the tissue during swelling. That this disruption is temporary was evidenced by the fact that it did not exist in the muscles of trained animals killed 24 h after exhaustion.

The massive swelling of the mitochondria may have metabolic significance for the working muscle. Studies with isolated mitochondria have shown that partial or complete uncoupling of oxidative phosphorylation is associated with swelling [2, 11, 12]. This would reduce the efficiency of the ATP produced per unit of oxygen consumed. Post-exercise oxygen uptake might also be adversely affected by such an uncoupling.

Acknowledgement

We express our sincere thanks to Dr. A. L. Cohen of the Electron Microscope Laboratory for his advice and consultation.

References

1. Arcos, J. C.; Sohal, S.-C.; Argus, M. F. and Burch, G. E.: Changes in ultrastructure and respiratory control in mitochondria of rat heart hypertrophied by exercise. Exp. Molec. Path. *8:* 49–65 (1968).
2. Burgos, M. H.; Aoki, A. and Sacerdote, F.: Ultrastructure of isolated kidney mitochondria treated with phlorizin and ATP. J. Cell Biol. *23:* 207–215 (1964).
3. Hearn, G. H. and Wainio, W. W.: Succinic dehydrogenase of the heart and skeletal muscle of exercised rats. Amer. J. Physiol. *185:* 348–350 (1956).
4. Holloszy, J. O.: The effects of exercise on mitochondrial oxygen uptake and respiratory activity in skeletal muscle. J. biol. Chem. *242:* 2278–2282 (1967).
5. Laguens, R. and Gomez-Dumm, C. L. A.: Fine structure of myocardial mitochondria in rats after exercise for one-half to two hours. Circulat. Res. *21:* 271–279 (1967).
6. Laguens, R. P.; Lozada, B. B. and Gomez-Dumm, C. L. A.: Effect of acute and exhaustive exercise upon the fine structure of heart mitochondria. Experientia. *22:* 244–246 (1966).
7. Paul, M. H. and Sperling, E.: Cyclophorase system. XXIII. Correlation of cyclophorase activity and mitochondrial density in straited muscle. Proc. Soc. exp. Biol., N.Y. *79:* 352–354 (1952).
8. Pease, D. C.: Histological techniques for electron microscopy. 2nd ed., p. 381 (Academic Press/New York 1964).
9. Reynolds, E. W.: The use of lead citrate at high pH as an electron-opaque stain in electron microscopy. J. Cell Biol. *17:* 208–212 (1963).
10. Watson, M. L.: Staining of tissue sections for electron microscopy with heavy metals. II. Applications of solutions containing lead and barium. J. biophys. biochem. Cytol. *4:* 727–730 (1958).
11. Weinbach, E. C.; Garbus, J. and Sheffield, H. G.: Morphology of mitochondria in the coupled, uncoupled and re-coupled states. Exp. Cell Res. *46:* 129–143 (1967).
12. Weinbach, E. C.; Sheffield, H. and Garbus, J.: Restoration of oxidative phosphorylation and morphological integrity to swollen, uncoupled mitochondria. Proc. nat. Acad. Sci., Wash. *50:* 561–568, (1963).

Authors' address: P. D. Gollnick and D. W. King, Exercise Physiology Laboratory. Dept. of Physical Education for Men and Electron Microscope Laboratory, Washington State University, *Pullman, Wash. 99163* (USA).

L'influence du travail musculaire systématique sur l'activité des ferments du métabolisme du glycogène et de G-6-P dans les muscles et dans le foie

N. N. YAKOVLEV

Institut Scientifique de Culture physique, Leningrad

Les recherches de l'école de A. PALLADINE [1] et de notre Laboratoire [2, 3] ont établi que sous l'influence du travail musculaire systématique a lieu un accroissement du potentiel énergétique des muscles et de l'organisme en tout; l'augmentation des possibilités de l'utilisation des sources d'énergie et de leur restitution, l'amélioration de la stabilité de l'homéostase en présence de l'activité musculaire intense [5]. Cela a permis dès 1953 de qualifier comme adaptifs les changements biochimiques qui surviennent à la suite de l'entraînement. Leur réalisation est due avant tout à l'accroissement de l'intensité d'un nombre de systèmes fermentatifs [2–4].

Pour compréhension plus profonde des voies de l'adaptation biochimique de l'organisme au travail musculaire chez les rats blancs adultes (poids 180–200 g) on a étudié l'activité des ferments suivants: hexokinase (selon STEINER et KING), phosphoglucomutase (selon CRANE et SOLS), UDPG-pyrophosphorylase (selon MUNCH PETERSEN), UDPG-glycogène-synthétase (selon LELOIRE), phosphorylase (selon CORI et al.). On a analysé aussi la teneur en G-6-P (selon STEINER et WILLIAMS) dans les muscles et dans le foie et l'activité de G-6-phosphatase et de G-6-P-déhydrogénase (selon STÉPANOVA) dans le foie.

On a partagé les animaux en deux groupes: un groupe témoin et un groupe de rats entraînés à la natation pendant un mois. Le premier jour la durée de l'effort est de 5 min, ensuite cette durée est augmentée d'une minute chaque jour. Les animaux sont testés au repos, après 15 min et après une heure de natation, et enfin après une heure de repos.

Il se dégage des résultats des recherches (tableau I) que l'entraînement amène dans les muscles l'accroissement de l'activité de l'hexokinase, des deux formes de la glycogène-synthétase, des deux formes de la phosphorylase, mais l'activité de la phosphoglucomutase et de UDPG-pyrophosphorylase reste la même. Le taux du glucose-6-phosphate baisse. Dans le foie l'activité de la hexokinase, des deux formes du phosphorylase et de la glucose-6-phosphatase s'accroît. L'activité sommaire de la glycogène-synthétase ne change pas, mais on constate l'accroissement de l'activité de sa forme

Tableau I. L'influence de l'entraînement sur l'activité des ferments (m M substrate/1 g protéine/h) et sur la teneur en G–6–P (mg%) dans les muscles et dans le foie (M ± m)

Les groupes des animaux	Tissu	Hexo-kinase	Phospho-glucomu-tase	UDPG-pyro-phory-lase	UDPG-glycogène-synthétase Forme I	l'activité total (I + D)	G–6–p-déhydro-génase	G–6–phospha-tase	Phosphorylase sans AMP	Phosphorylase avec AMP	G–6–p
non-entraînés n = 10	Muscle	1 131 ± 25	2 936 ± 38	1 639 ± 33	49 ± 0,6	240 ± 2,3	–	–	39,8 · 10³ ± 881	47,2 · 10³ ± 981	858 ± 11
	Foie	275 ± 3,8	2 120 ± 31	1 613 ± 28	57 ± 1,2	238 ± 3	6 929 ± 94	1 725 ± 19	3 652 ± 77	4 391 ± 90	53 ± 0,7
entraînés n = 10	Muscle	1 579 ± 26 p > 0,01	2 952 ± 36 p = 0,9	1 576 ± 23 p = 0,3	62 ± 1,4 p < 0,01	292 ± 4,7 p > 0,01	–	–	49,1 · 10³ ± 2 167 p < 0,01	60,7 · 10³ ± 1 546 p < 0,01	695 ± 14 p < 0,01
	Foie	345 ± 4,5 p > 0,01	2 037 ± 33 p = 0,3	1 671 ± 13 p = 0,3	69 ± 1,2 p < 0,01	235 ± 4,5 p = 0,7	6 832 ± 88 p = 0,7	2 230 ± 29 p < 0,01	4 985 ± 92 p < 0,01	6 057 ± 73 p < 0,01	45 ± 1,5 p = 0,3

ne dépendant pas du glucose-6-phosphate, dû à l'interconversion d'une partie de la forme D en celle I. L'activité de la phosphoglucomutase, pyrophosphorylase, glucose-6-phosphate-dehydrogénase et le taux du glucose-6-phosphate ne changent pas. L'augmentation de l'activité des ferments dans les muscles et dans le foie fait +20 +40%. Les expériences montrent que l'activité des ferments qui sont moins actifs chez les animaux de contrôle, augmente. Une seule exception: la phosphorylase dont l'activité est très haute par comparaison aux autres ferments. La phosphorylase mise à part, les changements obtenus peuvent être considérés comme élargissement des points difficiles de la synthèse du glycogène dans les muscles et dans le foie et de la glycogénèse hépatique.

Au travail musculaire d'une seule fois l'activité de la phosphorylase non-activée par AMP devient plus intense et se développe plus tôt chez les animaux entraînés. L'activité de la forme «I» de UDPG-glycogène-synthétase subit un abaissement. Au repos l'activité de la forme «I» de UDPG-glycogène-synthétase est fort augmentée ainsi que la teneur en G-6-P. La diminution de l'activité de phosphorylase non-activée par AMP est aussi exprimée plus nettement chez les animaux entraînés au repos.

Ainsi, les animaux entraînés sont caractérisés par des changements plus brusques concernant la corrélation des fractions plus actives et moins actives de la phosphorylase et de la glycogène-synthétase ainsi que par des variations plus brusques du taux du glucose-6-phosphate ce qui assure de grandes possibilités du glycogénolyse des muscles et du foie à la période de travail et sa resynthèse au repos.

Il est à remarquer que le travail d'une seule fois ne change presque pas l'activité des ferments. Ce n'est pas seulement l'intensification de l'interconversion des formes moins actives en formes plus actives qui a lieu sous l'influence du travail musculaire systématique, mais aussi l'accroissement de l'activité générale des ferments.

Ce dernier phénomène ne peut pas être expliqué par des changements des corrélations ferment-substrat ou du changement de la teneur en co-enzymes, parce que dans les conditions de l'analyse enzymatique tous les substrats et co-facteurs ont été ajoutés dans les quantités optimales. Ce qui paraît le plus probable c'est l'augmentation de la quantité des protides enzymatiques, mais cela doit être soumis à une vérification rigoureuse.

On peut résumer les résultats des recherches en constatant que sous l'influence de l'entraînement les possibilités de la participation de la glucose aux transformations métaboliques augmentent, ainsi que les possibilités de la glycogénolyse et resynthèse du glycogène dans le foie et dans les muscles, et du glycogénèse hépatique.

Tout cela contribue à l'élargissement des possibilités de travail de l'organisme et peut être considéré comme un des aspects de l'adaptation de l'organisme au travail musculaire plus intense et plus prolongé.

Bibliographie

1. PALLADIN, A. V.: Issledovanya po biochimii mychecnoi trenirovki. Fisiol. Z. SSSR *19:* 278–289 (1935).
2. YAKOVLEV, N. N.: Biochimiceskie osnovy trenirovki mychz. Usp. sovr. biol. (russ.) *27:* 257–271 (1949).
3. YAKOVLEV, N. N.: Ocerki po biochimii sporta (Fiskultura i Sport, 1955).
4. YAKOVLEV, N. N.: Problema biochimiceskoi adaptacii mycz. Z. obchtchei biol. (russ.) *19:* 417–427 (1958).
5. YAKOVLEV, N. N. i YAKOVLEVA, E. S.: O sakonomernostiach biochimiceskoi i morfologiceskoi perestroiki mychz pod vlijaniem ich sistematiceskogo upraznenija. Usp. sovr. biol. (russ.) *35:* 134–151 (1953).

Adresse de l'auteur: Dr N. N. YAKOVLEV, Institut Scientifique de Culture physique *Leningrad* (USSR).

Enzymatic Activity in Normal, Trained and Inactivated Muscle

D. BÖHMER

Department of Anaesthesia, Orthopaedic Clinic, University of Frankfurt/Main
(Director: Prof. Dr. E. GÜNTZ)

The enzymatic activity of each cell corresponds with its metabolic function. Does the trained muscle show an increased enzymatic activity, or does the immobilized muscle reveal a decrease therein?

In order to answer this question we have homogenised normal, trained, immobilized and denervated muscles of man and rat and have determined the enzymatic amount of aldolase (ALD), creatine phosphokinase (CPK), glutamate pyruvate transaminase (GPT), glutamate oxalacetate transaminase (GOT), lactate dehydrogenase (LDH), adenosine triphosphate (ATP).

Human muscle tissue was obtained in orthopaedic operations. Following osteotomy and after removal of fixating metals, muscle tissue was taken from the same place again. Between these two operations the musculature had been immobilized by means of a plaster cast. Another group of patients received no plaster cast, they were ambulant after the first operation and received additional physiotherapy.

Following immobilization the ALD and CPK activity decreased. After inactivity of several months duration the changes were significant. One patient had an atonic paralysis of the arm musculature for many years. In this case the enzymatic activity was decreased to very low values, with the exception of GOT (figure 1).

Among the patients, who were able to walk soon after their operations and received additional physiotherapy the enzymatic activity was similar to that of normal musculature.

In all operated patients the activity of the transaminase was decreased, according to the duration of inactivity. Even a short immobilization decreases the LDH activity, regardless of the duration of immobilization. The ATP in the immobilized musculature is also lower. The favourable influence of the physiotherapy, which was given intensively to the patients who were immobilized for a long period of time, can be seen. The ATP shows in these cases again a slight increase.

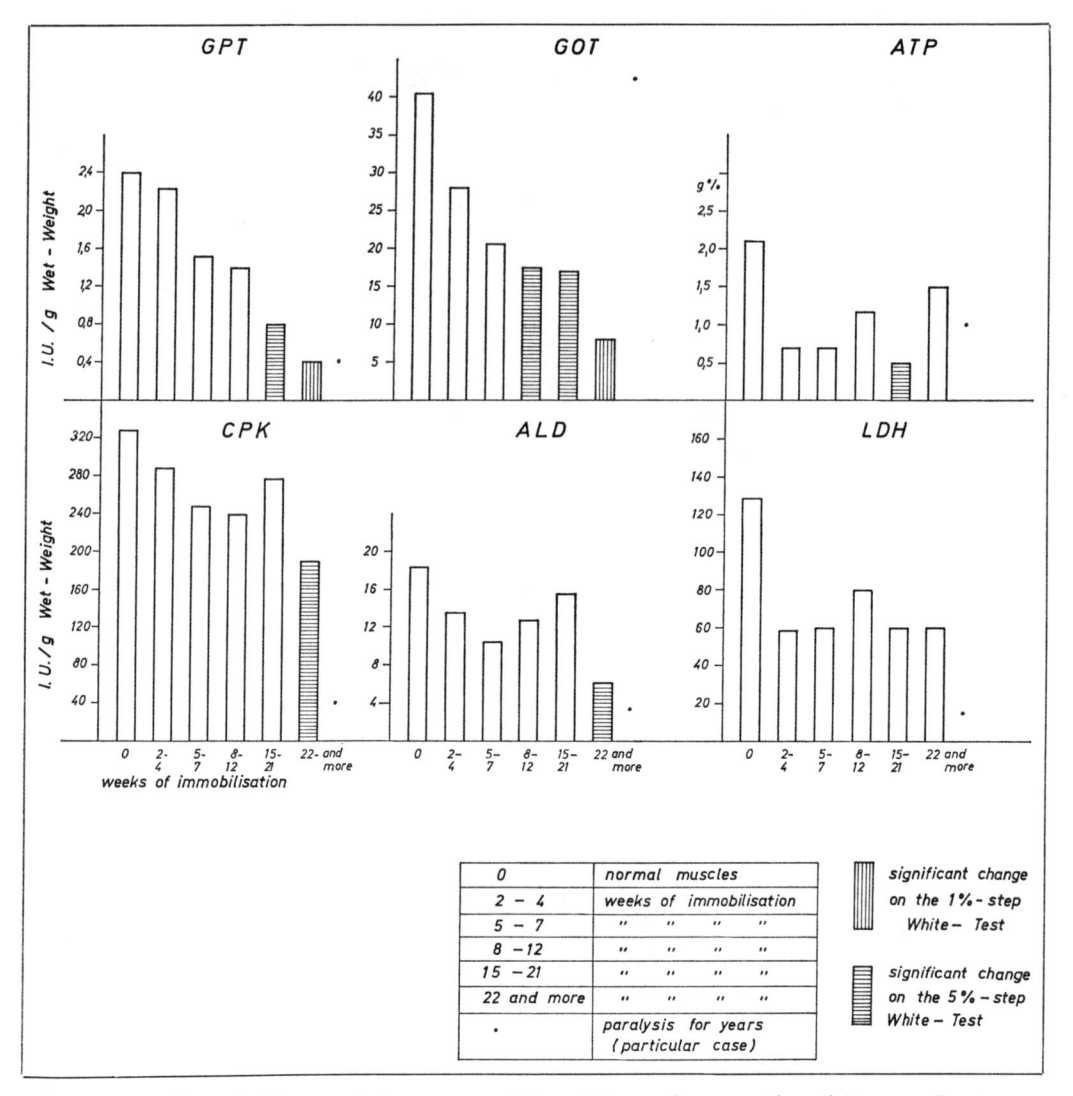

Figure 1. Enzymes in human musculature. Changes in enzymatic activity according to the duration of immobilisation.

The results, which were obtained from human showed variations, due to different basic conditions of each patient. We therefore undertook examinations on rats to support the results.

In one group of rats the posterior paw musculature was inactivated by denervation. In another group the rats went through a four weeks course

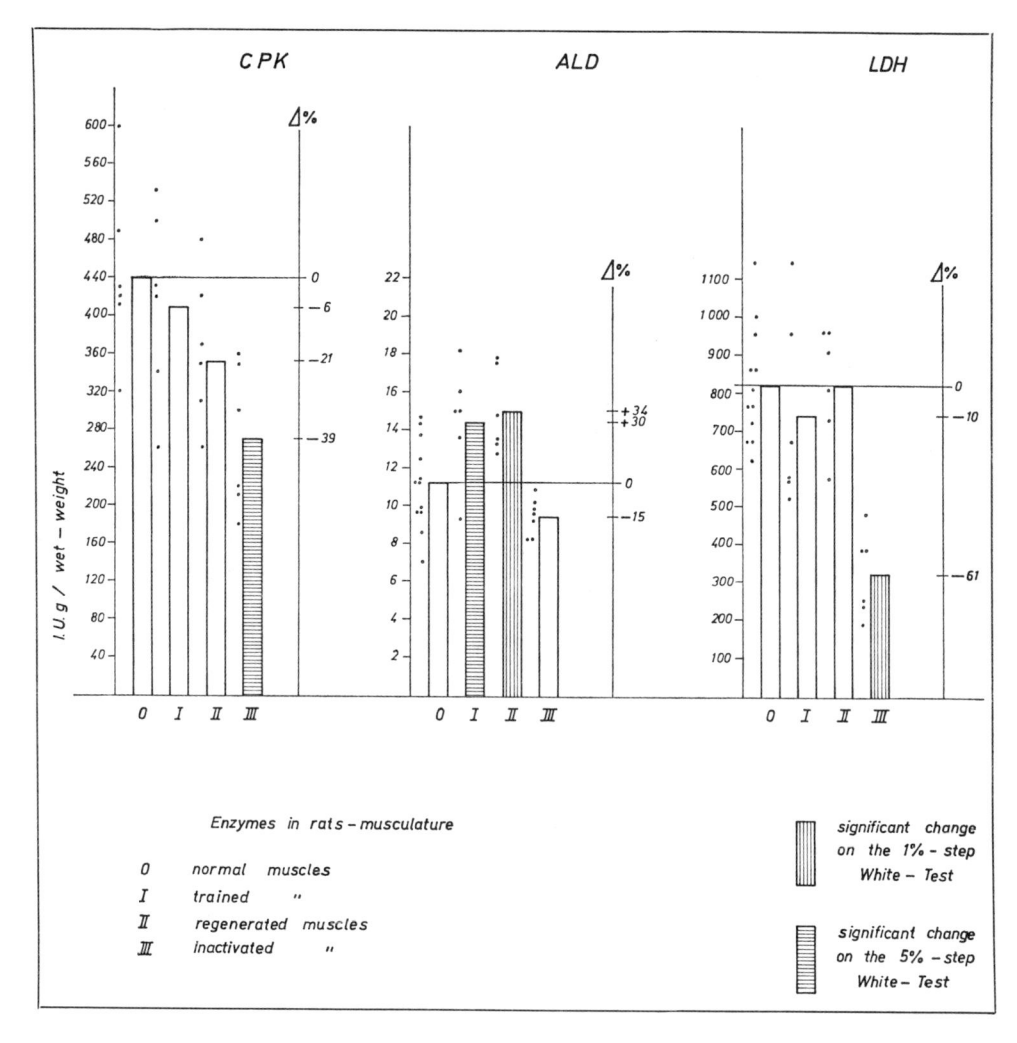

Figure 2.

of swimming, one hour daily. To be able to compare the results, as a standard, the musculature of the untreated animals of the same breed was taken.

From another group of rats a small piece of musculature was taken from the femoral muscle. After four weeks, musculature was taken again from the same place to show the influence of regeneration on enzymatic activity.

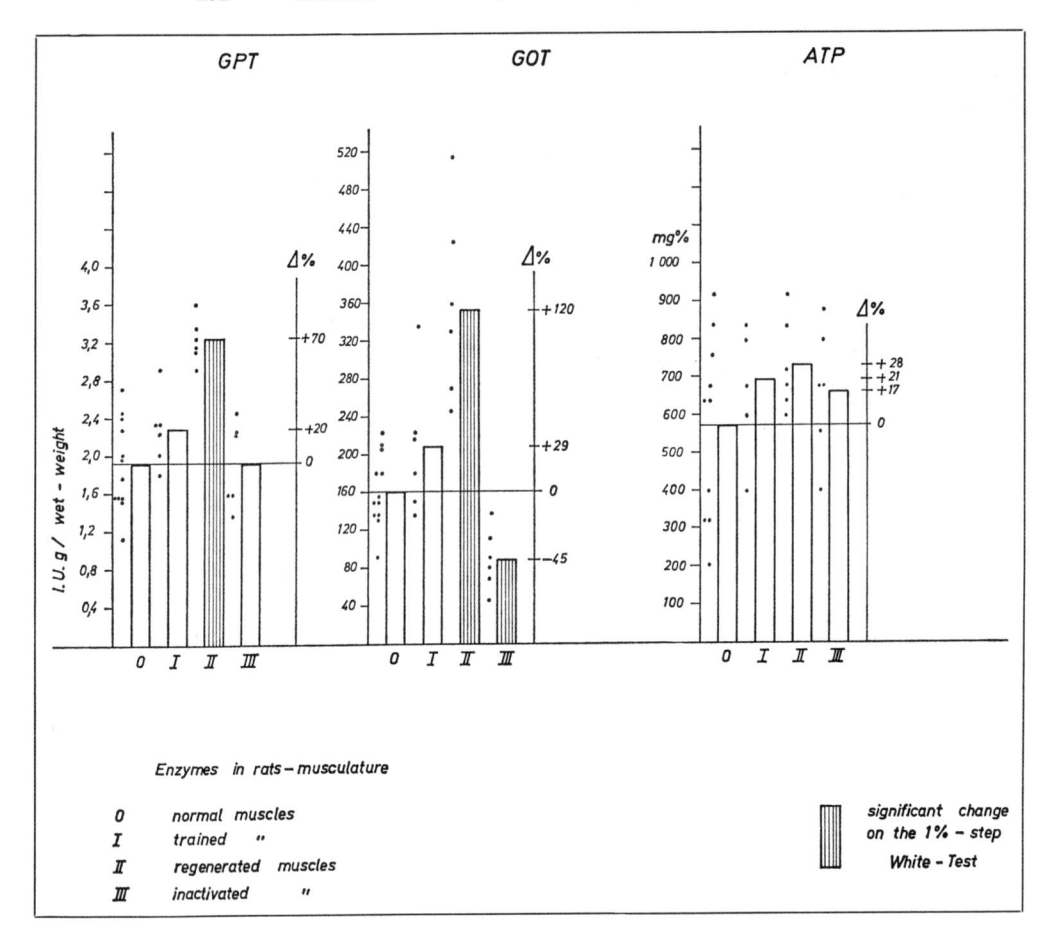

Figure 3.

In the trained musculature a significant rise in ALD activity was found, also the regenerated musculature showed a noticable increase. In the denervated muscle the activity slightly decreased. The CPK level did not show any significant changes, although the level was evidently decreased in the denervated muscle. The same applies for LDH activity (figure 2). The transaminases were a little higher on the trained rats, than on the control-group.

Significantly high values were found in the regenerated musculature. The ATP was almost equal in all groups (figure 3).

The experiments on rats show, that the swimming exercices were not very tiresome for the posterior paws. But the results support the opinion, gained on human musculature, that immobilization leads to a decreased activity in important cellular enzymes, apparently as a result of reduced metabolism.

Following longer training, an increase in enzymatic activity in the cell can be expected.

Summary

From orthopaedic patients, who had been operated twice, musculature was taken and examined. Between the two operations the patients were immobilized in a plaster cast. In these operated patients the enzymatic activity was decreased according to the duration of inactivity. Similar results were found on experiments with rats. With these rats we undertook swimming-exercises and came to the result, that some of the cell-enzymes increased due to the training. Significantly high values were also found in the regenerated musculature.

Author's address: Dr. DIETER BÖHMER, Chairman of the Department of Anaesthesia, Orthopaedic Clinic University of Frankfurt/Main, (Germany) *Frankfurt* – Niederrad, Marienburgstrasse 2.

Lactic Dehydrogenase Isoenzymes in Serum and Tissues after Exercise in Rats

J. Novosadová

Institute of Sports Medicine, Palacky University, Olomouc, Czechoslovakia

Serum enzyme levels rise markedly after strenuous exercise by men [2, 4, 6] and animals [1, 3, 5] untrained for such exertion. Exercise of lower intensity or exercise in trained subjects does not bring about such marked changes of serum enzymes. In the present paper the author tries to answer the question: what is the source of changed enzyme activity in dependence upon prior exercise? For this purpose the enzyme L-lactate: NAD oxidoreductase (lactic dehydrogenase, LDH) was used. It takes part in the metabolism, especially during the change of pyruvate into lactate, in working skeletal muscle under an absolute or relative shortage of oxygen during maximal stress.

Wieland [9], Wróblewski [11] and other authors have found by means of electrophoresis that in the liver, in the heart muscle and in the skeletal muscle the LDH fractions show specific qualities. Most often 5 of LDH isoenzymes which are specific for separate organs are described. Their picture changes in a characteristic manner in pathological conditions and is of diagnostic value. The isoenzymes LDH may indicate a potential tissue source of an increased level in the serum in dependence upon previous physical strain, which is accompanied by a relative hypoxia in working muscles.

Material and Methods

Groups of trained, control and untrained male rats of the Wistar strain with an initial weight of 160–180 g were used. The first group of 19 rats underwent a daily training on the treadmill for a period of 6 weeks. The velocity of the band was 15.7 m/min and the duration of exercises was increased up to 30 min. On the day of experiment the trained and untrained rats were exercised 30 min on identical velocity. Immediately after the exercise had ended, blood was withdrawn from the right heart under ether anaesthesia, the rats were killed, the heart muscle ectomized, as well as the liver and the gastrocnemius muscle.

LHD activity in the serum and in the homogenates of tissues was established by means of Boehringer's test and is expressed in miliunits/ml. An electrophoresis of the serum and the homogenates was made according to WIEME [10] in agar gel on a slide. The zones of LDH activity were visualised, according to VAN DER HELM [7], by using nitro-blue-tetrazolium. The values were estimated on a densitometer with the integrator ERI 65 at 560 nm and the percentage representation of fractions was calculated.

Results and Discussion

The serum and organ LDH values after exercise in trained and untrained rats in comparision with controls are demonstrated in table I. After a 30-min exercise there was a statistically significant decrease of LDH in the serum ($p<0.05$) in trained rats. In the untrained rats the same exercise brought about a statistically important increase of LDH activity ($p<0.05$). The greatest changes were manifested in the skeletal muscles. In both groups there was a decrease of LDH activity, which was significant in the trained animals ($p<0.01$). An almost identical and insignificant decrease of LDH was found in the heart muscle of both groups. The LDH activity decreased in the liver after exercise too, yet significantly only in the group of untrained rats ($p<0.05$).

This might indicate that the metabolism in active tissues is more economic in trained individuals following the same strain and the leakage of LDH from the cells into the outer environment, i.e. the blood serum through the cell barrier is intact during this type of stress.

Table I. Mean values with standard deviation of LDH activity in miliunits/ml in serum and organs in trained and untrained rats after exercise in comparison with controls

	N	Serum	Muscle	Heart	Hepar
I trained	19	100.82 ± 46.63	347.95 ± 71.24	307.24 ± 88.84	254.08 ± 63.90
II control	14	132.93 ± 36.50	425.10 ± 80.60	319.16 ± 50.75	278.20 ± 24.79
III untrained	14	168.02 ± 48.14	402.05 ± 81.99	313.62 ± 55.22	247.65 ± 39.17
p<		0.05	0.01		0.05

Table II. Mean values with standard deviation of % LDH isoenzymes in heart and skeletal muscle in trained and untrained rats after exercise in comparison with controls.

	N	%		Heart	Muscle
I trained	19	LDH	1	4.73	75.21 ± 8.56
			2	3.78	8.53
			3	16.22	5.37
			4	37.53 ± 3.62	5.89
			5	37.73 ± 5.87	5.00
II control	14	LDH	1	1.78	85.00 ± 9.17
			2	2.64	4.00
			3	17.00	3.64
			4	39.72 ± 6.95	3.58
			5	38.86 ± 3.81	3.78
III untrained	14	LDH	1	1.57	89.28 ± 9.76
			2	1.14	3.78
			3	13.00	2.36
			4	45.08 ± 3.36	2.36
			5	39.21 ± 5.54	2.22
$p<$				0.01	0.01

A similar finding in rats has been made by GARBUS et al. [3] who found in trained animals rather a decrease of LDH in the serum, whereas in untrained ones even a threefold increase. ALTLAND et al. [1] also found in untrained rats an increase of LDH and other enzymes after a prolonged exercise. They conclude on the basis of histopathological studies of organs, in which they had found slight to severe changes of transient character in hepatic cells, skeletal muscles and kidneys ranging from fatty changes to necrosis, that the serum LDH might come from different organs. They explain the cause of a changed permeability both by a relative hypoxia which develops in active organs, and further they take into consideration the role of the release of catecholamines from the adrenal medulla. ZIERLER [12] has demonstrated by his experiments *in vitro* that the cell permeability of the rat diaphragm and skeletal muscle increases for aldolase when there is a shortage of glucosis in an incubation environment. HIGHMAN et al. [8] have also demonstrated the effect of hypoxia on the increase of LDH in blood serum in the dogs, which were exposed to conditions of oxygen deprivation in a barochamber.

The changes of isoenzymes LDH in trained and untrained rats in comparision with controls are demonstrated in table II. Isoenzymogrammes of liver homogenates do not manifest any changes in the group of trained and untrained rats in comparision with the controls. Enzymogrammes of the blood serum show inconstant changes. In the skeletal muscle the decrease of the LDH_1 isoenzyme is significant ($p<0.01$) in the group of trained rats, whereas in untrained rats this fraction increases only insignificantly. It corresponds to the findings of the total LDH activity in the homogenate of the skeletal muscles. The heart muscle shows an insignificant decrease of the fraction LDH_5 and LDH_4 in trained animals. In untrained animals a significant increase of the fraction LDH_4 ($p<0.01$) has been found whilst the value of the fraction LDH_5 did not change.

GOLLNICK et al. [5] have also found an increase of LDH in the muscle of the heart chambers after physical exercise, whereas the LDH in the skeletal muscles remained unchanged. They show that the exercise which had been used was a higher stress for the heart muscle. The findings of GARBUS et al. [3] denote as possible source of an increased LDH activity in the serum of untrained individuals the isoenzymes from other organs as skeletal muscle, especially from the myocardium and kidneys.

The increase of LDH in the blood serum following physical exercise appears thus in individuals unadapted to such stress. The extent of changes depends upon the intensity and duration of exercise. This LDH has its origin in the active cells and its elimination is the manifestation of a changed permeability of the cell membrane which is caused by several factors which can be individual and specific.

Summary

1. A decrease of LDH activity in the blood serum and in the skeletal muscles and a decrease of the isoenzyme LDH_1 in the skeletal muscles were found in trained rats after exercise. In untrained rats after the same stress there was an increase of LDH activity in the blood serum, of the isoenzyme LDH_1 in the skeletal muscles and of LDH_4 in the myocardium.

2. The increased LDH activity in the blood serum of untrained subjects has its origin not only in the skeletal muscles, but especially in the myocardium.

3. The extent of changes depends upon prior adaptation to the stress that has been used and upon its duration.

4. The leakage into the serum through the cell membrane is caused by an increased permeability, the mechanism of which is discussed.

References

1. ALTLAND, P. D. and HIGHMAN, B.: Effect of exercise on serum enzyme values and tissues of rats. Amer. J. Physiol. *201:* 393–395 (1961).

2. Fowler, W. M., Jr.; Chowdhury, S. R.; Pearson, C. M.; Gardner, G. and Bratton, R.: Changes in serum enzyme levels after exercise in trained and untrained subjects. J. appl. Physiol. *17:* 943–946 (1962).
3. Garbus, J.; Highman, B. and Altland, P. D.: Serum enzymes and lactic dehydrogenase isoenzymes after exercise and training in rats. Amer. J. Physiol. *207:* 467–472 (1964).
4. Gardner, G. W.; Bratton, R.; Chowdhury, S. R.; Fowler, W. M., Jr., and Pearson, C. M.: Effect of exercise on serum enzyme levels in trained subjects. J. Sports Med. *4:* 103–110 (1964).
5. Gollnick, P. D. and Hearn, G. R.: Lactic dehydrogenase activities of heart and skeletal muscle of exercised rats. Amer. J. Physiol. *201:* 694–696 (1961).
6. Halonen, P. I. and Konttinen, A.: Effect of physical exercise on some enzymes in the serum. Nature, Lond. *193:* 942–944 (1962).
7. Helm, H. L. van der: A simplified method of demonstrating lactic dehydrogenase isoenzymes in serum. Clin. chim. Acta *7:* 124–128 (1962).
8. Highman, B. and Altland, P. D.: Serum enzyme rise after hypoxia and effect of autonomic blockade. Amer. J. Physiol. *199:* 981–986 (1960).
9. Wieland, T. und Pfleiderer, G.: Nachweis der Heterogenität von Milchsäure-Dehydrogenasen verschiedenen Ursprungs durch Trägerelektrophorese. Biochem. Z. *329:* 112–116 (1957).
10. Wieme, R. J.: An improved technique of agar-gel-electrophoresis on microscope slides. Clin. chim. Acta *4:* 317–322 (1959).
11. Wróblewski, F.: Multiple molecular forms of enzymes. Ann. N.Y. Acad. Sci. *94:* 655 (1961).
12. Zierler, K. L.: Muscle membrane as a dynamic structure and its permeability to aldolase. Ann. N.Y. Acad. Sci. *75:* 227–234 (1958).

Author's address: Dr. Jiřina Novosadová, tr. Spojencu 20a, *Olomouc* (Czechoslovakia).

The Effects of Exhaustive Effort on Serum Enzymes in Man

P. Block, M. Van Rijmenant, R. Badjou, A. Y. Van Melsem and R. Vogeleer

Laboratoire de l'effort (Prof. M. Segers)
Service de Médecine, d'Investigation clinique et de Chimie pathologique de l'Institut Bordet – Centre des Tumeurs de l'Université de Bruxelles
Faculté de Médecine de l'Université de Bruxelles
Laboratoire de Biologie clinique de l'Institut Médico-Chirurgical d'Ixelles (D^R. Vanderveiken) – Service de Médecine interne (D^R. Delcourt)
Centre d'Etude des Maladies des Artères Coronaires (CEMAC)

Introduction

This work was undertaken in order to assess the effect of an exhaustive effort on serum enzymes in healthy humans more than 40 years old, either sportsmen or not.

The following enzymes have been studied: serum glutamate-oxaloacetate transaminase (SGOT), serum glutamate-pyruvate transaminase (SGPT), creatine phosphokinase (CPK), lactic dehydrogenase (LDH) and the isoenzymes of LDH (LDH 1 to 5). The latter are numbered according to their electrophoretic mobility, the most rapid fraction being determined as LDH 1.

Laboratory Techniques and Norms

The determinations of SGOT and SGPT were done by colorimetry while U.V.-spectrophotometric methods were used for CPK and LDH. In all cases the Boehringer test combinations have been employed without modification.

For the electrophoresis of the LDH-isoenzymes, two techniques have been applied, both being slight modifications of the Agar gel electrophoretic method of Wieme [14]. In the first technique the nitro-blue tetrazolium (NBT) has been replaced by 2 (p-iodophenyl)-5(P-nitrophenyl)-5phenyl-tetrazoliumchloride (INT) and lactic acid enriched with the L (+) isomer is used as substrate. In the second technique the fractions are detected as described by Reesler and Joseph [11].

The normal values observed in 45 healthy subjects are as follows: SGOT: 30 W.U. (11–40), SGPT: 12 W.U. (8–24), CPK: 0.4 W.U. (0–1.3) and LDH: 89 I.U. (47–149). Slight differences have been noted in the LDH-isoenzymes according to the techniques employed; the second method seemed more sensitive for fractions 4 and 5. The following normal values were recorded: LDH 1: 32% (18.5–39.5), LDH 2: 48.3% (38.5–52), LDH 3: 14.3% (6–25), LDH 4 + LDH 5: 5.4% (0–13.4). The determination of the coefficient of variation, as determined on several samples of the same serum revealed maximal fluctuations of 10% for SGOT, SGPT, CPK and LDH and 15% for the LDH-isoenzymes. The enzymatic activities, as determined in 5 normal subjects under basal conditions for 3 consecutive hours remained unchanged. Thus, changes from the initial values of more than 10% for the enzymes and of more than 15% for the LDH-isoenzymes may be regarded as being significant.

Selection of the Subjects

The study of the enzymatic activities, as outlined above, has been done on clinically healthy subjects of 43 to 54 years old with a mean of 49 years. In every case they had been sportsmen, six of them pursuing an intensive training while the others only occasionally have intense physical activity.

Methods

Technique of the Exhaustive Effort Test

All of the volunteers were subjected to an effort test on a cycloergometer with a mean duration of 30 min (23–32 min). The power developed was increased stepwise as a function of heart frequency, the initial value being 100 W while the end value was between 170 and 230 W with an average of 200 W. At the end of the test, heart frequency reached values of 160 to 175 beats per min (mean frequency 171/min). It thus may be concluded that, considering the age, these heart frequencies are almost maximal. Furthermore, the determination of the ventilation and oxygen consumption at the end of the exercise revealed that this test was really an exhaustive effort. It should also be mentioned that in nearly every subject heart frequencies of more than 150 pulsations were observed during the final 10 min of the test. The electrocardiograms, as recorded during the test as well as within 15 min later, remained normal.

Blood Collection

Blood was collected on resting, at the beginning of the test and then 15, 30, 45, 60, 90 and 120 min after the end while in 6 patients blood was taken after 6 and 12 h and in 4 subjects after 24 h.

Results

In all subjects, a relatively important increase has been observed with an average of 53%, in SGOT ($\overline{X}$ rest: 30 U – $\overline{X}$ max.: 46 U; $P<0.001$). In seven subjects the maximal values were even slightly above the maximal physiological values (max. observed: 58 U).

Concerning SGPT, although the values never exceeded the maximal physiological limit, a mean increase of 20% has been detected, the increase being highly significant ($P<0.001$; $\overline{X}$ rest: 13.8 U – $\overline{X}$ max.: 27.5 U).

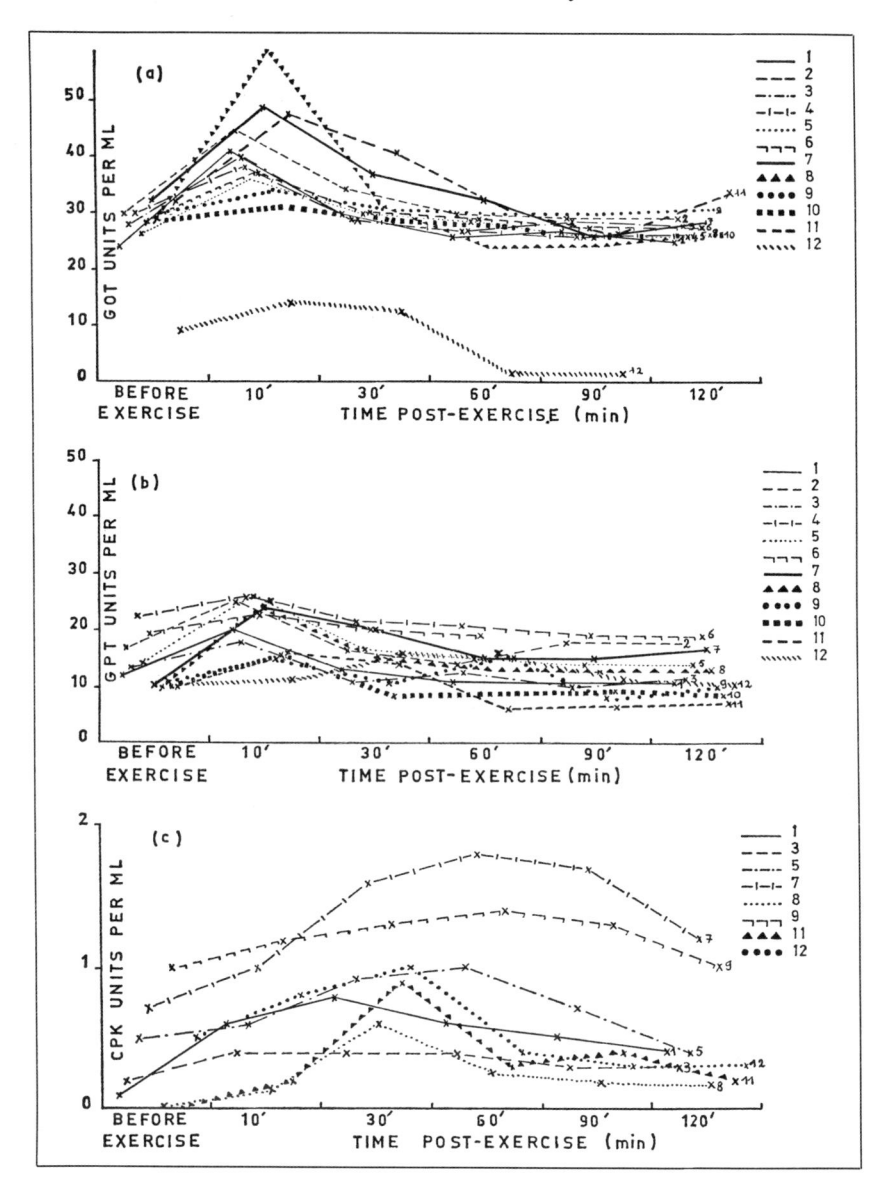

Figure 1. Serum enzyme values (units) in our subjects before and after exercise on a bicycle ergometer.

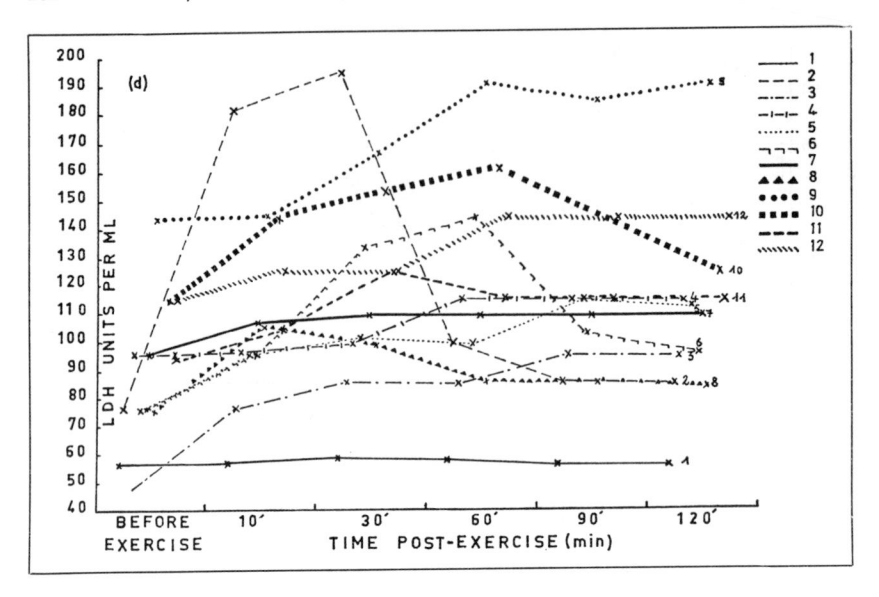

Figure 1.

For both transaminases the maximal values were always obtained within 15 min after the effort with a rapid decline towards the initial values (60–120 min) (see figure 1a and 1b). However, a second increase at 12–24 h was observed in 2 out of 6 cases which had been followed for a longer period. In 7 patients out of 15 who had been investigated, the rapid increase of SGOT and SGPT was followed by a return to values which were slightly (>10%) but significantly lower than the initial values within 2 to 4 h.

Concerning CPK, here also a significant increase could be noted ($P<0.001$) although the physiological maximum has been exceeded only once (CPK: 1.8 U) ($\overline{X}$ rest: 0.4 U – $\overline{X}$ max.: 0.95). Maximal values were reached within 30 to 60 min with a rather slow return to the initial values within 4 to 6 h (rarely within 2 h) (see figure 1c).

The elevation of LDH, which is significant also ($P<0.001$; $\overline{X}$ rest: 88.6 U – $\overline{X}$ max.: 129.8 U), is observed within 60 min and thus appears to be the slowest one. A complete return to the initial values requires a very long period and in 2 cases out of 4 this was not achieved within 24 h (see figure 1d).

Concerning the changes in LDH-isoenzymes, it could be seen that, when compared to the resting values, average increases took place of 23.5% (5–50) for LDH 1, 130% (10–800) for LDH 3 and 183% (15–500) for LDH 4 + LDH 5. The most rapid increase seemed to be in the LDH 1-

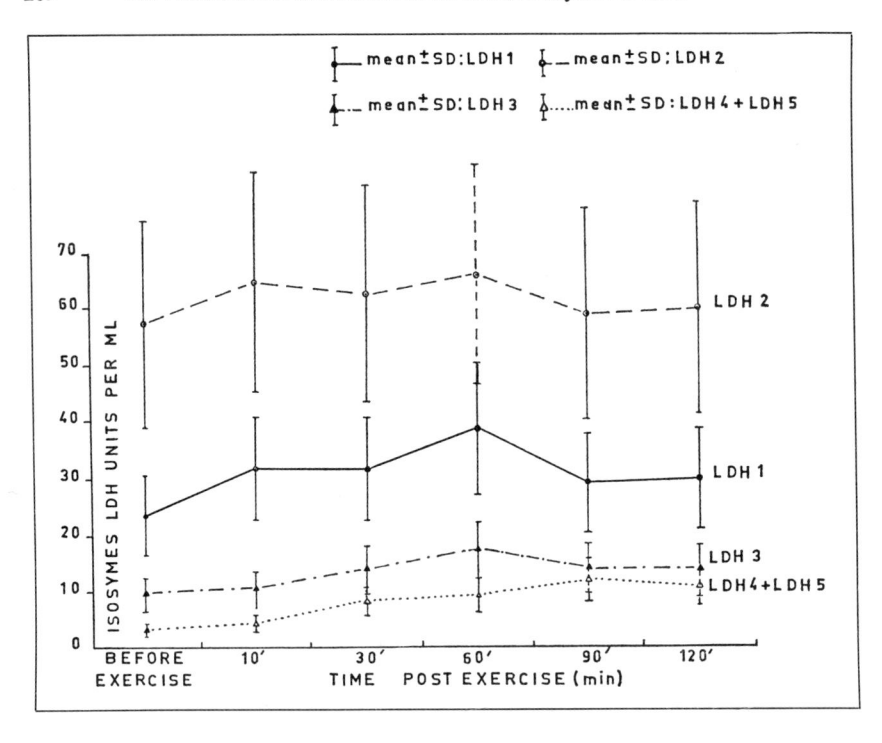

Figure 2. Variations of the mean values of the isozymes of LDH after exercise on bicycle ergometer.

fraction (30th–60th min) while for the other fractions they occurred within 60–90 min. Here also the values did not return completely to the initial low values within the experimental period especially not for LDH 3, LDH 4 and LDH 5 where they remained elevated even after 12 h in 4 cases out of 6 and after 24 h in 2 cases out of 4. As to LDH 2, a slight decrease was observed with a mean of 8% (–20 to + 15%). All of the values mentioned above, were expressed in terms of the relative values. If the absolute figures are considered, i.e. expressed in units, mean variations could be calculated of 39% for LDH 1, 15.5% for LDH 2, 78.5% for LDH 3 and 387% for LDH 4 + LDH 5, all of these changes being highly significant at the level $P<0.001$ except for LDH 2. ($\bar{X}$ LDH 1 rest: 23.5 U – $\bar{X}$ max. LDH 1: 38.9 U; $\bar{X}$ LDH 2 rest: 57.3 U – $\bar{X}$ LDH 2 max.: 66 U; $\bar{X}$ LDH 3 rest: 9.8 U – $\bar{X}$ LDH 3 max.: 17.5 U; $\bar{X}$ LDH 4–5 rest: 3.1 U – $\bar{X}$ LDH 4–5 max.: 12 U) (see figure 2).

We also investigated if, as reported by CRITZ [5] and AHLBORG [1], differences could be observed in the changes in enzymatic activities between trained subjects achieving a more intense effort (mean force: 220 W) and those less-trained who developed an average effort of only 170 W. Our results are completely in agreement with earlier observations in that we found a more important increase in SGOT and LDH in the first group, the difference being statistically significant ($P<0.015$). However, no significant difference could be stated regarding CPK while SGPT was even more elevated in the second group. Concerning the isoenzymes, the increase in LDH 3 and LDH 4–5 is greater in trained subjects while LDH 1 was less elevated in this group in comparison to the others, although the differences are not significant.

It should also be mentioned that the hematocrit values, as determined in some subjects prior to and 10 min after the test revealed an average hemoconcentration of 9% (7 to 11%).

Discussion

In view of the many discordances, not to say contradictions, encountered in the literature, it seems worthwhile to mention them briefly.

Several authors, such as FOWLER et al. [6], HALONEN and KONTTINEN [7], KONREICH and DENOLIN [9] and SCHLANG [12] reported that, following a moderate effort, rather important increases occurred in CPK (25–400%), SGOT and LDH (slightly above normal) and SGPT (only minor changes). The return to the initial values was achieved within 4 to 16 h. However, TOTARO et al. [13], only observed a significant increase in the aldolases of muscular origin. CASULA et al. [4] reported a slight increase in SGOT, SGPT and LDH only in some cases, this increase being attributed to the hemolysis and to some hemoconcentration following a physical effort. PEARCE and PENNINGTON [10] did not observe any modification in serum CPK and certainly not after a moderate effort while CRITZ and MERRICK [5] even reported a decrease in SGOT as a consequence of a physical exercise in untrained people while only slight variations occurred in sportsmen. A study from AHLBORG and BROHULT [1] on the effects of a prolonged (90 min) but not exhaustive effort (average absolute load in relation to W 170 = 80%) revealed a significant increase in SGOT, CPK and LDH during and shortly after the end of the experiment. This increase remained even for one day for SGOT and LDH, the latter returning to the initial value only on the 4th day. Here the elevation was more important and prolonged in untrained subjects than in sportsmen. Experiments of BEDRAK [3] in dogs, performing an intense exercise, are in complete agreement with these observations.

Finally, it should be mentioned that ATLAND [2] reported an increase in SGOT and serum aldolase in rats undergoing repetitive exercises of 6 h/24, those increases remaining for 4 days and being accompained by necrotic but reversible muscular lesions.

In order to add a small contribution to the resolution of a problem that seems to be rather confusing and where the origin of the enzymatic increases remains totally unknown, we investigated the modifications in SGOT, SGPT, CPK, LDH and the LDH-isoenzymes.

Concerning the classical enzymes we observed a significant elevation ($P < 0.001$) of SGOT, SGPT, CPK and LDH, those of SGOT and SGPT appearing slightly more rapidly than those ones of CPK and LDH. The latter, and especially LDH, returned more slowly to the initial values. However, the study of these modifications in serum enzymes shed no light on their probable origin.

It should also be noted that in some of our subjects a second elevation of SGOT and SGPT (more delayed) has been observed as well as a return to values being below the initial values within the 2nd and the 4th h. So far we cannot explain this phenomenon and the number of observations is too small to get a definite conclusion, but similar results have been published by CRITZ [5] and AHLBORG [1].

The examination of the isoenzymes may be of greater importance. Indeed, if we observed an increase in absolute figures for all of the 5 fractions, this increase is however more important and more prolonged for fractions 3, 4 and 5. The only reason why we preferred to express the values for the isoenzymes in units rather than in percentages is only because we felt that this way we would obtain more easily interpretable results. The more significant increase in fractions 3 to 5 may reveal that if the elevation of serum enzymes resulted from their release from the whole mass of tissues, the increase, here observed, is mainly from hepatic and muscular origin. Furthermore, the increase of LDH 1 being less important and of LDH 2 even being not significant, may exclude the hypothesis that the elevation of the classical enzymes should be regarded as a consequence of a hemolysis caused by the effort. The latter hypothesis also could not explain a change in CPK. Thus, if a hemolytic factor should be present, it should play only a secondary role. Furthermore, the hematocrit values revealed that the hemoconcentration could be only a minor factor in causing these changes in enzymatic activities.

Concerning the differences in enzymatic changes as observed between sportsmen and less trained people, it seems impossible to draw a conclusion. Indeed these differences are rather small especially if we keep in mind that the sportsmen performed a greater effort than the untrained subjects to attain maximal heart frequency (220 W versus 170 W).

Our investigations did not enable us to determine the intimate mechanisms responsible for the increases in serum enzymes. Therefore we will not discuss this problem that has been approached by several other authors [5, 7, 8, 12].

Conclusion

The increases in serum enzymes, resulting from an exhaustive effort, are significant at the level $P<0.001$ for all the enzymes studied (SGOT, SGPT, CPK, LDH and LDH-isoenzymes) except for LDH 2.

The study of the LDH-isoenzymes together with the results of the determinations of the hematocrit value permitted us, we believe, to minimize the role of the hemolysis and hemoconcentration as factors causing the changes observed. These elevations may thus be suggested to originate mainly from hepatic and muscular tissue. It is also likely that these enzymes might have been released from other tissues although to a lesser extent.

Acknowledgements

We are indebted to Dr. J. S'JONGERS and Dr. TRIBEL for the selection of the volunteers as well as to Mr. VAN BELLE, who translated the text.

Summary

The authors studied the changes in serum enzymes (SGOT, SGPT, CPK, LDH and LDH-isoenzymes) following an exhaustive effort in 15 healthy subjects aged 43 to 54 years. They observed a significant increase ($P<0.001$) of all the enzymes except for LDH 2, with a maximal increase being obtained most early for SGOT and SGPT. The return to the initial values was more delayed for CPK and especially for LDH and LDH-isoenzymes. Several considerations and hypotheses on the origin of this enzymatic changes have been discussed.

References

1. AHLBORG, B. and BROHULT, J.: Immediate and delayed metabolic reactions in well-trained subjects after prolonged physical exercise. Acta. med. scand. *182:* 1, 41 (1967).

2. ALTLAND, H. B.: Effects of exercise and training on serum enzymes and tissue changes in rats. Amer. J. Physiol 205: 162 (1963).
3. BEDRAK, E.: Blood serum enzyme activity of dogs exposed to heat, stress and muscular exercise. J. appl. Physiol 20: 587 (1965).
4. CASULA, D.; CHERCHI, P. and SPINAZZOLA, A.: The enzymoplastic features of muscular work. J. clin. Med. 42: 449 (1961).
5. CRITZ, J. B. and MERRICK, A. W.: Serum glutaminic-oxaloacetic transaminase levels after exercise in men. Proc. Soc. exp. Biol. Med. 109: 608 (1962).
6. FOWLER, W. M.; CHOWDHURY, S. R.; PEARSON, C. M.; GARDNER, G. and BRATTON, R.: Changes in serum enzyme levels after exercise in trained and untrained subjects. J. appl. Physiol 17: 943 (1962).
7. HALONEN, P. I. and KONTTINEN, A.: Effect of physical exercise on some enzymes in the serum. Nature 19: 942 (1962).
8. MCKECHNIE, J. K.; LEARY, W. P. and JOUBERT, S. M.: Some electrocardiographic and biochemical changes recorded in marathon runners. S. Afr. med. J. 41: 722 (1967).
9. KONREICH, F. et DENOLIN, H.: La créatine-phosphokinase dans le diagnostic de l'infarctus du myocarde. Acta cardiol. 19: 171 (1964).
10. PEARCE, J. M. S.; PENNINGTON, R. J. and WALTON, J. N.: Serum enzyme studies in muscle disease – Variations in serum CPK activity in normal individuals. J. Neurol. Neurosurg. Psychiat. 27: (1964).
11. REESLER, N. and JOSEPH, R.: Simple method for electrophoretic analysis of serum lactic dehydrogenase. J. lab. clin. Med. 60: 349 (1962).
12. SCHLANG, N. A.: The effect of physical exercise of serum transaminase. Amer. J. med. Sci. 242: 538 (1961).
13. TOTARO, S.; CURATELLO, G. e MANZO, F.: Effetti della fatica su alcune attività enzimatiche suriche. Sov. Murano 15: 372 (1963).
14. WIEME, R. J.: Studies on agar gel electrophoresis – Tech. Applications 155 (1959). – Agar gel electrophoresis: 115 (1965) (Elsevier Publishing Cy – Amsterdam/London N.Y.).

Author's address: Docteur P. BLOCK, Centre d'Etude des Maladies des Artères Coronaires (CEMAC), 61, rue Jean Paquot, *Bruxelles 5* (Belgique).

Studies on the Influence of the Diminished Atmospheric Pressure on some Enzymes

Part I. Serum activity of aldolase (ALD), phospho-hexose isomerase (PHI), glutamic-oxalacetic transaminase (GOT), glutamic-pyruvic transaminase (GPT) and alkaline phosphatase (alk. P) in athletes exercising in a low-pressure chamber

S. ŁUKASIK and B. BUŁA

Third Department of Internal Medicine, School of Medicine, Wrocław, and from the Physiology Department, University School of Physical Education, Wrocław

There have been several reports concerning the effect of physical effort on the activity of serum enzymes. In spite of some differences of results, it has been recently clearly established that a sufficiently hard and long lasting physical effort causes the increase of activity of most of the enzymes commonly used in clinical practice. This effect has been explained as a result of enhanced cell membrane permeability and moulting of the damaged cells.

The aim of this paper was to establish whether hypoxia due to the low atmospheric pressure may intensify the elevations of activity of serum enzymes caused by the physical exercise.

Material and Methods

The studies were performed on 8 well trained long-distance runners. Four of them comprised the experimental group, while the other four were used as a control group. Athletes of the experimental group were situated 3 times weekly for 2 h in a low-pressure chamber corresponding to the altitude of 3,000 m and performed exercises on the cycloergometer of the value of 9,000 kgm for 15 min. Athletes of the control group were subjected to the same exercises at normal atmospheric pressure.

All examined athletes in addition to these exercises trained as usual.

Experiments lasted 4 weeks. Blood samples were taken 4 times, namely: before and after the exercise, as well as at the beginning and at the end of the study. The activity of 5 serum enzymes: ALD, PHI, GOT, GPT and alk. P, was estimated.

Serum activities (in units)

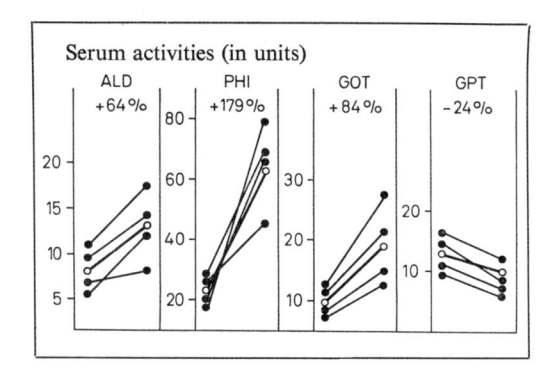

ALD +64%
PHI +179%
GOT +84%
GPT −24%

Figure 1. Activity of ALD, PHI, GOT and GPT in serum of 4 athletes before the experiment and after the four weeks of experiment in a low-pressure chamber. Black circles-individual values. Open circles-average values. The degree of changes is expressed as the percentage of initial average values.

Results

The initial values of the activity of the investigated enzymes were in normal range accepted in clinical diagnosis. After a single physical exercise in lowered atmospheric pressure, at the beginning as well as at the end of the study, only slight non-characteristic changes of activity were noted. The same results were obtained in the control group, exercising at normal atmospheric pressure. On the contrary, definite changes of activity of the studied enzymes were observed in the experimental group following 4 weeks experiment. Thus, the activities of ALD, PHI and GOT exhibited a marked increase as compared with the initial values. A decrease of GPT activity was found, while no changes of alk. P activity were detected.

Summary and Conclusions

1. No changes of activity of serum enzymes were found in single determinations following the experimental effort. The results obtained during a single experiment carried out at normal pressure did not differ from those obtained in the experiments performed in the low pressure conditions.

2. The physical exercise, repeated 3 times weekly in a four weeks period in the low pressure chamber conditions, resulted in an evident increase of activity of PHI, ALD and GOT, and the decreased GPT activity at the end of the study.

3. These findings do not seem to support the hypothesis of increased cell membrane permeability and cell moulting as the cause of the observed changes. On the

contrary, they suggest that an adaptational mechanism, in form of the enzymatic induction, might be a cause of these changes.

4. The evidence indicates that the increased serum enzymes originated from muscle tissue, since the elevation of ALD, PHI, GOT, but not of GPT was noted.

Author's address: Doc. dr S. ŁUKASIK, *Wrocław*, ul. Pasteura 4 (Poland).

Studies on the Influence of the Diminished Atmospheric Pressure on some Enzymes

Part II. The activity of aldolase (ALD), phospho-hexose isomerase (PHI), glutamic-oxalacetic transaminase (GOT) and glutamic-pyruvic transaminase (GPT) in serum and tissues of rabbits kept intermittently in a low-pressure chamber

S. Łukasik and B. Buła

Third Department of Internal Medicine, School of Medicine, Wrocław, and from the Physiology Department, University School of Physical Education, Wrocław

The results of the investigations presented in the first part of our paper have not established whether the cause of the observed increased activity of ALD, PHI and GOT, and decreased activity of GPT was due to adaptation to physical effort in hypoxia or to the hypoxia only. In order to obtain more information concerning this problem, experimental studies on rabbits were performed. The animals were placed in a low-pressure chamber, and the influence of this condition on ALD, PHI, GOT, and GPT activity in serum and in some tissues was studied.

Material and Methods

Eight rabbits weighing 2.5–3.0 kg were used for investigations. They were divided into two groups, experimental and control, of 4 animals each.

Rabbits of the experimental group were placed for 2 h daily in the low-pressure chamber (with a pressure corresponding to an altitude of 5,500 m) during a period of 3 weeks. Blood samples were taken twice a week from all animals. The enzyme determinations were performed additionally at the beginning of the study in 4 rabbits, before and after the first time-period in the low-pressure chamber.

After 3 weeks all the animals were killed and the estimation of the enzymes was performed in homogenates of the heart muscle, skeletal muscle and liver. Activity of ALD, PHI, GOT, and GPT was measured.

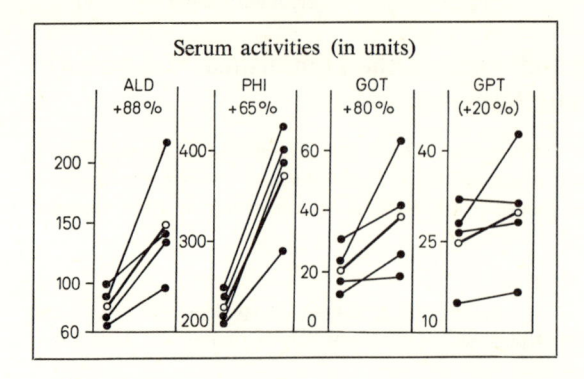

Figure 1. Serum activity of ALD, PHI, GOT and GPT in 4 rabbits before and after a single stay in a low pressure chamber. Black circles-individual values. Open circles-average values. Degree of activity increase is expressed by percentage of the initial middle value.

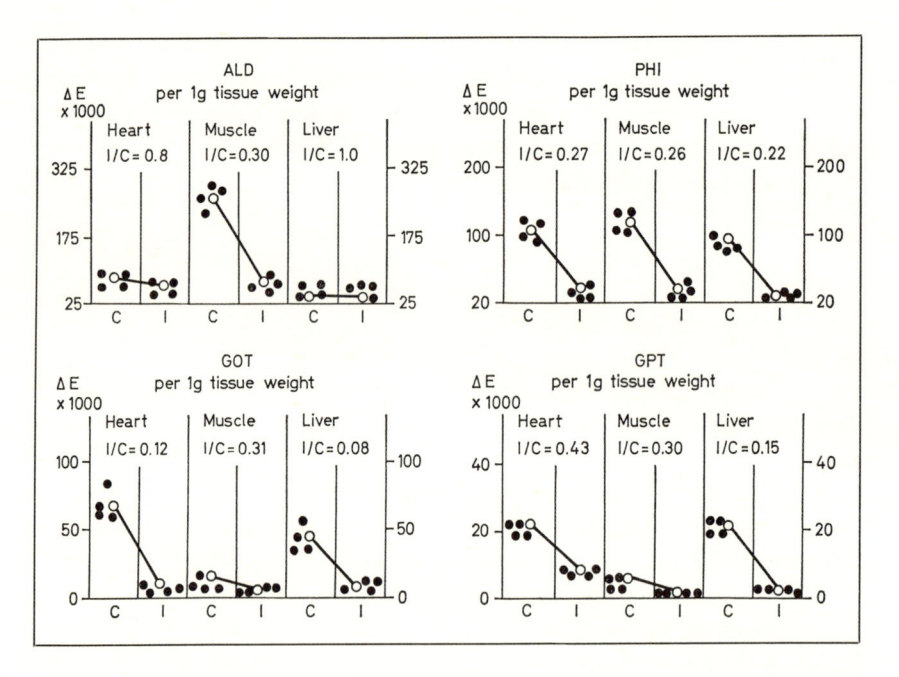

Figure 2. Tissue activity of ALD, PHI, GOT and GPT of heart muscle, skeletal muscle and liver expressed as optical density readings multiplied by 1,000 – in 4 rabbits of control /c/ and investigated group /I/. Other designations as in figure 1. Degree of decrease is expressed as the ratio of average value of the control and investigated group /C/I/.

Results

A single period in the low pressure chamber evoked in the serum of all the animals an evident increase of activity of ALD, PHI and GOT, and a rather doubtful increase of GPT activity.

The serum activity of all 4 enzymes, estimated repeatedly in the 3 weeks period in the experimental group, revealed changes remaining in the range of biological variability. Tissue activity estimated on animal specimens obtained at autopsy displayed the unexpected changes. All the enzymes except ALD in heart and liver homogenates, showed several-fold decrease of activity in all 3 examined tissues as compared to the control group.

Summary and Conclusions

1. A single 2-h-stay in a low pressure chamber caused transitory increase of activity of serum ALD, PHI and GOT in all examined rabbits.
2. Repeated periods in the low pressure chamber failed to cause in any animal constant serum activity changes of the investigated enzymes.
3. After 3 weeks of the experiment's duration, tissue activities of all enzymes, except heart and liver ALD, showed a several-fold decrease of activity as compared with controls.
4. The results give evidence of a complete lack of correlation between the tissues and serum activity of some enzymes.
5. Physiologic adaptation to high-altitude hypoxia is evidenced in rabbits by distinct decrease of activity of some enzymes in the heart muscle, skeletal muscle and liver.
6. The mechanism of the increase of activity following a single hypoxia could hardly be explained by increased permeability of cell membranes. This might be due to the active elimination of enzymic protein surplus.

Author's address: Doc. dr S. ŁUKASIK, *Wrocław*, ul. Pasteura 4 (Poland).

Amylasic Activity of the Blood During Physical Exercise

R. Dringoli, P. Ravaioli, P. L. Orsucci and E. Ciampolini

Istituto di Patologia Medica, Univ. of Siena Medical School, Siena

The present work is part of a series of research intended to individualise the factors responsible for the variations of the amylasic activity of the blood serum.

Ermini and Carboni [9, 10] were the first to demonstrate that an oral dose of glucose causes an increase of both the sugar level and the amylasic activity of the blood.

Some of us have been able to confirm these observations [6] and to ascertain that an increase of the amylase level can be obtained independently from the route of administration of the glucose. The blood amylase curves after the oral load of glucose, are in fact similar to those that can be obtained also with glucose administrated intravenously [7] and are, in any case, always parallel to the blood sugar curves.

More recently, on administration of two oral doses of glucose at a relatively short interval of time, we have had occasion to observe [8] that the amylase level after the second oral dose increases even if the level of blood sugar does not increase significantly. The above observations do not appear compatible with the hypothesis initially proposed, which indicated that hyperglycemia is responsible for the rise of blood amylase. We therefore proposed to observe the behaviour of amylasemia in some conditions where accelerated transport or utilization of glucose is not necessarily accompanied by high blood sugar levels: e.g. during muscular effort.

Method

We studied eight young males aged between 16 and 23, all belonging to a sports club, during a training period. All the subjects, at the start of the experiment had been fasting, for 12 hours. After a period of about 30 msin absolute rest, blood was drawn from the cephalic vein of the arm sufficient to determine blood sugar, amylase, NEFA and hematocrit. The same tests were made 10 min later, e.g. immediately before the effort. This

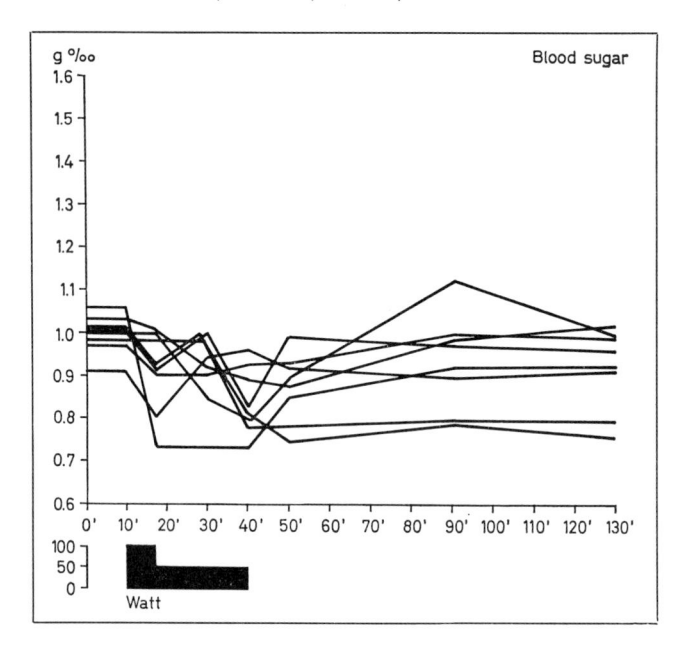

Figure 1.

was made by means of a Fleish universal cycloergostate. After some preliminary trials, we deemed it opportune to submit our subjects to a rather violent initial effort and then to a longer less intense effort. The athletes developed 100 watts during the 1st 7 min period and then 50 watts for 23 min. Blood samples were also drawn at the 7th, 20th, 30th min during effort, and at the 10th, 50th and 90th min after the cessation of the effort. During the withdrawals at the 7th and 20th minutes, the subjects ceased pedalling for a few seconds. The blood sugar level was evaluated after the Folin Wu method and the amylase level by using the enzymatic tests supplied by the STVT Institute 'A. Sclavo', Siena, Italy. NEFA levels were measured by a modified Ducombe method [15].

Results

Blood Sugar

Figure 1 clearly shows that the blood sugar level goes down during effort with some individual variability. In five cases in fact, the decrement is

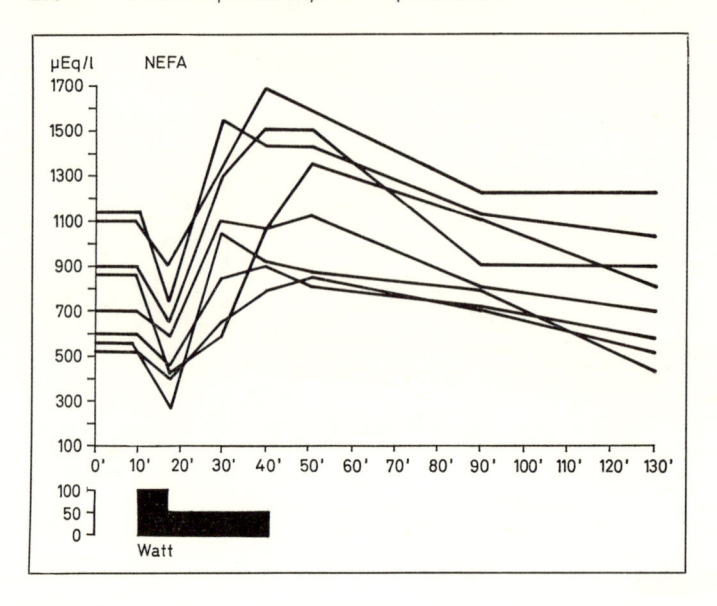

Figure 2.

already marked at the 7th min, namely at the height of the violent effort; in the other three subjects, the blood sugar level lowered only successively and namely during the second phase of the effort. At the cessation of the exercise, a rather rapid return of blood sugar to basic levels was observed in 5 cases, while in two cases, it did not go back to normal even 90 min after the cessation of the effort.

NEFA

Figure 2 shows that during the control period, NEFA concentration is steady. On the other hand, after a 7 min effort, namely at the height of the violent effort, NEFA level appears to be significantly reduced in all cases. The 4th and 5th tests, namely at the 20th and 30th min from the beginning of the effort show on the other hand a rapid increase of NEFA levels. The return to the initial values, however, does not occur at the same moment in all the subjects. In fact, 10 min after the end of the exercise, NEFA concentrations are still variably distributed; only the 7th blood sample, namely 50 min after cessation of the effort, presents in all the

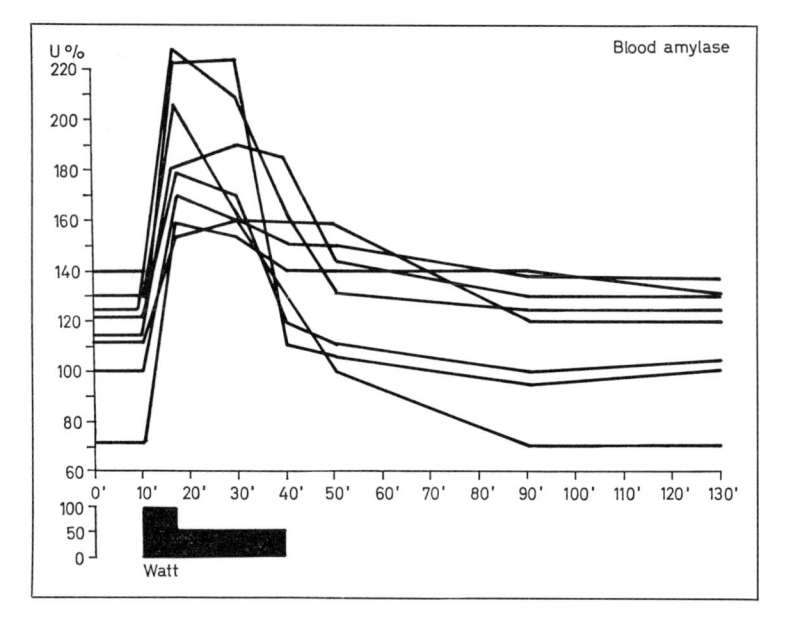

Figure 3.

subjects a clear reduction of NEFA, which at the 90th min have the same values like those before the start.

Blood Amylase

From figure 3 one can see clearly that the amylase level during the first 20 min of effort undergoes, in all cases, a noticeable increase. In the remaining 10 min of exercise, however, the amylase value reduces in measure more or less conspicuous. The return to the base-line value is then completed in the following period of rest.

The Hematocrit

The hematocrit made on samples drawn during and immediately after the effort showed variable increases between the 2 and 4%. These increases cannot alone explain the variations observed on the NEFA and the amylase.

Discussion

Blood sugar changes during effort in the subjects of our study are similar to those already observed by other authors [2, 12].

Also the observed changes of NEFA concentration do not differ from those previously reported by others [1, 3, 4, 5, 11, 12, 13].

We have therefore reason to assume that our experimental conditions are perfectly reliable and guarantee the primary results of our research which has proved the variations of the serum amylasic level during muscular effort. As it appears from the above reported results, we have indeed succeeded in recognizing a condition in which an unquestionable activation of the glucose metabolism is not accompanied by hyperglycemia and notwithstanding this, the amylase level rises. Amylase increments without parallel increase of blood sugar level we have already observed in other conditions [8], and namely when a second oral load of glucose was administered at a closer distance from a first one. All these observations together appear therefore to exclude that hyperglycemia is the factor responsible for the increase of the amylase level. Obviously, other researches will be necessary to establish if and when accelerated transport and utilization of glucose is responsible for the observed increase of blood amylase level.

Acknowledgment

The authors are greatful to Dr. A. GEROLA for his help.

References

1. BASU, A.; PASSMORE, R. and STRONG, J. A.: The effect of exercise on the level of non-esterified fatty acids in the blood. Quart J. exp. Physiol *45:* 312 (1960).
2. BUONI, M.: Il comportamento della glicemia durante i lavori pesanti. Folia med. *36:* 557 (1953).
3. CARLSON, L. A. and PERNOW, B.: Studies on blood lipids during exercise. I. Arterial and venous plasma concentrations of unesterified fatty acids. J. lab. clin. Med. *53:* 833 (1959).
4. CARLSON, L. A.; EKELUND, L. G. and ÖRO, L.: Studies on blood lipids during exercise. IV. Arterial concentration of plasma free fatty acids and glycerol during and after prolonged efforts in normal men. J. lab. clin. Med. *61:* 724 (1963).
5. CARLSON, L. A.; BOBERG, J. and HÄGSTEDT, B.: Handbook of physiology. V. Adipose tissue. (Ed.) RONOLD, A. E. and CAHILL, G. F., p. 625. American Physiological Society, Washington D.C. (1965).

6. CIAMPOLINI, E.; RAVAIOLI, P. e DRINGOLI, R.: Il test glico-amilasemico per lo studio della funzionalità pancreatica. Quaderni Sclavo di diagnostica (in press).
7. CIAMPOLINI, E. e DRINGOLI, R.: Il test amilasemico dopo carico venoso di glucosio (in press).
8. CIAMPOLINI, E.; DRINGOLI, R. e ORSUCCI, P. L.: Comportamento delle curve amilasemiche dopo doppio carico di glucosio (in press).
9. ERMINI, M. e CARBONI, M.: Metodo di valutazione della funzionalità pancreatica. Gazz. int. med. Chir. *16:* 1665 (1963).
10. ERMINI, M. e CARBONI, M.: Il valore del test glico-amilasemico nella pancreatite cronica. Atti del XVI Congresso della Soc. Ital. di Gastroenterologia (Bologna 1965).
11. FRIEDBERG, S. J.; SHER, P. B.; BOGDONOFF, M. D. and ESTES, E. H., Jr.: The dynamics of plasma free fatty acid metabolism during exercise. J. Lipid. Res. *4:* 34 (1963).
12. HAVEL, R. J.; NAIMARK, A. and BORCHGREVINK, C. F.: Turnover rate and oxidation of free fatty acids of blood plasma in man during exercise: studies during continuous infusion of palmitate – I-C^{14}. J. clin. Invest. *42:* 1054 (1963).
13. HAVEL, R. J.: Transport of fatty acids between adipose tissue and blood. Role of catecholamines and the sympathetic nervous system. Proc. First. int. Pharmacol. Meeting, Stockholm 1961. (Pergamon Press, London 1963).
14. HEBB, C. O.: Relation between blood sugar concentrations and exocrine function of pancreas. Arch. int. med. Pharmacodyn Therap. *52:* 33 (1965).
15. ITAYA, K.: Colorimetric determination of free fatty acids in biological fluids. J. Lipid Res. *15–16:* (1965).

Authors' address: R. DRINGOLI, P. PAVAIOLI, P. L. ORSUCCI and E. CIAMPOLINI, Istituto di Patologia Medica, University of Siena Medical School, *Siena* (Italy).

Modification enzymoplasmatiques causées par le travail musculaire chez des sujets d'âge moyen

G. C. Topi, L. Gandolfo d'Alessandro et G. Piovano

Istituto di Medicina dello Sport, Roma

Poursuivant les recherches sur les modifications métaboliques déterminées par différents types de travail chez des catégories diverses de sujets (athlètes et sujets non athlétiques d'âges divers) nous avons étudié le comportement des activités aldolasique, lactique-déhydrogénéasique, malico-déhydrogénéasique, créatine-phosphochinasique, glucose-6-phosphate-déhydrogénéasique du sérum chez un groupe de sujets non entraînés, soumis au travail au cyclo-ergomètre.

Nous avons pris en considération six sujets âgés de 30 à 50 ans, exerçant des professions libérales, non entraînés, un peu trop lourds, à diète mixte équilibrée, présentant des valeurs normales, en conditions de repos, des paramètres considérés.

Le travail musculaire a été effectué au cyclo-ergomètre (Elema-Schollander avec contrôle électronique de la charge) préparé pour une charge de 565 kgm/min. Etant donné que les sujets ne devaient pas atteindre un état de fatigue, le travail a été effectué par périodes variant de 15 à 30 min, le travail extérieur total étant de 5 250 à 16 950 kgm.

En même temps et pendant toute la durée de chaque expérience l'on a effectué les relevés du volume respiratoire, de la consommation de O_2, de la production de CO_2, en employant un appareil de Hartmann-Brown modifié, à circuit ouvert.

Les prélèvements de sang ont été effectués avant l'effort (après 30 min de repos absolu), immédiatement après l'effort et après 30 min de repos.

L'on a employé les méthodes suivantes: pour l'aldolase, la méthode de Bruns; pour la lactico-déhydrogénase la méthode de Wroblewski et La Due; pour la malicodéhydrogénase, la méthode des mêmes AA.: pour la créatine-phosphochinase la méthode de Forster; pour la G-6-P-déhydrogénase la méthode de Kornberg et Horecker.

Les résultats sont rapportés au tableau I.

Le tableau permet d'observer que l'activité aldolasique du sérum est augmentée, après l'effort principalement aérobie réalisé par le sujet

Tableau I.

Cas	Temps	Aldolase mU/ml serum	LDH mU/ml	MDH mU/ml	CPK mU/ml	G-6-Ph-D mU/ml
1	A	3,40	45,48	184,50	0,00	0,00
	B	4,24	65,69	181,38	0,67	0,00
	C	3,52	54,57	182,42	0,22	0,00
2	A	1,47	113,69	32,31	0,11	0,00
	B	1,23	126,32	39,61	0,17	0,00
	C	1,29	113,69	40,65	0,06	0,00
3	A	2,79	69,73	39,92	0,00	0,00
	B	9,19	93,99	79,74	0,00	0,00
	C	3,02	78,83	42,53	0,00	0,00
4	A	2,84	82,52	164,70	0,00	0,00
	B	3,38	89,24	180,33	0,00	0,00
	C	2,61	76,60	174,08	0,00	0,00
5	A	3,63	30,32	47,95	0,00	0,00
	B	3,63	36,18	52,12	0,00	0,00
	C	3,18	29,46	46,91	0,00	0,00
6	A	3,45	59,78	41,70	0,00	0,00
	B	4,95	71,55	42,53	0,00	0,00
	C	5,03	71,55	32,11	0,00	0,00

A = en condition de repos; B = aussitôt après l'effort; C = après 30 min de repos. Valeurs normales: ALD = 1–3,5; LHD = 96–241; MDH = 50–104; CPK = jusqu'à 1; G-6-Ph-D = 0 mU/ml.

examiné, en quatre cas sur 6; l'augmentation, faible d'ailleurs, a disparu en trois cas après la période de repos.

L'activité lactique-déhydrogénasique du sérum s'est avérée constamment augmentée après l'effort; l'augmentation, d'importance variable selon les sujets, a tendance à s'annuler après la période de repos.

L'activité malicodéhydrogénasique présente une augmentation inconstante et d'importance variable aussitôt après l'effort, et une tendance à diminuer après la période de repos.

L'activité créatine-phosphochinasique a présenté une augmentation très faible après l'effort dans deux cas; chez les autres sujets, l'activité enzymatique n'a pu être démontrée en aucun des prélèvements. De même, aucune activité glucose-D-phosphate-déhydrogénasique dans le sérum n'a été démontrée, même après l'effort.

Les différences de la casuistique et du travail accompli ne permettent pas de faire des comparaisons critiques des résultats obtenus avec ceux de la littérature; néanmoins, sur la base du travail d'autrui et du nôtre, il nous semble que des possibilités remarquables se présentent pour la diagnostique enzymatique, soit en ce qui concerne les recherches sur les répercussions métaboliques du travail, soit pour juger du degré d'entraînement à l'exercice physique.

Adresse des auteurs: Prof. G. C. Topi, Dr L. Gandolfo d'Alessandro et Dr G. Piovano, Istituto di Medicina dello Sport, *Roma* (Italie).

V. Electrolytes

Modifications des électrolytes au cours des activités physiques

G. Rougier et J. P. Babin

Les variations des électrolytes à l'effort ont suscité de nombreux travaux: nous avons lu plus de 300 publications mais en avons certainement omis plusieurs. La difficulté d'une mise au point sur une question pourtant si étudiée nous est apparue tout de suite. C'est donc avec beaucoup de réserves que nous présentons les conclusions qui vont suivre. Les résultats des auteurs sont en effet souvent divergents voire contradictoires; ceci tient à de multiples causes. La nature, la durée et l'intensité des exercices demandés sont difficilement comparables, parfois mal précisées. L'état d'entraînement des sujets, de même que les conditions propres de l'expérience (température, hygrométrie, altitude, heure, sujets à jeun ou non, absorbant ou non des liquides ou des aliments, fréquence et horaire des prélèvements, techniques de recueil et de dosage des échantillons...) sont susceptibles, à travail égal, d'influer sur l'importance des réactions. Enfin les caractéristiques individuelles des sujets jouent d'autant plus que leur nombre souvent restreint ne permet pas de les fondre dans celles de la masse.

Le petit nombre de pages qui nous est imparti ne nous permet pas de donner pour chaque électrolyte et chaque milieu autre chose qu'une synthèse très succinte des conclusions des publications les plus sérieuses. N'ayant pas la place d'en citer tous les auteurs nous avons choisi avec regret de n'en mentionner aucun. Tout en ne perdant pas de vue que l'homéostasie fonctionne comme un tout il nous a paru utile de séparer l'étude des différents liquides. Nous envisagerons successivement le plasma auquel s'associent obligatoirement les liquides du muscle squelettique, l'urine, la sueur et la salive. Les variations du liquide céphalo-rachidien ont été peu étudiées mais il y a tout lieu de croire qu'elles sont semblables à celles du plasma. L'évolution des différents électrolytes sera aussi donnée séparément. Cette manière de procéder que d'aucuns trouveront illogique nous a paru la plus expéditive permettant plus aisément de dégager quelques conclusions dont il convient seulement de se rappeler le caractère parcellaire étant données les interférences électrolytiques. Nous avons borné notre étude à celle des électrolytes usuellement dosés dont nous avons écarté le carbonate monosodique étudié dans un autre rapport. Nous avons classé les résultats suivant qu'ils se rapportent à des efforts brefs (inférieurs à 15 min), de durée moyenne (entre 15 et 30 min) ou longue. Cette classification est évidemment arbitraire et artificielle (le groupe des efforts longs comporte notamment des travaux de moins d'une heure ou de plusieurs jours); nous l'avons adoptée car elle correspond souvent à des modalités réactionnelles différentes. Pour alléger notre exposé nous n'avons pas non plus donné de chiffres (il aurait fallu alors en donner beaucoup) et nous nous sommes bornés à indiquer un pourcentage moyen de variations.

Ce rapport, qui nous a pourtant donné beaucoup de mal, comporte donc de nombreuses imperfections. Certaines nous sont imputables, nous n'avons probablement pas su extraire de chaque article la quintessence et avons dû parfois manquer d'objectivité. Nous sollicitons l'indulgence du lecteur compte tenu des conditions qui nous ont été imposées.

I. Sang – plasma – muscle

a) Potassium. Plusieurs facteurs sont susceptibles à l'effort de modifier (habituellement pas plus de 35%) en plus ou en moins la kaliémie; leur interférence et leur importance variable expliquent les divergences des publications. Le métabolisme glucidique accru retentit sur la kaliémie. Il est admis que la glycogénolyse musculaire et la sortie du glucose des cellules hépatiques s'accompagnent d'une perte cellulaire en K. Or la compétition sportive engendre souvent une forte hyperglycémie. Les mécanismes régulateurs sont d'ailleurs similaires dans l'hyperkaliémie et l'hyperglycémie provoquées. L'acidose métabolique (lactique) ou gazeuse (CO_2) accompagnant en général une activité même brève rend compte d'une extrusion cellulaire potassique. La stimulation des surrénales par l'effort est prouvée par un accroissement de l'excrétion urinaire de tous les corticoïdes. On connaît l'action de l'aldostérone sur l'excrétion urinaire du K, celle des glucocorticoïdes sur la déplétion potassique cellulaire, et le rôle diphasique de l'adrénaline freinant ou facilitant sa libération du muscle. Les contractions musculaires répétées peuvent aboutir à une baisse du rapport K_i/K_e par retour incomplet du K dans la cellule. Une partie serait transportée avec l'acide lactique et sous forme de phosphates dans la cellule hépatique, participant à la resynthèse du glycogène, puis serait restituée au muscle avec le glucose qui lui est fourni. La libération des métabolites durant le travail musculaire, augmentant les molécules osmotiquement actives et la pression osmotique intracellulaire, entraîne en compensation un transfert rapide du K, ion très mobile, vers le plasma. Les nombreux systèmes enzymatiques pour lesquels le K paraît indispensable, notamment la pyruvate-kinase, sollicités au cours de l'exercice musculaire, consomment du K.

Les résultats observés peuvent s'interpréter comme suit: Les répercussions déclenchées dans l'organisme par des activités physiques mêmes modérées, se traduisent par des mouvements rapides et complexes du K aboutissant à des modifications variables suivant l'importance relative des différents processus et le moment précis du prélèvement sanguin. Dans l'ensemble on constate une hyperkaliémie (majorée par une hémoconcentration de 5 à 10%) pour les efforts brefs avec retour plus ou moins rapide à la normale. En ce qui concerne les efforts moyens et surtout longs, il semble bien que les nombreux partisans de l'hyperkaliémie n'aient observé là qu'un temps intermédiaire, préparatoire au temps suivant. Il n'y faut voir (indépendamment d'un processus possible d'hémolyse) qu'une décharge fugace précédant l'hypokaliémie (minimisée par l'hémoconcentration). Avant de fuir dans les urines, le K provenant de la déplétion cellulaire passe dans le plasma. Une hypokaliémie, témoin pour certains d'un début d'épuisement cellulaire (mais ce mécanisme est discuté) paraît en définitive se manifester après un effort tant soit peu prolongé. Elle peut même s'accentuer, avant de s'estomper, lors du repos consécutif, traduisant probablement la recharge cellulaire, puis elle se compense ensuite en faisant appel aux réserves de K de l'organisme, voire aux apports extérieurs (intérêt d'une ingestion modérée de K).

Certains auteurs pensent avoir démontré que l'hypokaliémie permettrait une meilleure économie des pertes d'eau, et partant, une meilleure adaptation à l'hyperthermie.

b) Sodium. Le Na est un cation stable, même à l'effort. Les variations de la natrémie portent sur quelques mEq, et n'excèdent jamais les limites physiologiques, pour ne pas dire les erreurs de laboratoire. Le problème du Na est lié à celui de l'eau ce qui ne fait que compliquer les interprétations étant données les opinions divergentes émises sur les mouvements hydrosodés à l'intérieur du muscle lui-même. Suivant les opinions, il existe une hypertonie cellulaire par excès de métabolites acides avec élévation de l'eau I.C. et gonflement de la cellule, une augmentation de l'eau E.C. du muscle, une déshydratation I.C. avec liquide E.C. non modifié, une perte du Na_i avec élévation du Na_e du muscle, une élévation du Na_i du muscle, des variations de l'eau et du Na avec l'âge...

Très nombreux sont ceux qui, en admettant la modicité des variations, trouvent une hypernatrémie. Ils s'appuient sur l'intervention de facteurs de rétention sodée (aldostérone) ou de résorption tubulaire (ADH), sur la perte d'eau supérieure à celle du sel, responsable de l'hémoconcentration (sudation, polypnée). Le passage, au cours des activités physiques, de liquide plasmatique vers les liquides intersticiels du tissu musculaire, passage supérieur à celui du Na, rendrait compte en outre de l'hypertonie plasmatique.

Bien qu'ils soient en moins grand nombre, il semble que l'on puisse accréditer les partisans de l'hyponatrémie. Très souvent l'élévation du Na est moins importante que celle de l'hématocrite ou que celle de l'osmolarité globale. L'hyponatrémie correspondant à l'abaissement du gradient Na_e/Na_i au cours de la contraction, est confirmée par ceux qui ont étudié le muscle lui-même dans lequel ils ont trouvé une élévation du Na. Quoiqu'il en soit, ces échanges complexes et quasi individuels n'intéressent qu'une proportion apparente de moins de 5% du Na sérique.

c) Chlore. Le chlore, qui est loin d'être exlusivement extracellulaire, paraît subir des déplacements à travers les différents secteurs du muscle. Le taux de la chlorémie de base est diversement apprécié. Compte tenu de l'hémoconcentration, les variations sont faibles ou nulles, mais non forcément parallèles à celles du Na. Les partisans de l'élévation (compensation d'une baisse des CO^3H) ou de la baisse (pertes par la sueur) admettent la limitation extrême des changements. Pour les efforts très prolongés (plusieurs jours), une légère tendance à l'hypochlorémie se dégage.

d) Calcium. C'est un des électrolytes les plus stables, les variations de la calcémie à l'effort ne sont pas importantes, les modifications des quelques 300 mg plasmatiques ne reflétant pas les changements au niveau du bloc calcique. Pour les efforts moyens ou surtout brefs, on observe une tendance discrète mais nette à l'élévation de la calcémie (moins de 20 mg/l). Pour les efforts prolongés ou très prolongés et épuisants, une baisse légère peut se manifester, avec balance calcique négative.

Les interprétations physiologiques des modifications sont sommaires, les parathyroïdes ont un rôle mal défini. Les mouvements transmembranaires du Ca sont complexes. Le Ca, essentiellement ionisé, serait capté transitoirement par la fibre musculaire, entraînant pour certains une baisse du Ca ionisé sérique. La fatigue inhiberait ces mouvements. Le Ca lié aux protides, augmenterait avec eux et avec l'hémoconcentration qui joue naturellement un rôle important. Mais le parallélisme entre la calcémie et la teneur en protides ne se vérifie pas toujours.

L'entraînement est un facteur important d'annulation des oscillations calciques.

e) Magnesium. Mal connue au repos, la destinée du Mg au cours des activités physiques est encore plus imprécise. Le Mg plasmatique ne reflète que de très loin le métabolisme du Mg total. Les modifications semblent très modérées ou nulles, perturbées par d'importantes variations nycthémérales. On note cependant une tendance à l'hypermagnésiémie au cours d'efforts brefs et intenses. L'hémoconcentration l'explique aussi bien que des mouvements d'eau intracellulaires ou que l'acidose. Les variations du Mg sont bien moindres que celles du K, l'autre cation intracellulaire.

f) Phosphore et *phosphates.* Certains notent une hypophosphorémie (pénétration des ions Po^4 dans la cellule grâce à l'hyperinsulinisme provoqué par l'hyperglycémie, blocage par les hexoses, phosphorylation du glycogène). La plupart signalent une hyperphosphorémie, parfois importante (30%), quelle que soit la durée de l'effort mais fonction de son intensité. Elle peut se manifester très vite après le début, et ne plus guère se modifier, ou se prolonger au repos, ou retomber à des chiffres inférieurs à ceux du départ. Cette élévation serait expliquée, outre l'hémoconcentration, par la migration plasmatique du K sous forme de phosphates, et par la libération musculaire de composés phosphatés riches en énergie. La réintégration cellulaire aurait lieu au repos. Ces variations témoignent de l'importance du P dans le métabolisme énergétique.

g) Fer. Si quelle que soit la durée de l'effort une élévation du Fer sérique est toujours notée, les variations interindividuelles sont très grandes (supérieures à 100%). L'élévation paraît plus importante chez les sujets entraînés, la récupération du taux normal, quoique demandant plusieurs jours, plus rapide que chez les sédentaires. Le mécanisme le plus logique serait celui d'une hémolyse, plus nette chez les sportifs. La ferritinine pourrait aussi relarguer une partie de son stock ferrique.

h) NH^{4+}. L'ammoniémie veineuse s'élève, souvent considérablement (de 50 à 800%), surtout au cours des efforts brefs, les plus fréquemment étudiés. L'hyperammoniémie semble essentiellement locale, bien que pouvant se manifester dans la circulation générale. Le chiffre de repos est indispensable à connaître, puisqu'avec le perfectionnement des techniques, le taux normal d'ammoniémie a pu baisser de 1 mg/100 ml jusqu'à 15 ou 10 γ/100 ml. Les modalités d'apparition et d'évolution de l'hyperammoniémie varient : d'emblée ou rapidement, délai après la fin de l'effort, disparition en quelques secondes, persistance pendant des heures.

Ces faits suggèrent l'intervention de mécanismes différents. Ils sont nombreux et d'ailleurs incertains : épuration insuffisante par les muscles débordés, désamination excessive (discutée), court-circuits musculaires, perméabilité membranaire modifiée par des variations de pH, des gaz...

L'entraînement stimule les processus enzymatiques épurateurs, en abaissant aussi bien l'ammoniémie de base que celle d'effort.

i) De nombreux *oligoéléments*, l'*iode*, les *sulfates* subissent des variations. Les valeurs du pH et des CO^{3}H sont pour la plupart modérément perturbées, mais paraissent parfois défier les lois de l'équilibre acido basique.

II. Urine

La fonction rénale subit de grosses perturbations à l'effort, les réactions sont très éloignées de celles du repos, l'exploration fractionnée (surtout menée pour le Na) difficile. La correlation entre débit urinaire et excrétion est discutée. Une baisse modérée de la filtration glomérulaire et une diminution du flux rénal plasmatique sont admises (vasoconstriction artériolaire) avec le plus souvent réduction de la diurèse.

Il importe de distinguer l'élimination, seule digne d'intérêt, de la concentration trop souvent étudiée. Les variations à l'effort sont fortement influencées par la sueur qui modifie considérablement les rapports du Cl Na et K urinaires.

a) Potassium. Voie primordiale d'excrétion, l'élimination urinaire est pour la plupart augmentée. Rares sont les partisans de la baisse, qui est beaucoup moins marquée que celle du Na (rétention maintenant l'isoosmolarité, compétition entre H et K, l'acidité urinaire entravant l'excrétion du K qui réintègre le tubule distal à la place des ions H).

L'hyperkaliurie est parfois très importante (jusqu'à décupler) et particulièrement nette au cours des efforts de longue durée, souvent d'apparition décalée. Elle est rapportée :

à l'élimination de l'excès plasmatique du K d'origine cellulaire ;

à l'hémolyse et aux microhématuries;

à l'intervention de mécanismes hormonaux: aldostérone, 17 OH (plus accessoire). A la fin de l'exercice, la baisse de sécrétion d'aldostérone permet la réintégration cellulaire et la diminution de l'excrétion (délai très variable). Les mécanismes sont rendus complexes par l'intervention d'un processus d'excrétion tubulaire corticale, indépendant de la filtration.

Les variations individuelles sont considérables, des variations nycthémérales peuvent perturber des exercices très prolongés. L'entraînement freine les pertes en K (le contraire pour certains, par hypersurrénalisme).

b) Sodium. Les modifications signalées sont très variables. Les moins nombreux notent une hypernatriurie, toujours peu marquée. Certains y voient, pour des efforts prolongés, une action des 17 OH inhibiteurs de l'ADH à effets natridiurétiques, d'autres un simple effet de la concentration.

La plupart constatent une réduction importante de l'excrétion (jusqu'au triple), pour tous les types d'effort, surtout pour les longs. Le rapport K/Na s'élève considérablement. L'exercice (polypnée, sudation) crée une hypertonie plasmatique d'où sécrétion d'ADH, affaisse les espaces E.C., stimulant le système rénine angiotensine et – après un temps de latence – la sécrétion d'aldostérone, qu'une certaine tension émotionnelle favorise. Le Sodium Extracting Factor serait inhibé. La fraction excrétée du Na filtré diminue (baisse de la clearance), avec augmentation de la réabsorption tubulaire maintenant l'isoosmolarité (indépendance entre le Na excrété et la clearance de l'inuline). La part réciproque revenant au glomérule, à la zone proximale et perméable au Na, et à la zone distale de réabsorption active, n'est pas bien déterminée dans l'excrétion qui est d'une extrême souplesse.

Au repos, la disparition rapide de l'aldostérone ramène la Natriurie aux valeurs de départ. Mais parfois les modifications peuvent persister plusieurs heures ou plusieurs jours. L'entraînement amortit les variations en plus ou en moins.

c) Chlore. Au repos la chlorurie des sportifs est importante (gros consommateurs de sel). A l'effort la baisse de l'excrétion est forte, perturbée au cours d'exercices prolongés par des variations nycthémérales, mais dans l'ensemble le rapport Na/Cl diminue (perte supérieure en Cl) à la fin d'un effort important. Du $ClNH_4$ se forme. Bien que partiellement dissociée de celle du Na, la réduction chlorurée est sous la dépendance de l'aldostérone.

d) Calcium. Les variations de la calciurie, comme celles du métabolisme calcique en général, sont, selon les auteurs, très sensibles aux exercices ou non. La calciurie dépend d'un rythme circadien, de l'alimentation, du jeûne. Dans l'ensemble les activités physiques entraînent une baisse de l'excrétion (jusqu'au quart). Les partisans de l'hypercalciurie, modérée et s'épuisant dans les efforts très prolongés, la rapportent à l'acidose provoquant la libération des ions Ca fixés aux protéines. Les partisans de l'hypocalciurie (un effort bref étant suffisant pour certains, un effort prolongé nécessaire pour d'autres) l'interprètent comme une meilleure fixation tissulaire (les exercices corrigent les pertes dues au décubitus prolongé). L'inhibition de la sécrétion gastrique par l'activité musculaire crée un pH intestinal trop alcalin freinant l'absorption et partant l'excrétion urinaire. La balance calcique et la calciurie de l'adulte sont plus stables à l'effort que celles des sujets jeunes ou âgés.

e) Magnésium. Les efforts étudiés sont tous de longue ou très longue durée. Quantitativement, les partisans de l'hypermagnésiurie l'emportent. Un travail sérieux note une excrétion diminuée de moitié. Rythme circadien et alimentation jouent un rôle important. Les mécanismes paraissent inconnus (intervention probable des parathyroïdes, compétition avec le Ca).

f) Phosphore et *phosphates.* Quelle que soit la durée, les modifications sont très variables, souvent importantes (quadruples), les partisans de l'hyperphosphaturie, de l'hypo, de l'absence de changements dans l'excrétion sont en nombre égal. L'hyperphosphaturie serait le témoin de la libération de radicaux phosphates, l'hypophosphaturie s'expliquerait par la resynthèse de composés phosphatés riches en énergie.

Rythme nycthéméral et excrétion intestinale retentissent sur les modifications urinaires à l'effort. Celui-ci entraînerait des modifications des mécanismes parathyroïdiens de filtration, réabsorption et sécrétion tubulaires des phosphates.

g) L'NH^{4+}, les *sulfates* et l'*iode inorganique* ont une excrétion augmentée.

III. Sueur

Les pertes de ce liquide difficile à prélever sont d'appréciation délicate. La sueur thermique, presqu'obligatoirement associée, masque partiellement les réactions à l'effort. Les variations interindividuelles et topographiques chez un même individu (sueur des mains très concentrée par rapport au reste du corps) sont grandes. Il n'est pas possible d'étudier les efforts brefs.

a) Potassium. Pour la majorité la concentration s'élève. Son origine est à la fois plasmatique et cutanée. Pour certains elle baisse beaucoup (50%). L'accord n'est pas réalisé quant à la concentration ou la dilution en K lorsque l'exercice se prolonge. L'entraînement (efforts prolongés) ou l'adaptation (efforts plus brefs) amortissent les variations. La fatigue sévère accentue la déperdition.

b) Sodium. La concentration augmente à l'effort, surtout prolongé. Toujours plus marquée que celle du K, elle peut quadrupler chez le sédentaire non entraîné. Le rapport Na/K s'élève. Certains signalent une baisse relativement faible (10%) et moins marquée que celle du K dans la vraie sueur ergique. Certains notent cependant une baisse de Na/K (aldostérone). L'accord n'est pas fait sur la diminution ou l'augmentation de la concentration lors de la prolongation de l'effort, ni sur une réabsorption partielle, en relation avec une hypothétique résorption aqueuse.

Il existerait un antagonisme entre aldostérone (rétention) et ADH (déperdition). L'augmentation concomittante paradoxale de l'excrétion du Na et du K serait due à une réaction d'hyperthyroïde. L'entraînement abaisse la concentration (baisse Na/K) malgré une sudation plus abondante. Fatigue et surentraînement accentuent les pertes (capacité de rétention débordée).

c) Chlore. Malgré l'absence d'un rapport quantitatif rigoureux, les conclusions tirées pour le Na peuvent s'appliquer au Cl. Le rapport Na/Cl baisse ou s'élève légèrement selon les auteurs. La nécessité d'un apport modéré en sel paraît admise.

d) Les activités physiques augmentent, dans la sueur ergique, les pertes en *Calcium* (origine partielle dans la desquamation). L'entraînement et l'acclimatement (sueur thermique) les diminuent. Les *phosphates*, l'NH^{4+} et l'*iode* subissent une élévation appréciable.

IV. Salive

Le nombre de travaux est restreint, les résultats contradictoires. Certains signalent une augmentation du débit mais l'hémoconcentration le diminue et la sécrétion est tarie quand la déshydratation atteint 8% du poids. En outre l'hyperventilation assèche la sécrétion et rend le recueil difficile.

a) Potassium. En général considéré comme inchangé au cours d'exercices prolongés, une augmentation importante a pu être observé par un auteur.

b) Sodium. La concentration de la salive, source importante d'élimination, est très variable, l'excrétion très élevée, inchangée ou très abaissée selon les auteurs, de même que le rapport Na/K. L'hyperconcentration paraît l'emporter (double), avec élévation de Na/K: par défaillance cortico surrénale, augmentation de la perméabilité de la barrière plasmo salivaire (ischémie), évaporation.

c) Les *chlorures* s'élèvent faiblement (efforts longs), les *iodures* davantage et les *phosphates* très fortement (une seule publication pour chacun).

Conclusion

Les activités physiques s'accompagnent de mouvements rapides et complexes des électrolytes aboutissant à des modifications humorales qui, comme on pouvait s'y attendre chez des sujets sains, sont habituellement peu importantes et sans retentissement majeur sur l'homéostasie. Ceci peut expliquer les nombreuses divergences notées dans la littérature.

Adresse des auteurs: Dr G. ROUGIER et Dr J. P. BABIN, Faculté de Médecine, Université de Bordeaux, Institut d'Education Physique, 3, place de la Victoire, *Bordeaux* (France).

Difference in the Quantity and Concentration of Sweat Produced on the Same Place of the Forearm

J. A. Král, J. Kopecká and A. Ženíšek

Institute of Sports Medicine, Medical Faculty of Charles University, Prague

The aim of this paper is to demonstrate that different factors changing the amount and concentration of sweat excreted on the same forearm under different influences, and the unacceptability of the supposition that on homologous places of extremities its quantity and concentration are identical.

Quantity

Asymmetry

The secretion of sweat is not symmetrical. In 95% of cases (men and women) an asymmetry in the amount of sweat (exceeding ± 5 mg) could be demonstrated.

Sex differences

A difference in the amount of sweat between men and women was found. In men, the quantity of induced sweat was 247.4 mg on the right and 264.9 mg on the left forearm. In women it was significantly lower, 201.6 mg on the right and 207.1 mg on the left side [3].

Crossed locomotor and sudomotor dominance

The quantity of induced sweat in the left-handed was greater on the contralateral than on the left forearm in 78,1 % of cases. Only 18,7 % of the left-handed had a greater amount of sweat on the forearm corresponding with their handedness. Among right-handed the percentage of those having a greater amount on the opposite forearm was equal to 60.0 % and on the same forearm to 40.0 % [3].

Influence of acute muscular work

Pilocarpine iontophoresis was performed before and after physical work. In all cases acute muscular work increased the amount of sweat [4].

Also the comparison of the influence of pilocarpine and of muscular work showed a significantly greater amount of effort sweat [5].

Influence of training

After a 2-months intensive power training the amount of sweat induced by pilocarpine at rest in wrestlers increased from 279.7 ± 97 mg to 318.0 ± 77 mg, whereas after an endurance training of cyclists it decreased from 392.9 ± 68 mg to 265.0 ± 150 mg [6].

Concentration

Difference between thermal and work sweat

In work sweat, the concentration of electrolytes (Na, K), urea and citrulline are higher than in thermal sweat; the concentration of amino-acid nitrogen, histidine and urocanic acid were the same as in thermal sweat.

The fractionated collection of sweat showed an increase of concentration of sodium during the three first 10-min periods in thermal sweating and its decrease in work sweating. This observation was done on sweat from the back [1, 2].

Acute muscular work

In the concentration of electrolytes in sweat there are differences. In a short work, we found an increase by 51.8% and 6.0%, in an exhausting work of longer duration a decrease of 9.4% and 8.2%. This decrease of concentration could perhaps be explained by a 'fatigue of sweat gland' after a previous sweating [5].

Training

After 2 months of power-training the concentration of Cl' in two groups of wrestlers decreased by 5.2 meq/l and after 1 month by 17.9 meq/l in endurance training of cyclists.

Although the chloride concentration of the rest sweat declined significantly under the influence of training, it remained within the limits of normal concentrations.

The study of the amount and concentration of sweat gives us much information about the irritability of sweat gland and indirectly about the changes of the tissue fluid, but if some comparison is done, it is necessary to be aware of differences due to sex and laterality.

Summary

The difference in quantity and concentration of eccrine sweat were studied. A difference between the sweat produced by thermal and chemical influence was found. An asymmetry in sweat gland secretion was found in 95 % of subjects. A crossed locomotor and sudomotor dominance was detected. A difference exists between the amount of sweat in men and women. Right-handed people sweat more then lefthanders. The concentration of sweat in trained athletes does not differ significantly from that of untrained ones, but there is a difference in the amount and concentration of induced sweat before and after muscular work.

References

1. HAIS, I. M.; KRÁL, J. A.; ŽENÍŠEK, A. and KREJČÍ, E.: Composition of thermic perspiration and perspiration after strenuous work in fractionated specimens. II. Effort Sweat. Vnitřní Lék. *5:* 1305–1315 (1959).
2. KRÁL, J. A.; HAIS, I. M.; KREJČÍ, E. and ŽENÍŠEK, A.: Composition of thermic perspiration and perspiration after strenuous work in fractionated specimens. I. Thermic perspiration. Čas. Lék. čes. *98:* 1268–1275 (1959).
3. KRÁL, J. A.; KOPECKÁ, J. and ŽENÍŠEK, A.: The physiological dissociation of motor and visceral nerve dominance. Vnitřní Lék. *13:* 726–730 (1967).
4. KRÁL, J. A.; KOPECKÁ, J. and ŽENÍŠEK, A.: The influence of an acute effort on the quantity of sweat and on the concentration and quantity of chlorides in induced-sweat. Čas. Lék. čes. *104:* 901–906 (1965).
5. KRÁL, J. A.; KOPECKÁ, J. and ŽENÍŠEK, A.: A different reaction of the sweat gland on the motoric load of different intensity. (In press.)
6. KRÁL, J. A.: KOPECKÁ, J. und ŽENÍŠEK, A.: Unterschiede der Adaptation des Chloridenhaushaltes beim Ausdauer- und Krafttraining; in Kongressbericht des XVI. Weltkongresses für Sportmedizin in Hannover 1966, pp. 524–528 (Deutscher Ärzte-Verlag, Köln–Berlin 1966).

Author's address: J. A. KRÁL, Institute of Sports Medicine, Medical Faculty of Charles University, Salmovské 5, *Prague* (Czechoslovakia).

Potassium and Physical Exercise

M. Mitolo† and D. Leone

Istituto di Fisiologia Umana, University of Bari, Bari

As the conclusion reached in a previous work [1], we have already reported that 10 albino rats (Wistar), by means of successive swimming tests performed at average intervals of 24 hours, can be trained to endure progressively longer periods of physical exercise; this duration is always greater when a solution of KCl is administered orally immediately before swimming.

In the present study our intention has been to define the experimental conditions better, not only as regards the diet of the rat (in view of the close relationship between potassium (K), glucide metabolism and adrenal glands), but also with regard to the mechanism by which the element acts upon the performance of the muscles. For this purpose we experimented on 8 albino rats (Wistar), of the male sex and weighing about 200 g, keeping them on a synthetic diet either with or without glucides: 4 rats (lot A) were given a food mixture containing pure starch (and consisting of raw casein 30%, gluten of raw maize 30%, rice starch 20%, butter 1 g *pro die* – about 15% – and Briggs saline mixture 5%); the other 4 rats (lot B) were given a diet composed of raw casein 35%, gluten of raw maize 35%, butter 2 g, *pro die* – about 25% – and Briggs saline mixture 5%. Each rat of lot A consumed, daily, an average of 6.66 g of the synthetic food; each rat of lot B consumed 8 g *pro die*. Briggs saline mixture was used since, among the saline mixtures used in synthetic diets, it is the one that contains the lowest amount of K; in fact, each rat of lot A consumed (*pro die*) 28.3 mg of K (in the form of K_2HPO_4) and each rat of lot B consumed (*pro die*) 32.8 mg (in the same form). Vitamins were not added, since casein and maize gluten, both administered in the raw state, contain factors B_1, B_2, B_6, PP, pantothenic acid, biotin, folic acid, and vitamins A and E, while butter contains vitamin A, D and E; the quantities of these vitamin factors ensured that the animal's relative daily need was satisfied. Each rat was kept, separately from the others, in a double-bottomed circular metal cage and the urine was collected (under toluene). In 3–5 days it was possible to collect 80–100 ml of urine, or more, on which to make the relative analyses.

At the beginning of the experiment, each rat was kept at rest in its cage for 4–5 days, during which time the urine was collected; the period of rest was then continued for a further 4–5 days (without collecting the urine). This was followed by the period of physical exercise, consisting of swimming in a rectangular reservoir of galvanized sheet iron, 4 m long, 40 cm deep and 14 cm wide, which had smooth walls in order to avoid the clinging of the animal. The water, which was frequently renewed, was at a temperature of 33–34°C and filled the reservoir to a depth of 30 cm. The physical exercise took place in a half-darkened laboratory; at the opposite end to that from which the animal started, an electric lamp (Philips 150 W) was placed, which acted as an attraction for the rat, which, on being thrown into the water at the other end (from a constant height), swam towards the lamp, also stressed by a jet of air issuing from bellows placed just above the surface of the water and moved along in the track of the animal. On the rear part of the rat's body, almost at the root of the tail, a small 10 g lead plate was tied, in order to prevent the animal from floating passively. As soon as the rat had swum the distance of 4 m, it was picked up with a large pair of forceps and returned to the starting-point; it was induced to swim once more, and so it continued until clear signs of fatigue appeared, first revealed as a decrease in speed, then as a tendency to swim *sur place* and finally as brief submersion. When this submersion lasted for 10 seconds it was thought as well to conclude the experiment, the total duration of which was noted (in minutes). Throughout the experiment, two swimming sessions were held every day: one in the morning and one in the afternoon, always at the same times.

The animal was then kept at rest for a week, during which time the effect of the training (which revealed itself as a period of endurance to swimming that generally lasted longer, each time, than the time before) passed off completely (see also [1]). Subsequently, the swimming sessions were resumed; this time, however, after the oral administration, *immediately before each session*, of 0.5 ml (45 mg of K) of a solution of KCl (16.96 g dissolved in H_2O to make 100 ml). In this second series of swimming experiments, each session was interrupted at the expiration of the time in which, in the first series, the animal had reached the stage of showing clear signs of fatigue, even if, as a result of the K consumed, the animal was either still swimming well or else was only slightly fatigued. Also in these experiments with K, two swimming sessions were held every day, one in the morning and one in the afternoon, at the same times. Throughout this period the urine was collected.

The total volume (in ml) of the urine collected in the three series of experiments (with a constantly alkaline reaction) was determined; it was then centrifuged, and albumin, if present, was separated after previous boiling and filtration (through a Schleicher-Schuell filter paper no. 589). The following tests were carried out on the filtrate: a) biuret test; b) qualitative glycosuria test (Trommer's reaction); if this was found to be positive, the urinary sugar was determined (Fehling's reaction); c) after previous acidification with HCl 1 N and prolonged boiling, Bial's test was carried out in order to check the presence of pentose (ribose or deoxyribose), resulting from the hydrolysis of nucleoproteids eventually present in the urine; d) the Elson-Morgan's test for amino-sugars, carried out on a sample of urine (of a volume always proportional to the total volume) acidified with HCl 2 N and passed through a Dowex-50 ion exchange column (in order to clear the excretum and separate out the amino-compounds that might give the colouring, even if glucosamine or galactosamine is not present); this test served to check whether mucopolysaccharides were or were not present in the urine; e) Donaggio's 'obstacle phenomenon' test, which, as is well-known, constitutes an excellent test of fatigue. For details of the results, see table in [2].

Conclusions

a) By means of successive daily swimming sessions (morning and afternoon), rats kept on a suitable synthetic diet can become trained to physical exercise, which generally increases progressively. When the synthetic diet is devoid of glucides (that is to say, devoid of rice starch) the progressive increase in the duration of the swimming sessions is not always very evident, so that the result of the training is fairly moderate compared with that of animals receiving the same diet, but also containing starch.

b) Comparing the results obtained with and without the oral administration of KCl (45 mg of K, just before swimming), it is observed that, at the expiration of the time in which, in the first series of sessions without K, the clear signs of fatigue were reached, the same rat is still capable of giving a good performance (at times, very good) or, at the most, shows only the first signs of fatigue. Consequently, if the experiment had not been interrupted, the animal would have gone on swimming.

c) The longer duration of the physical performance is due to the edlaying of the phenomenon of fatigue, as is shown by the analytical tests on the urine, which were carried out, for each rat, during the rest period, the swimming period without K and the swimming period with K. The behaviour of the Donaggio's 'obstacle reaction' is very significant, since it reveals the presence of mucoproteins in the urine of fatigued rats (in the second series of experiments), whereas, in the condition of rest and of swimming with K, these mucoproteins were either completely absent or else present in more or less limited quantities. The Elson-Morgan's reaction for the amino-sugars shows a similar behaviour even if this test and the Donaggio's reaction do not always show clearly parallel results. Both reactions give similar results, both for the rats kept on a synthetic diet containing starch and for those deprived of glucide.

d) In some cases the mucoproteinuria is associated with nucleoproteinuria, without there being, however, a similar behaviour of the Donaggio's reaction; this is a sign that the 'obstacle reaction' is found to be positive only when there are mucoproteids in the urine. In fact, nucleoproteinuria may occur even when the rat is not fatigued (having been treated with K).

e) Glycosuria may appear both in fatigued rats (without K) and in those that are still swimming well at the end of the experiment with K. Indeed, at times, the glycosuria either is present only in the series of experiments with K or else reaches higher values when K is administered (therefore, no clear fatigue appears). Evidently, the glycosuria resulting from effort is not directly related to the state of fatigue, nor does it express it, since it depends on other factors (metabolic, circulatory etc.); it is not even related to the presence or absence of starch in the synthetic diet of the rats.

f) The positive results of the biuret reaction is the generic expression not only of the mucoproteinuria but also of the nucleoproteinuria; it therefore cannot be considered any urinary biochemical criterion on the condition of fatigue, even if the reaction is performed on dealbuminized urine.

References

1. MITOLO, M.; LEONE, D. e VITELLIO, E.: Potassio ed esercizio fisico. Boll. Soc. ital. Biol. sper. *42:* 881–885 (1966).
2. MITOLO, M. e LEONE, D.: Ulteriori ricerche sperimentali sul potassio ed esercizio fisico. Boll. Soc. ital. Biol. sper. *43:* 807–810 (1967).

Author's address: Dr. D. LEONE, Physiological Institute, University of Bari, Policlinico, *70124 Bari* (Italy).

Enzymatic and Ionic Changes in Man Associated with Physical Work

Guy Metivier

Director, The Biokinetics Laboratory and Graduate Studies, The University of Ottawa, School of Physical Education and Recreation

Introduction

Work efficiency, a product of a multitude of physiological changes, has been analysed from various points of view by numerous investigators and by a multitude of methods, under various situations, both in normal, well trained and pathological subjects [2].

The capacity for prolonged muscular work is contingent upon the ability of the circulatory system to transport nutritive elements, oxygen and rid of the waste products. The organic efficiency required for sustained work, however, depends upon the functional capacity of the cell. Therefore, in order to better understand the physiology of work stamina one will ultimately seek the answers at the molecular level. The more vigorous the exercise, the more strain and stress will be placed upon the cell and the more efficient will enzymatic and endocrinological mechanisms will have to be.

In order to continue the rate of work, the cells will need an increased permeability. This necessitates either an increased concentration gradient of the substance across the membrane, a change in electrical gradient across the same or a difference in pressure gradient. It is a well known fact that decrease calcium in the extracellular fluid causes an increase in cell permeability [24]. Also, during prolonged exercise considerable dehydration results through sweating and lung ventilation. This, of course, causes a loss of water from the blood plasma causing a reduced circulating blood volume, and circulatory deficiency ensues. The elevated heart rate during this state is due to the circulatory strain [28].

The Aim

The purpose of the present investigation was to shed more light on the effects of exercise at the cellular level and especially to investigate the effects of a prolonged work period on the sodium, potassium, chlorine and calcium ions. A secondary purpose was to observe the variation, if any, of serum glutamic-oxalacetic transminase during this physical stress.

Method

Five young male physical education students in good physical condition were selected for the experiment. Each was requested to report in a post absorptive state at our laboratory three mornings during one week at which time a 30 cc sample of blood was taken from the brachial vein. The sodium, potassium, chloride and calcium and SGOT levels were determined by means of a technicon sequential automatic analyzer.

The following weeks each subject was requested to report to the laboratory in a similar state and at the same time. Following a resting period of 30 min, a catheter was introduced in any large peripheral vein of the subjects' arm. The catheter remained in the arm for as long as 1 h following the exercise bout. The subject was then made to run on a motor driven treadmill (0° inclimation) for 30 min at 7 mph. Blood samples were collected every ten min during the run, 30 min following it, one h and two h after. Each subject was tested a second time the week which followed. Following the collection of blood, the serum was frozen and stored to be analyzed the following day. The 't' test for the difference between means was applied to the data.

Results

Exercise caused an increase in all ions studied but the highest concentrations were observed 20 min after the exercise had begun and consequently a gradual decline appeared in the Cl^-, $K+$ and $Na+$ respectively. The $Ca++$ level increased until the end of the work bout. There was a sudden drop in all of the ions studied following exercise. (*Graph 1, 2, 3, 4*).

Serum glutamic-oxalacetic transaminase (SGOT) increased for the first 10 min of exercise, decreased somewhat during the middle of the run to subsequently increase to the termination of the work period. Following exercise it showed a decline for one h and increased thereafter (*Graph 5*).

Discussion

The ions here studied have a predominant role to play during activity. The excitability, contractility and permeability of muscle are strongly

Table I. Ionic and enzymatic values associated with exercise

	R	A	B	Time C	D	E	F	G
			Parameters					
Na	143.4	143.9	144.7	145.2	145.0	143.9	143.9	144.4
K	4.27	4.29	4.69	4.91	4.69	4.42	4.37	4.34
Cl	105.7	104.0	105.9	106.5	105.9	105.3	105.6	105.0
Ca	9.66	9.68	10.0	10.1	10.2	9.46	9.60	10.0
SGOT	24.3	31.0	31.9	30.3	32.9	31.5	31.6	33.0

R: Average of 3 samples, 1 week before exercise
A: Immediately before run
B: After 10 minutes of exercise
C: After 20 minutes of exercise
D: Immediately after exercise
E: 30 minutes after exercise
F: 60 minutes after exercise
G: 120 minutes after exercise

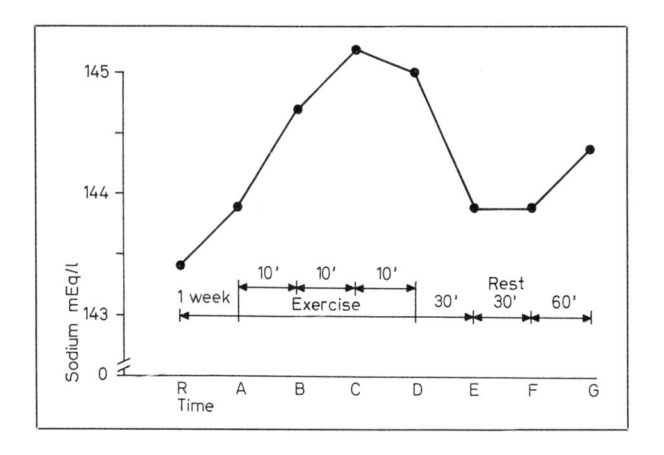

Graph 1 Sodium changes associated with physical exercise

influenced by the presence of K+ and Ca++ within and outside of the muscle cells. Depolarization of the muscular membrane is a consequent of its increased permeability to Na+ ions and repolarization a result of outward flow of K+ ions [16]. It was also reported by GROB [23] that the increase in serum K+ during repeated muscle contraction was roughly proportional to the work done.

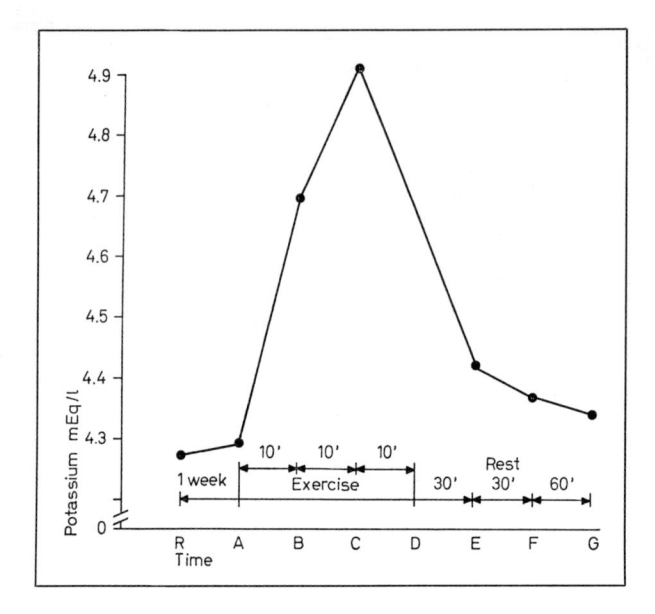

Graph 2 Potassium changes associated with physical exercise

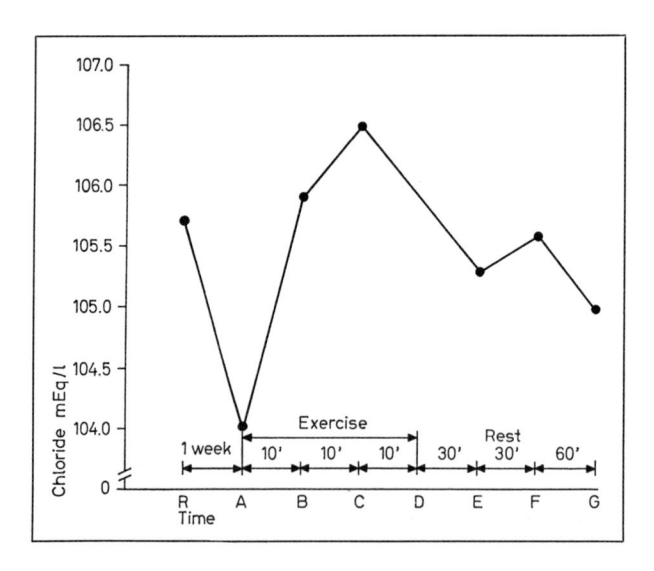

Graph 3 Chloride changes associated with physical exercise

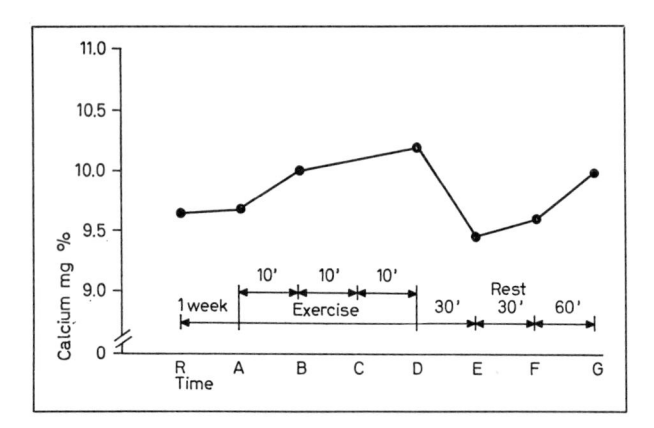

Graph 4 Calcium changes associated with physical exercise

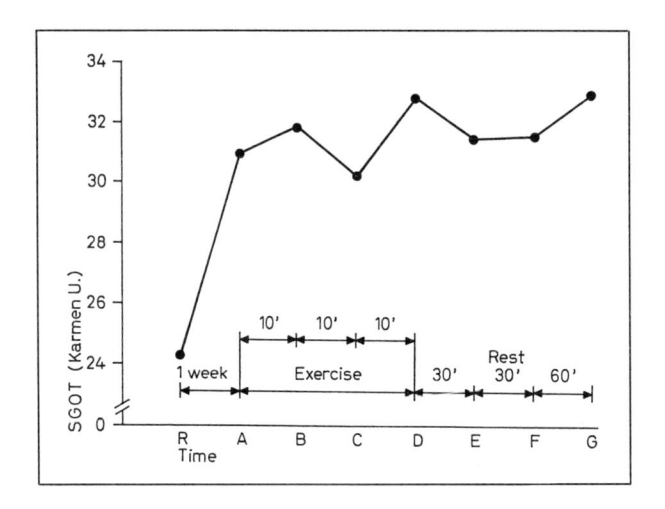

Graph 5 Changes in SGOT associated with physical exercise

Also numerous studies *in vitro* have demonstrated that glucose enters the cells of both muscle [18] and liver [19] with K+ ions, and that this transfer is followed by a deposition of glycogen [17, 8]. It seems also probable that *in vivo* this occurs. BOYER and co-workers [4, 10] showed that K+ is employed in the phosphorylation of hexose and in the transfer of high energy phosphate from phosphopyruvate, to adenosine diphosphate (ADP) ot

Table II. Values of t ($p < \cdot 0.5$)

	M-X$_1$	M-X$_2$	D	t
Na	143.7	145.24	-1.54	-2.6688
K	4.282	4.690	-0.408	-1.0840
Cl+	104.820	105.920	-1.10	-0.6815
Ca	9.678	10.210	-0.532	-3.0477*
SGOT	27.680	32.900	-5.22	-0.8466

* Significant

adenosine triphosphate (ATP) and perhaps to creatinine to form creatinine phosphate [5].

GROB [23] suggested also that these organic phosphate compounds may be present in the cell as the K+ salts. Also he continues in saying that the release of K+ during muscular exercise may be the result of their dephosphorylation as well as of glycolysis. An increase in the amount of diffusible K+ in muscle after prolonged activity has been demonstrated [34].

DE LANNE [14] and colleagues observed that following a 30 min work bout on a bicycle ergometer, set at 540 KPM, Na+ and Ca++ and K+ increased, but K+ more so than the two others. They suggested that according to their finding of a proportional increase in plasma phosphate, there is the probability of K+ leaving the muscles bound to phosphates.

The increase in Na+ and Cl- ions in the serum does in fact reflect an increased permeability of the muscle cell membrane; whereby these ions are liberated into the interstitial fluids and eventually into the blood stream through diffusion to maintain osmotic equilibrium [14]. The state of hyperchloremia occurring during exercise can be accounted for by the increased CO_2 production and its rapid elimination through hyperventilation. Changes in chlorides and sodium in the body occur simultaneously and in the same direction, except under certain conditions [22, p. 175]. The high concentration of protein in the cells limits the amount of base available for combination with electrolytes and ions [22, p. 175].

Cases of hyperchloremia may reflect in part the lack of tubular filtration by the renal tubule. This state of vasoconstriction of renal blood vessels during work is well known, and the slow rate of Na+ absorption by the renal tubule has been demonstrated during work [35], therefore explaining also its high concentration in the serum.

The increase in Ca+ during the work period could be caused by a hypersecretion of the parathyroid glands [36]. Turner states that during periods of parathyroid hypersecretions, hypercalcemia and demineralization of the skeleton develops. Also the alkaline phosphatase concentration of the serum is increased indicating heightened osteoblastic activity or the retention of Ca++ within the plasma during work was probably caused by an increased protein binding as suggested by Ewig and Weiner [15].

In 1937 Braunstein and Kritsman [6] opened up the field of transamination. Since then the interest of SGOT has been focussed on its presence in the serum accompanying myocardial infarction [29]. Some investigators [31, 7] were of the opinion that the aforementioned enzyme was liberated into the blood because of damaged tissue of the myocardium. It was also suggested by Agress [1] and colleagues that the serum content of the enzyme was proportional to the degree of the infarct.

There seems to be conflicting evidence as to the variation of this enzyme during physical exercise [11, 13, 30, 32]. One has to take, however, into consideration that exercise tolerance from one subject to the next is not the same and investigators have reported their findings in accordance with various work loads.

Critz [12] found in his work that the duration of exercise in rats determined the SGOT response. Swimming rats for 1 min caused a decline in SGOT activity while a 5 min swim resulted in elevation of the activity.

During very long exercise the SGOT activities increased. According to this investigator the elevated enzyme activity was a result of a hypoxic condition developing in the active muscle. This would increase the cellular membrane's permeability thus releasing the enzyme in the serum. This increased permeability is a result of catecholamine secretion initiated by the hypoxic condition [27].

Cohen [9] suggested that GOT in the serum may play a role in muscle contraction and could enter the Krebs cycle. Since trained subjects have usually a higher VO_2 capacity, and also capable of encountering a greater O_2 debt than untrained athletes, it follows that this last hypothesis may hold true. Inference to this effect may be made in respect to the work of Fowler et al. [20], where it was found that the increase in serum activity was related to the previous training of the person and the severity of the exercise over a 15 min period.

Pearson [33] inferred also that during long sustained exercise there was a change in the cellular structure of the liver. This cellular change could be associated with the release of this enzyme into circulation. Also since during prolonged exercise there is a serious depletion of liver glycogen, this would mean a greater cellular permeability of the cells of the organ which could account for the high concentration of SGOT in the blood plasma [3, 25, 26].

Conclusion

Even if the changes associated with a work bout of 30 min on a motor driven treadmill at 7 mph did not prove to be statistically significant in young trained subjects, it remains that these variations indicate some physiological modifications. In accordance with our data and that of others, we are of the opinion that during physical exercise, the increase in electrolytes in the serum is a resultant of increased celullar permeability Grought about by catechol amine release. This condition serves as a protective mechanism to retain blood osmolality hence controling plasma volume. Potassium ions are moving along with the glucose molecules and suggest an increase hepatic activity.

The increased glutamic-oxalacetic transaminase in the serum, we believe, is a result of either increased permeability or traumatized cells. The latter hypothesis needs verification.

Acknowledgement

Acknowledgement is made to Dr. W. Poznanski and Dr. D. Strikland of the Ottawa Civic Hospital for their valuable contribution toward the project.

References

1. Agress, C.; Jacobs, H.; Glassner, H.: Serum transaminase levels in experimental myocardial infarction. Circulation *11:* 711–713 (1955).
2. Ahlborg, Björn: Capacity for prolonged exercise in man. Forsvarsmedicin *3:* Suppl. 1 (1967).
3. Bedrak, E.: Blood serum enzyme activity of dogs exposed to heat stress and muscular exercise. J. appl. physiol. *20:* 587–590 (1965).
4. Boyer, P. D.; Lardy, H. A. and Phillips, P. H.: Further studies on the role of potassium and other ions in the phosphorylation of the adenylic system. J. biol. Chem. *97:* 62 (1932).
5. Boyer, P. D.; Lardy, H. A. and Phillips, P. H.: The role of potassium in muscle phosphorylations. J. biol. Chem. *146:* 673 (1942).

6. Braunstein, A. and Kritsman, M.: Decomposition and synthesis of amino acids by conversion of amines, studies on muscle tissues. Enzymologia 2: 129–146 (1937).
7. Brouhon, N.: Clinical interest in the determination of serum transaminase and lactic dehydrogenase. J. Pharmacol. Belg. 16: 286–300 (1961).
8. Buchanan, J. M.; Hastings, A. B. and Nesbett, F. B.: The effect of the tonic environment on the synthesis of glucogen from glucose in rat liver slices. J. biol. Chem. 180: 435 (1949).
9. Cohen, P.: Transamination with purified enzyme preparations (Transaminase). J. biol. Chem. 136: 565–601 (1940).
10. Conway, E. J. and Boyle, P. J.: A mechanism for the concentrating of potassium by cells with experimental verification for muscle. Nature 144: 709 (1939).
11. Critz, J. and Merrick, A.: Serum Glutamic-oxalacetic transaminase levels after exercise in men. Proc. Soc. exp. Biol. Med. 109: 608–610 (1962).
12. Critz, J. and Merrick, A.: Transaminase changes in rats after exercise. Proc. Soc. exp. Biol. Med. 115: 11–14 (1964).
13. Critz, J.: Heart disease, exercise and serum glutamic-oxalacetic transaminase. S. Dak. Jour. Med. 20: 27–30 (1967).
14. De Lanne, R.; Barnes, J. R. and Brouha, L.: Changes in osmotic pressure and ionic concentrations of plasma during muscular work and recovery. J. appl. Physiol. 14: 804–808 (1959).
15. Ewig, W. and Wiener, R.: Z. ges. exper. Med. 61: 562 (1928).
16. Fatt, P.: Biophysics of junctional transmission. Physiol. Rev. 34: 674 (1954).
17. Fenn, W. O.: The role of potassium in physiological processes. Physiol. Rev. 20: 377 (1940).
18. Fenn, W. O. and Haege, L. F.: The deposition of glycogen with water in the liver of cats. J. biol. Chem. 136: 87 (1940).
19. Fenn, W. O.: The deposition of potassium and phosphate with glycogen in rat livers. J. biol. Chem. 128: 297 (1939).
20. Fowler, W. M.; Chowdhury, S. R.: Changes in serum enzymes levels after exercise in trained and untrained subjects. J. appl. Physiol. 17: 943 (1962).
21. George, W. K.; Dotson, D. A.: A comparison of the changes of serum calcium during exercise and hyperventilation. Clin. Res. 14: 62 (1966).
22. Gradwohl's Clinical Laboratory Methods and Diagnosis, p. 175 (C.V. Mosby Company, Saint Louis 1963).
23. Grob, David; Liljerstrand, A. and Johns R. J.: Potassium movement in normal subjects; effect on muscle function. Am. Journ. Med., pp. 340–355 (1957).
24. Guyton, A. C.: Textbook of medical physiology, p. 48 (Saunders Co., Philadelphia and London).
25. Halonen, P. I. and Konttinen: Effect of physical exercise on some enzymes in the serum. Nature 193: 942–944 (1962).
26. Highman, B. and Altland, P. D.: Serum enzyme and his topathologic changes in rats after cold exposures. Proc. Soc. expl. Biol. Med. 109: 523–526 (1962).
27. Highman, B.; Mal'ng, H. and Thompson, E.: Serum transaminase and alkaline phosphatase levels after large doses of morepinephrine and epnephrine in dogs. Am. J. Physiol. 196: 436–440 (1959).
28. Johnson, W.: Science and Medicine of Exercise and Sports, p. 226 (Hayer and Brothers Publ., New York 1960).

29. LA DUE, J.; WROBLEWSKI, F. and KARMEN, A.: Serum glutamic-oxalacetic transaminase activity in human acute transmural myocardial infarction. Science *120:* 497–499 (1954).
30. LAETS, G. J.: Variations of serum transaminase activity during labour. Proc. IV. Intern. Congr. clin. Chem., p. 172 (Livingstone, Edinburgh and London 1961).
31. LEMLEY-STONE, J.; MERRILL, J.; GRACE, J. and MC-NEELY, G.: Transamination in experimental myocardial infarction. Am. J. Physiol. *183:* 555–558 (1955).
32. NERDRUM, H. and NORDOY, S.: Changes of serum glutamic-oxalacetic transaminase following exercise in patients with and without coronary disease. Scand. Jour. clin. Lab. Invest. *16:* 617–623 (1964).
33. PEARSON, C. M.: Histopathological features of muscle in the preclinical stages of muscular dystrophy. Brain *85:* 169 (1962).
34. REGINSTER, A.: Recherches sur le potassium diffusible et non diffusible du muscle. Arch. int. Physiol. *45:* 69 (1937).
35. SHEER, R.: Studies on the renal concentrating mechanism. J. clin. Invest. *38:* 8 (1959).
36. TURNER, D. C.: General Endocrinology, p. 161 (Saunders Co., Philadelphia and London 1961).

Author's address: GUY MÉTIVIER, Ph.D., F.A.C.S.M., Director, Department of Kinanthropology, University of Ottawa, School of Physical Education and Recreation, *Ottawa 2* (Canada).

VI. Proteins in Biological Fluids

Influence of Physical Exercise on Proteins in Biological Fluids

J. R. POORTMANS[1]

Laboratoire de l'Effort, Université Libre de Bruxelles, Bruxelles[1] (Director: Prof. M. SEGERS)

Proteins have a particular significance in biology in that they constitute one of the indispensable components of living matter. Since an enormous number of proteins is known, and since their properties vary considerably, many attempts have been made to classify proteins systematically. Most of the classifications are unsatisfactory. In view of the present lack of a structural basis for the classification of proteins, it seems suitable to arrange the proteins according to their biological distribution and function.

It is well known that, generally, proteins do not belong to substances which contribute as a source of energy for muscular activity. However, they may reflect modifications in membrane permeability, for example in the kidney, an increased metabolism or a tissue breakdown, as in the connective tissue. Therefore, the study of protein distribution, especially in the body fluids, might shed light on some feature connected with muscular exercise.

In the present report, we will emphazise the changes which occur in the protein distribution in blood, urine and to a lesser extent in sweat secretion.

The plasma proteins comprise a dynamic system with varied functions. They are properly considered together as a system of proteins because of their similar biosynthetic origin, their participation in common processes, and their occurrence together as the major extracellular components of the circulatory system. Plasma is also an important medium to investigate, since it is a common denominator to interstitial tissue fluids or extravascular circulation. This extravascular portion is biologically the most important one, since it represents the very medium in which the body cells live and with which they exchange nutrients and wastes. The primary functions of the plasma proteins include the maintenance of the colloid osmotic pressure, pH and electrolyte balance; the transport of metal ions, fatty acids, steroids, hormones, etc.; their ready availability as a nutritional source of amino acids

---

[1] This work has been supported by a grant of the Fonds National de la Recherche Scientifique.

for the tissues; hemostasis and prevention of thrombosis; regulation of cellular activity and function via the hormones and defense against invasion through the action of antibodies and other serum factors.

Some proteins are capable of performing an exclusive function, i.e. without the assistance of any other plasma protein. For instance, free iron is transported by transferrin and by no other protein, in man. In contrast to this are the functions requiring a number of factors, i.e. the function of complement which is dependent on the sequential action of a series of proteins. The above considerations have conducted FREEMAN [7] to elaborate a distinction between *biophilic proteins* that survive after performing their function and *suicidal* ones that are destroyed in the process of their function.

The identification, characterization and separation of the plasma proteins has been greatly facilitated by zone electrophoresis. Paper electrophoresis has established five conventional zones: albumin, a_1-, a_2-, β- and γ-globulins. However, the introduction of immunological techniques give a new dimension to the electrophoresis of serum, through the identification of components with the a-, β- and γ-areas. In the case of normal serum, up to 30 independent proteins can be distinguished.

Immunoelectrophoresis not only offers the specificity of immunoprecipitation, but also achieves a separation of components based on their rate of diffusion and initial concentration in serum. This technique offers a very sensitive test for homogeneity and identification of serum proteins.

After these preliminary considerations, the perturbations which occur in blood during exercise may be analysed.

It is well recognized that strenuous exercise enhances the level of plasma proteins in serum (table I). Generally there is an increase up to 15%. However, one of the problems to be solved was: Is this increase in relation to a phenomenon of hemoconcentration which might occur after strenuous exercise? Studies on a comparison of proteinemia and hematocrit do not reveal a complete relationship between these two factors (table II). Generally,

Table I. Variation of proteinemia during exercise: g/100 ml

	Rest	Exercise	Authors
Untrained	6.55	6.92	R. DELANNE (1957) [5]
Cyclists	7.83	8.49	P. CHAILLEY-BERT, F. PLAS (1959) [3]
Gymnasts	7.38	8.10	B. DELFORGE, E. DELFORGE, J. R. POORTMANS (1968)
Olympic athletes	7.01	7.56	J. R. POORTMANS (1968)

Table II. Variation of proteinemia and hematocrit during exercise (difference in percent between exercise and rest)

No	Hematocrit	Proteinemia	Authors
36	+ 8.7	+ 11.0	R. Delanne (1957) [5]
10	+ 7.1	+ 11.6	J. R. Poortmans (1968)
4	0	+ 4.8	
1	− 2.0	+ 7.0	

Table III. Determination of plasma proteins in serum of 31 athletes, during exercise: statistical validity
A. Rest   B. after exercise   C. 30 min after exercise

Components	B/A	C/A
Total protein	+ + +	NS
Perchlorosoluble proteins	NS	NS
Thermosoluble proteins	NS	NS
Albumine	+ +	+
a_1-acid-glycoprotein	NS	NS
a_1-antitrypsin	NS	NS
Transferrin	NS	NS
γA-globulin	NS	NS
γM-globulin	NS	NS
γG-globulin	+	NS

$P < 0.0005$: + + +
$P = 0.005$: + +
$P = 0.05$: +
NS: non significant

the variation between exercise and rest is greater for proteinemia than for hematocrit. Therefore, the next step was to investigate the electrophoretic pattern of serum proteins during muscular activity. Statistical analyses have not revealed any variation in the relative proportion of the peaks of albumin, a_1-, a_2-, β- and γ-globulins, compared between rest and exercise. Knowing that the previous technique remains a rough method, immunological quantitative determinations of several individual serum components were persued on athletes who underwent a maximal effort on a ergometric cycle (table III).

Only albumin and γG-globulin follow a statistically valuable increase after exercise, as compared to rest. This represents nearly 11% for both proteins.

However, when athletes who had the highest proteinemia variation between rest and exercise were tested, a decrease of the a_1-acid-glycoprotein was found in addition to the previous results immediately after stopping the exercise. It must then be proposed that, in addition to the hemoconcentration phenomenon, strenuous exercise brings into the plasma a supplement of albumin and γG-globulin, while the content of a_1-acid-glycoprotein is reduced in severe exercise.

These results have probably to be related to changes in the membrane permeability of capillaries. Nevertheless, the theory of PAPPENHEIMER [15] on the exchange of macromolecules through the capillary walls is to be applied with great care, since generally the values of all the parameters included in his formula are not known. However, it was found in dogs that while the flow of lymph was much increased by exercise, its protein content declined and then remained constant as long as exercise continued. The elevations of capillary blood pressure and of interstitial fluid pressure during exercise have also been described.

Few authors have taken their attention to the variations induced by exercise on the level of glycoproteins in serum. Serum glycoproteins are usually designated as components which reflect disturbances of connective tissue. Here, some discrepancies appear in the results obtained by different workers, who found no variation or an increase in the plasma level of glycoproteins, following muscular activity.

An interesting finding was that of HARALAMBIE who points out that overtraining may influence the level of plasma proteins and glycoproteins. Usually, overtraining reduces the level of proteinemia and rises those of glycoproteins and urea [9]. This author therefore suggests that strenuous exercise and overtraining induce perturbations at the level of connective tissue. Meanwhile, this hypothesis remains to be prooved by suitable methods, such as by turnover studies.

The metabolism of proteins may be appreciated in some extent by the determination of amino-acids, ammonia and urea in blood (table IV).

These results reveal that amino-acids are presumably not important as energy supply during exercise. However, the increase in urea and ammonia indicates that the catabolism of proteins and amino-acids might be enhanced under strenuous physical activity.

Several authors have attempted to describe the modifications involved in blood coagulation during and after exercise. Difficulties arise from the fact that many substances are utilized during the normal process of

Table IV. Variations of amino acids, urea and ammonia during exercise

	Amino acids mg/100 ml	Urea mg/100 ml	Ammonia µg/100 ml	Authors
R	–	32	–	P. Chailley-Bert and Plas (1959) [3]
Ex	–	61	–	
R	–	38	–	G. Haralambie (1966) [9]
Ex	–	58	–	
R	–	–	70	H. McCullough (1968) [17]
Ex	–	–	280	
R	5.23	–	275	J. Keul, E. Doll et al. (1968) [13]
Ex	5.72	–	358	

R: Rest
Ex: After Exercise

coagulation. Generally, the amount of thrombocytes, of fibrinogen, of factors V, VII and VIII are increased during exercise and these results have led to the conclusion of an excessive process of clotting.

It has been suggested by Sarajas, Konttinen and Frick [27] that hypercoagulability associated with exercise might possibly be ascribable to thrombocytosis rather than to any increase in the level of the coagulation factors in the plasma. These authors suggest that, on acceleration of circulation leucocytes and platelets, an altered fragility and adhesiveness of these cellular blood elements may come into play. Besides this phenomenon, it has been shown that the fibrinolytic response to exhaustive exercise appears to be impaired in some normal subjects. Cash [1] has described that exercise induces an increase of fibrinolytic activity. However, some subjects may present a poor fibrinolytic response to exercise. This differentiation may prove to be relevant when further thought is given to the physio-pathological significance of the poor fibrinolytic response.

The next medium to be analyzed for its protein content is urine. One knows that normal human urine contains, under rest conditions, a small quantity of proteins, amounting to nearly 40 mg per 24 hours. It has been recognized as early as 1878 by von Leube, that strenuous exercise induces a rise in urinary protein excretion [16]. Several authors have presented the variations of proteinuria produced during muscular activity [see 22]. It has been shown that urinary protein excretion may be enhanced up to one hundredfold during and after exercise.

It was of great interest to investigate the qualitative aspect of exercise proteinuria, and to compare it to normal proteinuria at rest. For this purpose, several techniques are available: agar gel electrophoresis, immunoelectrophoresis, immunodiffusion, gel filtration and ultracentrifugation.

All these methods reveal fundamental differences between normal proteinuria and exercise proteinuria. Agar gel electrophoresis gives a better resolution of the globulin fraction in the latter case than in the former one.

In immunoelectrophoresis, a higher number of precipitin lines are obtained in urine collected after exercise than in urine collected at rest. Up to 25 components are found, as compared to 15 in normal urine (fig. 1).

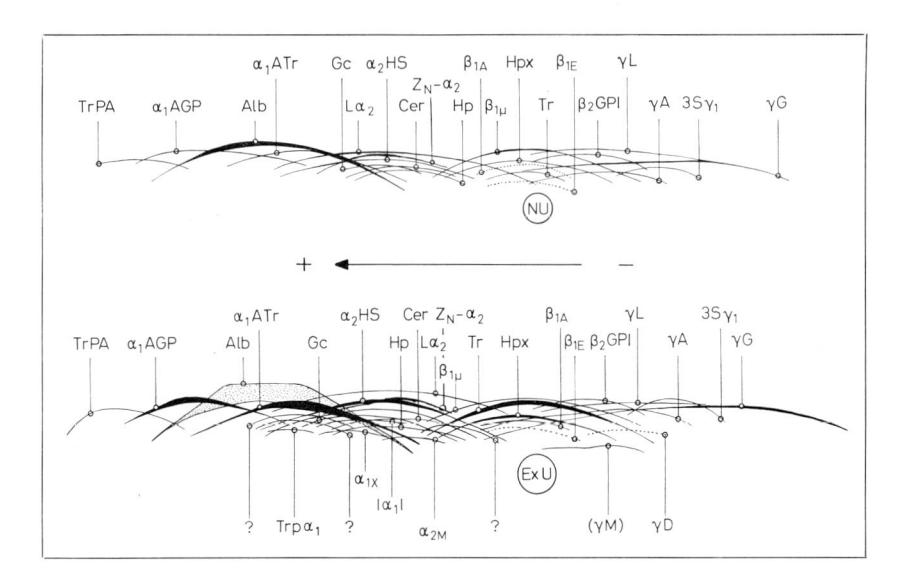

Figure 1. Immunoelectrophoresis pattern of plasma proteins in normal human urine, before and after exercise.

The following abreviations are used: Tr PA, tryptophan-rich prealbumin; a_1AGP, a_1-acid glycoprotein; Alb. albumin; a_1ATr, a_1-antitrypsin; Trpa_1, tryptophan poor a_1-glycoprotein; Gc, a_2Gc-globulin; a_2HS, a_2HS-glycoprotein; Hp, haptoglobin-a_{1X}, a_{1X}-glycoprotein; Cer., Ceruloplasmin; I a I, inter- a trypsininhibitor; Zn-a_2, Zn-a_2; glycoprotein; La_2, long a_2-globulin; a_2M, a_2-macroglobulin; β_{1u}, β_1-microglobulin; Tr., transferrin; Hpx, hemopexin; β_{1A}, β_{1A}-globulin; β_{1E}, β_{1E}-globulin; β_2GPI, β_2-glycoprotein I; γL, light chain; (γM), γM-subunit; 3Sγ_1, 3Sγ_1-globulin; γA, γA-globulin; γG, γG-globulin.

The pattern of 'exercise urine' (Ex U) shows in its lower part the proteins which are not found in normal urine at rest (NU).

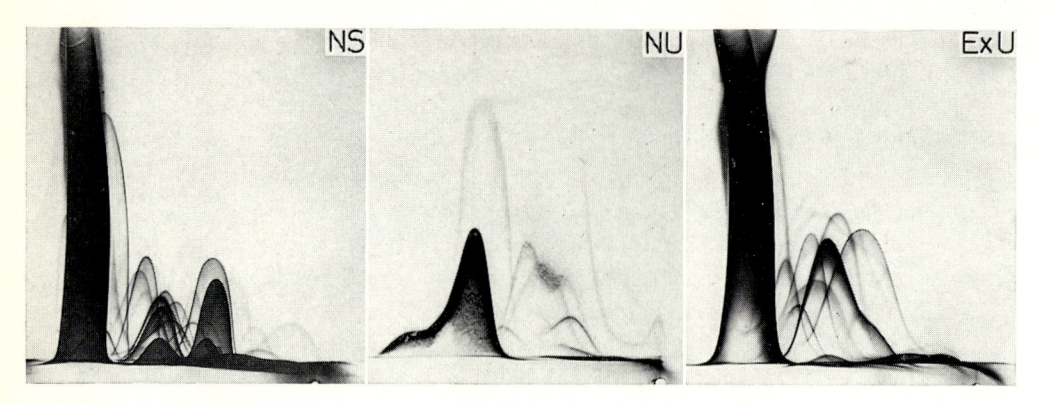

Figure 2. Quantitative immunoelectrophoresis of normal urine collected at rest and after exercise.

By use of an antiserum against plasma proteins, this technique reveals that normal serum (NS) contains numerous proteins. Normal urine (NU) gives an entirely different pattern where it can be shown that this medium contains only few proteins in the globulin fractions. On the contrary, urine collected after strenuous exercise (Ex U) exhibits a unique distribution which is not related to normal serum and normal urine. More proteins are quantitatively and qualitatively detected in exercise urine.

A new technique, named quantitative immunoelectrophoresis, also shows the differences in the protein pattern of normal serum, normal urine and exercise urine (fig. 2).

Figures 1 and 2 reveal that the normal urine pattern is not related to normal serum, and most important, that exercise proteinuria is not comparable to a more concentrated normal urine. To argue on this latter point, the level of 15 plasma proteins has been investigated in normal urine and in urine collected after exercise. The single radial immunodiffusion technique stresses that the urinary excretion of plasma proteins is increased from an average of 2- to 40-fold, depending on the protein investigated (table V).

If the quantitative data concerning the plasma proteins are cumulated, one comes to the conclusion that they represent nearly 55% of the non-ultrafiltrable proteins of normal urine, while this percentage reaches a value of 82% after strenuous exercise.

These results suggest that exercise proteinuria is mainly due to an accentuated penetration of plasma proteins through the glomerule. At this point, the next question to solve was: Does exercise increase the glomerular permeability, or, in other words, are higher molecular weight proteins found in exercise urine than in normal urine?

Table V. Excretion of plasma proteins in the urine of normal subjects at rest and after exercise. (Marathon race of 42.5 km)

Plasma proteins	At rest µg/min	After exercise µg/min
Tryptophan-rich prealbumin	0.02	0.26
Albumin	8.84	126.70
a_1-acid glycoprotein	0.29	11.83
a_1-antitrypsin	0.21	2.04
Ceruloplasmin	0.04	0.39
a_2HS-glycoprotein	0.75	2.88
Zn-a_2-glycoprotein	0.93	18.00
Haptoglobin type 1-1	0.13	0.79
Gc-globulin	0.02	0.37
Transferrin	0.15	3.31
Hemopexin	0.14	1.21
β_2-glycoprotein I	0.23	0.34
3Sγ_1-globulin	0.02	0.35
γA-globulin	0.35	1.18
γG-globulin	1.71	20.09

This problem was investigated by gel filtration on Sephadex G150 and G200. Comparing normal urine and exercise urine it was found that the protein distribution differs for both fluids. Immunoelectrophoresis shows that more γG-globulin was present in the 7S peak of urine collected after exercise. Generally, more proteins are present, especially in the peaks 7S and 4.5S (fig. 3, 4).

Moreover, it was also demonstrated that haptoglobin type 2-1 of 200,000 of molecular weight was present in some exercise urine, while haptoglobin type 1-1 of 100,000 of molecular weight only could be found in normal urine [25].

Finally, gel filtration experiments are capable to elucidate more or less the problem of immunoglobulins and their subunits in normal and exercise urines. Concerning the subunits of γG-molecule, no qualitative variation was identified between normal and exercise urines. It is to say that Fab- and Fc-fragments as well as light and heavy chains are detected. Also urine collected after exercise presents special interest for its content of γM- and γD-related substances. Using specific antiserum, it was possible to detect a precipitin line related to the μ-chain. This component was present in the 4S peak of Sephadex G 200 gel filtration [24]. Some exercise urines also show a precipitin reaction against an anti-γD-globulin.

Normal Urine: Sephadex G 200

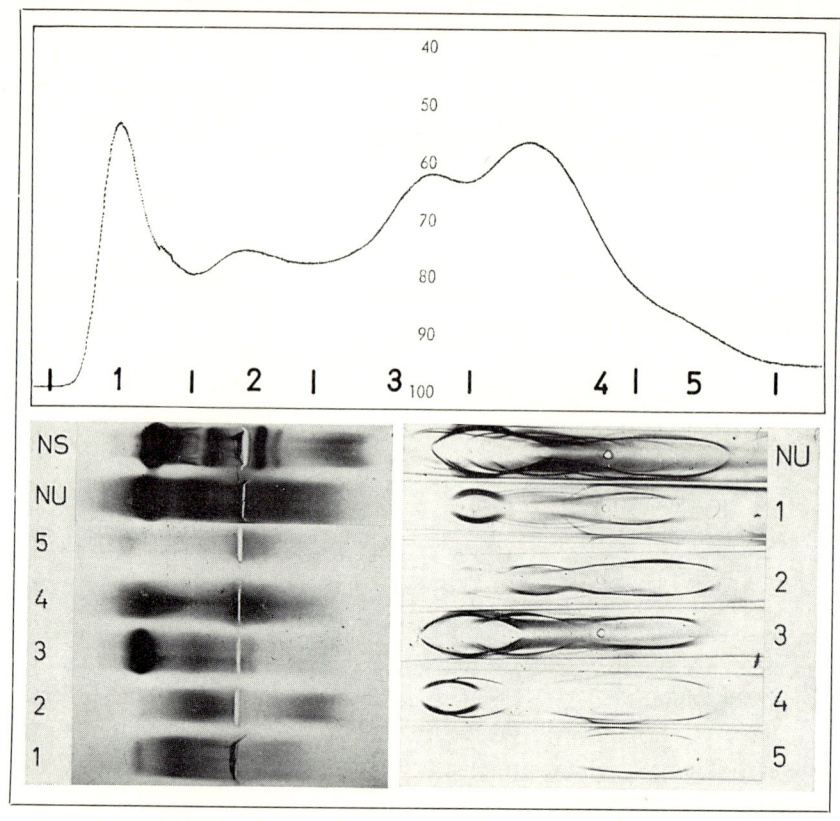

Figure 3. Gel filtration of concentrated normal urine on Sephadex® G 200.
    The upper part shows the optical density curve at 280 mμ which reflects the gel filtration of urinary proteins according to their decreasing molecular weight distribution from left to right.
    The lower part indicates the agar gel electrophoresis (at left) and immuno-electrophoresis (at right) of the 5 collected fractions isolated after gel filtration.

Comparing exercise proteinuria with pathological proteinuria we are able to answer that the perturbations observed in urine after strenuous physical exertion are of glomerular origin. Indeed, it has been shown that pathological proteinuria may originate from glomerular and/or tubular disturbances. The presence of high level of tubular proteins in urine are detected by bidimensional starch-gel electrophoresis and analytical ultra-centrifugation. This discrepancy is based on the low molecular weight of

Exercise Urine: Sephadex G 200

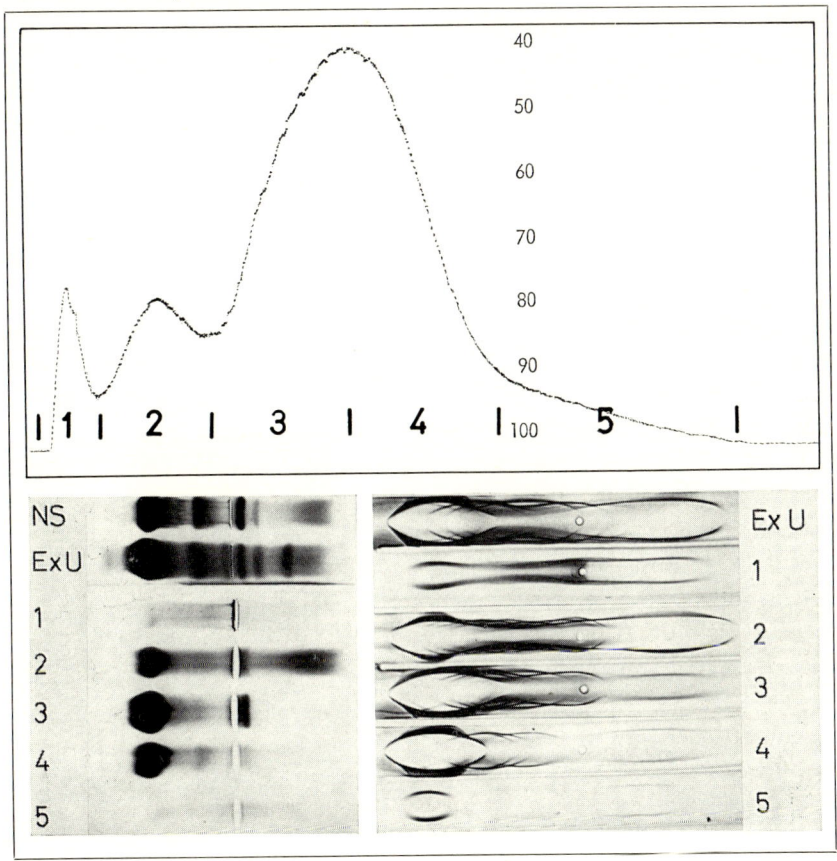

Figure 4. Gel filtration of concentrated exercise urine on Sephadex® G 200 (same legend as for figure 3).

tubular proteins. Using both criteria, it may be concluded that exercise proteinuria is of glomerular origin. All the above data support the hypothesis that during physical exertion the kidney permits free egress to plasma proteins of high molecular weight than those normally found in urine.

The accuracy of the immunological determination of plasma proteins in both plasma and urine allow the calculation of the renal clearance of individual plasma proteins at rest and after exercise. It was shown by HARDWICKE, SOOTHILL, *et al.* [10] that, under pathological conditions, the kidney handling of plasma proteins was related to their molecular weight.

That is to say the urinary excretion of a protein is related in an inverse ratio to its molecular weight. Using plasma and urine values, we previously mentionned [23] that this relation was not entirely exact for physiological proteinuria. In addition, the data obtained after strenuous exercise are not comparable to normal urine. Some proteins revealed a higher increase of their renal clearance than others, and there was no strict relationship due to molecular weight.

We have now to turn to sweat secretion, at least where proteins are concerned. JIRKA and MASOPUST [12], MANUEL [4], REMINGTON [20], VAN-FRAECHEM and POORTMANS [28] have detected and analysed the presence of plasma proteins in normal sweat. Our laboratory has investigated the perturbation induced by exercise on plasma proteins in sweat (see p. 353 and p. 356). It has been shown that, during exercise, the protein secretion of the sweat gland was increased as expressed in terms of mg/min. This necessitates that the skin clearance of plasma proteins is enhanced during exercise. Furthermore, it was found that the electrophoretic distribution of sweat secretion gives merely an identical protein pattern before and after exercise, except for the post-γ-globulins, which are not related to any plasma proteins (fig.5).

Before leaving the analysis of the incidence of physical exercise on proteins in humoral secretions we have to consider the somewhat perturbing

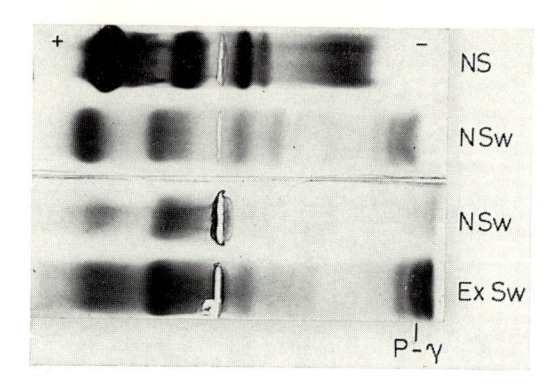

Figure 5. Agar gel electrophoresis of concentrated sweat collected at rest and after exercise.

As compared to normal serum (NS), normal sweat (NSw) shows a particular distribution, especially in the post-γ position (p-γ). Sweat collected after exercise (Ex Sw) has a pattern similar to normal sweat, though the proteins in the post-γ position seems to be reinforced.

feature of what is called 'Donaggio Substances'. A precipitate appears upon mixing solutions of thionine and ammonium molybdate. DONAGGIO discovered that normal urine had no effect upon this reaction, while urine from physically tired or pathologic subjects inhibited it [6]. The reaction of Donaggio, also called 'obstacle phenomenon', is thus said to be positive when most or all the dye is allowed to remain in solution. Increased values in serum, in urine appeared to be characteristic of the acute phase of the General Adaptation Syndrome of SELYE. Therefore, a theory has been presented which deals with connective tissue damage occuring during strenuous physical exercise. JAYLE has proposed that Donaggio substances are in fact hydrosoluble glycoproteins of the connective tissue [11]. Under the influence of stress, these substances pass into the blood stream, and thereafter into the urine. It was believed, at that time, that the Donaggio substances were one type of glycoproteins. By isolation of these substances from blood and urine, we are now convinced that most of the Donaggio substances are identical with several plasma proteins. Furthermore, although the type of reaction is similar for serum and urine, the identification of the components reveals that the Donaggio substances are fundamentally different in both fluids.

Therefore, even if we know what type of substances we are analyzing, namely thermosoluble proteins, we do not know what we are investigating. The cycle of JAYLE [11] which represents a schematic view of the hypothesis concerning the degradation of glycoproteins of connective tissue has to be taken with great care, concerning strenuous exercise.

We have now to try to elaborate a general concept on the incidence of physical exercise on proteins in biological fluids (fig.6).

In muscle, exercise induces an increase of acid metabolites which, by their low molecular weight, enhance the intramuscular osmotic pressure. To neutralize the latter, water is withdrawn from the plasma and hemoconcentration occurs. Some proteins might come from the extravascular bed and contribute to the rise of the level of proteins in plasma. DE LANNE [5] and RAISZ et al. [26] have established that during exercise the blood osmotic pressure rises from 2.0 to 2.5 per cent. This change of osmotic pressure stimulates the osmoreceptors and enhances the release of antidiuretic hormones (ADH) in the blood [21]. The classical studies of VERNEY [29] have established that secretion of ADH depends on changes in the osmotic pressure of the blood. KOSLOWSKI et al. have investigated the relations between the blood antidiuretic activity, the changes of osmotic pressure in blood and the water diuresis during physical exercise [14]. It was reported

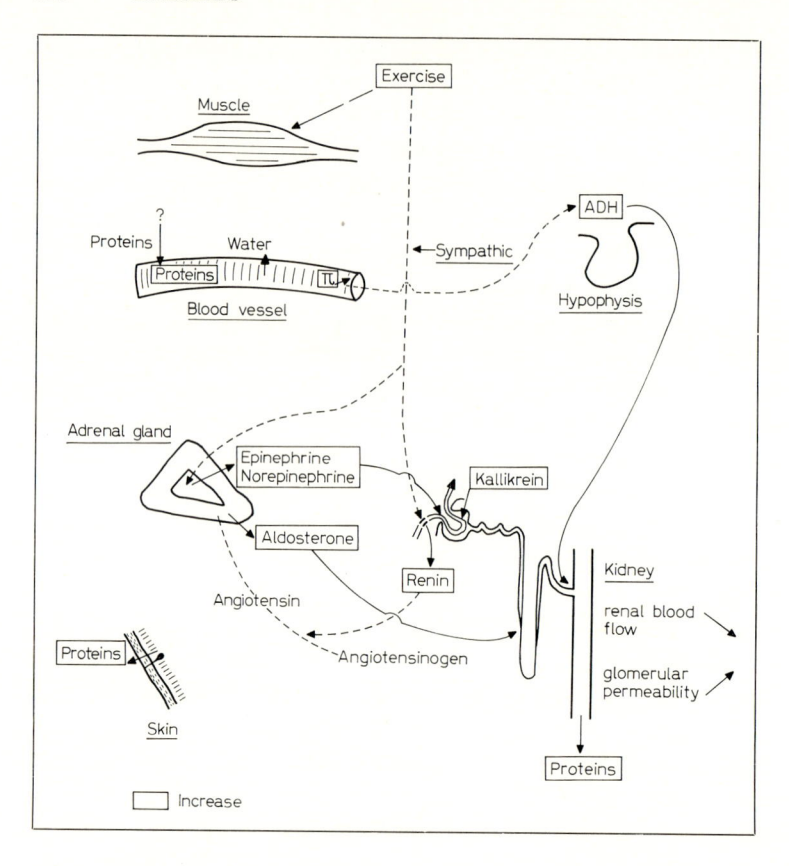

Figure 6. General concept leading to modifications occurring under physical activity in the protein distribution in biological fluids.
　　See text.

that strenuous physical exercise causes a rise in plasma ADH activity amounting up to 3-fold the resting value. This produces a consequent decrease of water diuresis to as much as 75% of the level at rest. Inactivation of ADH activity by drinking ethylalcohol before the exercise abolishes the rise of ADH in blood and causes a slighter reduction in water diuresis. Besides ADH, water diuresis is also controlled by an adrenocortical hormone, i.e. aldosterone. The level of this hormone in blood is increased during muscular activity [18]. One may propose that this increase is induced by the renin-angiotensin system. In fact, CASTENFORS has reported that during prolonged heavy exercise there was a mean increase of plasma renin activity of 4-fold that of the resting level [2]. On the basis of several experimental evidences, this author proposes that the increased renin activity in blood during exercise is caused by a direct sympathetic nervous stimulation of the juxtaglomerular apparatus which controls the degree of constriction of the afferent arteriole of the glomerule. It is also suggested that vasoconstriction of renal glomerular arterioles occurs during exercise. Arguments to the above hypothesis are given by some workers who showed that a reduction of renal plasma flow is induced by a plasma increase of 1-norepinephrine and epinephrine [8] the level of which may be elevated 3-fold during the exercise. The sluggish flow of blood in the glomerule probably enhances the diffusion process of macromolecules into the tubular lumen. Furthermore, an increase of the glomerular permeability presumably reinforces this phenomenon and gives a glomerular ultrafiltrate rich in proteins. It has been shown that an increased protein excretion in urine has been produced experimentally by i.v. injection of renin [2] and of kallikrein [19], the latter being an enzyme which enhances membrane permeability. Moreover, if we assume that the tubular mechanism of reabsorption of proteins is saturated, this contributes to an elevated urinary content in proteins which occurs during and after exercise.

The analysis of the study of clearance of plasma proteins in urine and in sweat reveals that this phenomenon is raised in both fluids, as a consequence of muscular activity. However in this case, renal clearance of plasma proteins is not just a simple accentuation of what is found at rest. Exercise proteinuria is therefore a unique concept which is not related to physiological, orthostatic or pathological proteinurias. Concerning sweat clearance of plasma proteins, little is known, but we may assume that this process is also perturbated by exercise.

It is now time to conclude this review with some aims of future research which should be performed on animals or on man.

For example:

1. *Increase of membrane permeability*
    by – clearance studies of (^{131}I)-labelled plasma proteins
       – immunofluorescent studies of plasma proteins in kidney, sweat glands

2. *Turnover studies of plasma proteins*
    by – (6-^{14}C) arginine

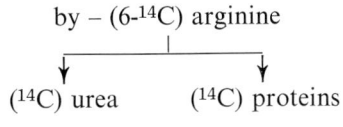

    (^{14}C) urea   (^{14}C) proteins

3. *Blood coagulation and fibrinolytic processes*

4. *Tissue breakdown*
   by detection in blood and urine of – myoglobin
                                – hydroxyproline – containing peptides
                                – acid glycosaminoglycans.

Acknowledgment

We are indebted to Mrs. O. RUBIN for her kind technical assistance.

References

1. CASH, J. D. and WOODFIELD, D. G.: Fibrinolytic response to moderate, exhaustive and prolonged exercise in normal subjects. Nature *215:* 628–629 (1967).
2. CASTENFORS, J.: Renal function during exercise. Acta Physiol. Scand. *70:* suppl. 293 (1967).
3. CHAILLEY-BERT, P. et PLAS, F.: Modifications du sang au cours des efforts prolongés. Méd. Ed. Phys. Sport, *numéro spécial:* 5–14 (1959).
4. CIER, J. F.; MANUEL, Y. et LACOUR, J. R.: Etude électrophorétique des protéines de la sueur humaine. Electrophorèse sur papier, immuno-électrophorese et électrophorèse en gel d'amidon. C. R. Soc. Biol. *157:* 1623–1626 (1963).
5. DELANNE, R.: Variations provoquées dans le sang veineux par l'activité musculaire. p. 174 (Impr. des Sciences/Bruxelles 1957).
6. DONAGGIO, A.: Un phénomène particulier ('phénomène d'obstacle') provoqué par l'urine et le liquide céphalorachidien dans les conditions diverses: procédé pour sa démonstration. Rev. Neurol. *2:* 155–160 (1933).
7. FREEMAN, T.: The function of plasma protein. In PEETERS, H. (Ed.): Protides of the Biological Fluids, Proceedings of the 15th Colloquium, Bruges 1967; p. 1–14 (Elsevier Publ. Co., Amsterdam 1968).
8. GRAY, I. and BEETHAM, W. P.: Changes in plasma concentration of epinephrine and norephinephrine with muscular work. Proc. Soc. exper. Biol., N.Y. *96:* 636–638 (1957).
9. HARALAMBIE, G.: Valeurs biochimiques sériques et syndrome de suprasollicitation chez le sportif. Acta biol. med germ. *17:* 34–43 (1966).
10. HARDWICKE, J. and SOOTHILL, J. F.: Glomerular damage in terms of 'pore size' In Ciba Foundation Symposium on Renal Biopsy, G. E. W. WOLSTENHOLME and M. D. CAMERSON (Edit.) p. 32 (Little, Brown and Co., Boston 1961).
11. JAYLE, M. F. et BOUSSIER, G.: Les séromucoides du sang: leurs relations avec les mucoprotéines de la substance fondamentale du tissu conjonctif. Exp. ann. Bioch. Méd. *17:* 157–194 (1955).
12. JIRKA, M. and MASOPUST, J.: Immunochemical behaviour of proteins in human sweat. Biochim. biophys. Acta *71:* 217–218 (1963).
13. KEUL, J.; DOLL, E.; ERICHSEN, H. und REINDELL, H.: Die arteriellen Substrat-

spiegel bei Verminderung der Sauerstoffkonzentration in der Inspirationsluft während körperlicher Arbeit. Int. Z. angew. Physiol. *25:* 89–103 (1968).

14. KOZLOWSKI, S.; SZCZEPANSKA, E. and ZIELINSKI, A.: The hypothalamo-hypophyseal antidiuretic system in physical exercises. Arch. Internat. Physiol. Biochi. *75:* 218–228 (1967).

15. LANDIS, E. M. and PAPPENHEIMER, J. R.: Exchange of Substances through the capillary walls. In VISSCHER, M. B.; HASTINGS, A. B.; PAPPENHEIMER, J. R. and RAHN, H.: Handbook of Physiology, *Section 2, Circulation, Vol. II:* 961–1034 (Amer. Physiol. Soc./Washington D.C. 1963).

16. LEUBE, W. VON: Über Ausscheidung von Eiweiss im Harn des gesunden Menschen. Wirchows Arch. *72:* 145–147 (1878).

17. MCCULLOUGH, H.: A simple microtechnique for the determination of blood ammonia and a note on the effect of exercise. Clin. chim. Acta *19:* 101–105 (1968).

18. MULLER, A. F.; MANNIG, E. L. and RIONDEL, A. M.: Influence of position and activity on the secretion of aldosterone. Lancet *1:* 711–712 (1958).

19. MURAKAMI, N.: Exercise proteinuria and proteinemia induced by kallikrein. Nature *218:* 481–482 (1968).

20. O'NEAL, C., Jr., and REMINGTON, J. S.: Immunologic studies in normal human sweat J. lab. clin. Med. *69:* 634–650 (1967).

21. POORTMANS, J.: La protéinurie physiologique au repos et à l'effort. Ann. Soc. royale Sc. Méd. et Natur. de Bruxelles *17:* 89–188 (1964).

22. POORTMANS, J.: Exercise proteinuria. In JOKL and HEBBELINCK, M. (Ed.): International Research in Physical Education (C. Thomas Publ., Springfield, in press).

23. POORTMANS, J. R. and JEANLOZ, R. W.: Quantitative immunological determination of 12 plasma proteins excreted in human urine collected before and after exercise. J. clin. Invest. *47:* 386–393 (1968).

24. POORTMANS, J. R.: Immunology evidence of a γM-subunit in exercise proteinuria. Nature *221:* 376–378 (1969).

25. POORTMANS, J. and SEGERS, M.: Haptoglobinuria following muscular activity. Experientia *20:* 44 (1964).

26. RAISZ, L. G.; AU, W. and SCHEER, R. L.: Studies on the renal concentration mechanism. III. Effect of heavy exercise. J. clin. Invest. *38:* 8–13 (1959).

27. SARAJAS, H. S. S.; KONTTINEN, A. and FRICK, M. H.: Thrombocytosis evoked by exercise. Nature *192:* 721–722 (1961).

28. VANFRAECHEM, J. et POORTMANS, J. R.: Les protéines plasmatiques de la sueur humaine normale. Rev. fr. ét. cl. et biol., 13: 383–387 (1968).

29. VERNEY, E. B.: La régulation de l'excrétion hydrique. Triangle (Sandoz) *3:* 307–312 (1958).

Author's address: Dr. J.R. POORTMANS, Laboratoire de l'Effort, Université Libre de Bruxelles, *Bruxelles* (Belgium).

Tableau biochimique sérique chez la femme sportive

G. Haralambie et G. Jeflea

Laboratoire de Physiologie et de Biochemie du Centre de Recherches
Scientifiques au domaine du Sport, Bucarest

Ce travail présente les résultats d'une investigation concernant l'équilibre humoral de repos de la sportive, en pleine période de préparation physique. Les facteurs étudiés, dont le niveau normal et les modifications chez le sportif ont fait l'objet de plusieurs publications [1, 2, 3, 4, 5, 10], permettent certaines conclusions concernant la réponse humorale tardive à l'effort, l'équilibre alimentaire et l'état de santé des sportives.

Sujets et méthodes

On a dosé: dans le sérum du sang veineux récolté sans stase, le matin au repos et à jeun, les protéines et leurs fractions électrophorétiques, les glycoprotéines (hexoses, acide sialique, séromucoïde), l'urée, le cholestérol et la lipémie, dans le plasma, le potassium (photomètre à flamme) et dans le sang l'hémoglobine, par des méthodes déjà décrites [1, 3, 5, 10]. Les 73 sportives étudiées étaient pour la plupart membres des équipes représentatives roumaines. Dix ont été examinées après 48 à 72 h de repos et considérées comme témoins, le reste après plusieurs jours d'entraînement, toutes entre le 7e et le 25e jour du cycle menstruel. Dans le dernier groupe, dix sportives pouvaient être considérées, tenant compte de leur programme de travail très chargé, des données physiologiques et du mauvais rendement sportif, comme en état de suprasollicitation.

Résultats

Les données humorales des sportives-témoins se situent dans l'ensemble au domaine considéré en physiologie comme optimal, sauf peut-être une tendance à l'augmentation du séromucoïde.

Certaines déviations peuvent au contraire être observées dans les groupes examinés 14 à 18 h après le dernier entraînement. Concernant le tableau protidique, 5 cas présentent une nette hypoprotéinémie et les valeurs moyennes sont généralement plus basses que celles du sportif. Le rapport A/G est cependant assez élevé (albumines sériques entre 56–59,2%), de sorte que la valeur absolue des albumines se situe à un niveau supérieur en général

Tableau

Groupe	No cas	Prot. tot. [g%]	Albumines [g%]	Glyco-protéines [mg%]	Ac. sialique [mg%]	Séromucoide [mg%]	Lipémie [mg%]	Urée [mg/l]	Hémoglobine [g%]
Témoins	10	6,75 ± 0,27	4,01 ± 0,21	122,9 ± 15,1	55,4 ± 6,3	98,5 ± 15,3	595 ± 63,7	245 ± 59,2	13,1 ± 0,99
Volley-ball 1964	11	6,63 ± 0,31	–	138,7 ± 7,17	57 5,55	–	630 ± 54,2	280 ± 67,5	11,9 ± 0,97
Volley-ball 1965	10	6,81 ± 0,29	3,97 ± 0,23	136,8 ± 11,1	63,8 ± 7,5	108 ± 11,8	570 ± 55,4	370 ± 89,7	–
Basket-ball	11	6,71 ± 0,21	3,85 ± 0,28	133 ± 15,2	62 ± 6,5	85 ± 12,9	575 ± 46,7	360 ± 77	12,8 ± 0,76
Athlétisme sprint	12	6,54 ± 0,36	3,72 ± 0,17	140 ± 12	67,9 ± 7,8	118 ± 29	580 ± 90	332 ± 89,3	12,9 ± 0,96
Aviron	9	6,92 ± 0,32	3,87 ± 0,28	142,5 ± 14,8	67 ± 8,7	106 ± 18,2	560 ± 71	327 ± 68,7	12,8 ± 0,98
Suprasollici-tation	10	6,42 ± 0,32	3,55 ± 0,17	147 ± 7,5	68,5 ± 4,9	–	–	415 ± 65	–

à celui trouvé chez la femme non-sportive [9]. La proportion des sportives dont la fraction a_2-globulines est légèrement augmentée est comparable à celle trouvée par nous chez le sportif.

La tendance à l'augmentation de l'urée sérique est nettement moins marquée que chez l'homme; toutefois, dans 24,5% des cas, la valeur de ce facteur dépasse 400 mg/l, fait très peu commun chez la non-sportive.

A deux exceptions près, le niveau des hexoses liés et celui de l'acide sialique est significativement plus élevé chez tous les groupes, comparé aux témoins. Dans quelques cas seulement ce fait s'explique par l'existence d'une infection ou inflammation (γ-globulines dépassant 20%). Pour le reste, nous pouvons supposer que, tout comme chez l'homme, l'hyperglycoprotéinémie modérée est en rapport avec la récupération incomplète après l'effort. Dans de tels cas, nous avons trouvé chez la femme aussi, le rétablissement des facteurs déviés après 2 à 4 jours de repos.

Les valeurs moyennes des fractions électrophorétiques sont très rapprochées de celles admises comme normales pour les européens sains, déterminées par une méthode similaire [11].

Le groupe considéré en état de suprasollicitation présente des modifications humorales de la même nature que celles décrites pour le sportif [2], mais cependant plus atténuées. Les examens répétés montrent, ici aussi, l'amélioration du tableau humoral lors des périodes d'activité réduite.

Les valeurs moyennes de la lipémie et du cholestérol sont nettement plus basses que chez le sportif; trois sportives seulement dépassent une lipémie de 700 mg% et respectivement une cholestérolémie de 230 mg%.

Pour 38 dosages, il y a 11 sportives dont l'hémoglobine est inférieure à 12 g%, limite minimum admissible pour une sportive de performance; la proportion est sensiblement plus élevée que celle trouvée chez des jeunes étudiantes présumées saines, non sportives [7]. Pour 87 cas examinés il y a 41,4% avec kaliémie légèrement augmentée (17 à 19 mg%) et 13,8% avec hyperkaliémie. Ce fait doit être rapproché des observations de Jones [6], concernant la perte rénale élevée de potassium chez la femme après l'effort, pour laquelle il fournit peut-être une explication indirecte.

Discussion

Comme on a affirmé dans un travail récent, concernant des joueuses de basket-ball, le sport de performance effectué par des femmes bien entraînées, sous stricte surveillance médicale, y compris des examens de laboratoire complexes, ne paraît pas déterminer, du moins pour les domaines étudiés, des modifications humorales traduisant un déséquilibre grave [8]. Les déviations observées montrent cependant que la récupération n'est pas, dans tous les cas complète d'un jour d'activité à l'autre. Tant dans notre laboratoire, que dans certains investigations faites en collaboration avec PARTHENIU (non publiées), nous avons aussi trouvé des modifications de l'excitabilité neuromusculaire et de la réactivité végétative, et notamment chez des sujets – hommes ou femmes – qui présentaient aussi des déviations humorales notables. Pratiquement dans tous les cas il s'agissait d'un effort fourni, supérieur à la capacité d'adaptation, d'un état sous-clinique fruste ou d'une alimentation mal dirigée, trop riche, et moins souvent trop pauvre en protides.

Il est probable que, pendant les périodes de sollicitation accrue, il est nécessaire d'enrichir artificiellement la teneur en fer et en certaines vitamines (surtout B_6 et B_{12}) de la ration alimentaire de la sportive. A ce sujet, nous devons mentionner les observations faites par des auteurs japonais [12] concernant «l'anémie d'effort» chez les femmes qui suivent un programme d'entraînement physique dur.

Significance des différences entre les groupes «d'entraînement» et les témoins (valeur du facteur «p»)

Groupe	Urée sérique	Glycoprotéines	Acide sialique	Hémoglobine
Volley-ball 1964	n.s.	< 0,01	n.s.	< 0,02
Volley-ball 1965	< 0,005	∼ 0,03	< 0,02	–
Basket-ball	∼ 0,001	n.s.	∼ 0,03	n.s.
Sprint	< 0,02	< 0,01	< 0,001	n.s.
Aviron	< 0,02	∼ 0,01	< 0,005	n.s.
Suprasollicitation	<< 0,001	< 0,001	<< 0,001	–

Bibliographie

1. HARALAMBIE, G.: La valeur de certaines constantes biochimiques du sérum chez les sportifs en régime d'entraînement intense. Acta biol. med. german. *13:* 30 (1964).
2. HARALAMBIE, G.: Valeurs biochimiques sériques et syndrome de suprasollicitation chez le sportif. Acta biol. med. german. *17:* 34 (1966).
3. HARALAMBIE, G. et JEFLEA, GENOVEVA: Indices biochimiques du sérum et la récupération après l'effort physique. Int. Z. angew. Physiol. *20:* 515 (1965).

4. HARALAMBIE, G. et MURESANU, I.: Le tableau biochimique en relation avec l'activité sportive dans le pentathlon moderne. Méd. éduc. phys. Sport *41:* 141 (1967).
5. HARALAMBIE, G.: Le dosage des glycoprotéines sériques dans l'investigation de laboratoire du sportif. Schweiz. Z. Sportmed. *15:* 41 (1967).
6. JONES, CH.: La déficience potassique et la suralimentation protéique: un danger pour la femme sportive. Méd. éduc. phys. Sport *37:* 145 (1962).
7. MARKWARDT, J. und COUTELLE, CH.: Eisenmangel als Ursache für die Häufung erniedrigter Hb-Werte bei jungen Frauen. Dtsch. Gesundheitsw. *22:* 1033 (1967).
8. PARTHENIU, AL.; HARALAMBIE, G. und CHIRIAC, D.: Beobachtungen über den biologischen Zustand der rumänischen Basketballspielerinnen vor Beginn der Europameisterschaften 1964. Sportarzt u. Sportmed. *18:* 161 (1967).
9. STEINFELD, J.: Difference in daily albumin synthesis between normal men and women as measured with I^{131}-labeled albumin. J. labor. clin. Med. *55:* 904 (1960).
10. ULMEANU, FL. C. et HARALAMBIE, G.: La récupération après l'effort physique: Manifestations humorales. Apuntes Med. Deport. *4:* 103 (1967).
11. WUNDERLY, CH.: Die Papierelektrophorese, 2. Aufl. (Sauerländer & Co., Aarau – Frankfurt/Main 1959).
12. YOSHIMURA, H.; YOSHIOKA, T.; YAMADA, T. and MAMOTA, J.: Studies on the prevention of anemia due to hard physical training. Abstr. of Papers pres. at the Int. Congr. Sport Sci., p. 128: Tokyo (1964).

Adresse des auteurs: Dr G. HARALAMBIE et Dr GENOVEVA JEFLEA, Laboratoire de Physiologie et de Biochimie du Centre de Recherches Scientifiques au domaine du Sport, *Bucarest* (Roumanie). Bd. Muncii 37–39.

Exercise Proteinuria in Monozygotic and Dizygotic Twins[1]

I. LILJEFORS, M. PISCATOR and C. RISINGER

Department of Internal Medicine, Karolinska Institutet at Serafimerlasarettet, Institute of Hygiene, Karolinska Institutet, Department of Environmental Hygiene, National Institute of Public Health, Stockholm, and Department of Internal Medicine, University Hospital, Uppsala

Introduction

In studies on proteinuria after prolonged heavy exercise CASTENFORS, MOSSFELDT and PISCATOR [1967] found that when the same subjects repeated the exercise after one year both protein excretion and percentage of albumin in the urinary proteins were correlated. It was also found that though glomerular proteinuria with predominance of albumin was the most common finding there were exceptions, so that in some cases there was mainly an increase in proteins with β- or γ-mobility, as in tubular proteinuria. It was concluded that some individual factor could be responsible for the magnitude and type of proteinuria and this factor was more important than the intensity of the exercise. To obtain more information the present investigation was undertaken. In Sweden a twin register comprising about 10,000 pairs of twins has been built up for the study of constitutional factors in chronic diseases, for details see CEDERLÖF [1966] and twins were now used to study the influence of constitutional factors on exercise proteinuria.

Material and Methods

The total material consisted of about 100 pairs of monozygotic and dizygotic twins, who participated in an investigation of some factors contributing to the etiology of coronary heart disease. Here only these investigated in spring 1967 will be presented, 20 monozygotic pairs and 34 dizygotic pairs, between 42 and 67 years of age. They were grouped according to the order of birth, so that the first born in each pair was called A and the second born B. Three urine samples were obtained. One morning sample, one pre-exercise sample after a standardized breakfast and one post-exercise

[1] This work was supported by grants from the Folksam Insurance Company and the Swedish National Association for the prevention of Heart and Chest Diseases.

sample. Exercise was performed on a bicycle ergometer, beginning with six minutes at a load of usually 300 kpm/min. The load was increased every sixth minute by a further 300 or 150 kpm/min. The exercise continued until they either complained of chest pain or were exhausted. The twins were usually examined on separate days to avoid confusion.

In the urine, protein was determined by a biuret method described by Piscator [1962] and creatinine by the method of Hare [1950]. Protein excretion was expressed as mg of protein per g of creatinine. Urines[1] were concentrated 100–1,000 times in collodion bags and the concentrates were separated by paper electrophoresis in barbital buffer at pH 8.6, and in some cases also by electrophoresis in agarose. To test the reliability of electrophoretic determinations of albumin, it was in 20 urines quantitatively determined by the immunochemical method of Glass, Risinger, Wide and Gemzell [1963].

Data on previous diseases, blood pressure, serum creatinine etc. were obtained from the clinical records.

Results

There was a high incidence of hypertension (systolic blood pressure > 170 or diastolic blood pressure > 95 mm Hg) as shown in *table I*, where also age and exercise loads are presented. There was no correlation between exercise loads in the two monozygotic groups, but there was in the dizygotic groups.

Table I. Age, blood pressure and exercise load

	n	Age		Blood pressure Systolic	Diastolic	Maximum exercise load
Mz	20	56 ± 6	A	160 ± 23	95 ± 10	968 ± 236
			B	154 ± 19	94 ± 10	975 ± 209
			r	0.49	0.56	0.11
Dz	34	55 ± 6	A	139 ± 20	88 ± 11	968 ± 290
			B	143 ± 23	88 ± 11	980 ± 296
			r	0.25	0.37	0.53

[1] In some cases very small urine volumes were obtained and it was impossible to obtain sufficient amounts of protein concentrates.

Table II. Protein excretion in monozygotic and dizygotic twins

		n	Morning	r	Before exercise	r	After exercise	
Mz	A	19	70 ± 43	0.80	107 ± 57	0.51	177 ± 122	
	B		62 ± 29	0.66	101 ± 72	0.46	183 ± 130	Total material
	r		0.42		0.56		0.51	
Dz	A	31	59 ± 21	0.28	79 ± 25	0.03	187 ± 279	
	B		68 ± 30	0.65	97 ± 41	0.69	150 ± 96	Total material
	r		0.11		0.35		0.27	
Dz	A	23	56 ± 18	0.26	79 ± 28	0.19	157 ± 123	
	B		64 ± 27	0.63	98 ± 34	0.61	143 ± 86	Normotensive
	r		0.32		0.63		0.47	

In one monozygotic pair and in three dizygotic pairs one or both excreted more than 200 mg protein in the morning urine. These pairs were excluded from the statistical treatment.

In all groups protein excretion increased from morning to after breakfast, as seen in *table II*. In both monozygotic groups morning values were correlated to pre-exercise values, whereas only one of the dizygotic groups showed a correlation. The same was found for pre-exercise values compared with post-exercise values. When monozygotes A and B were compared, correlations were found both pre- and post-exercise, whereas the morning values differed more. The dizygotic twins A and B did not show correlation at any time. However, when only normotensive dizygotes are compared, also shown in *table II*, protein excretion was correlated both pre- and postexercise. There was no difference between hypertensive and normotensive monozygotes.

Protein excretion after exercise showed large variations, in some cases it was unchanged or even lowered compared with pre-exercise values, and in others relatively large amounts were excreted. The percentage of albumin also showed a big variation, as seen in *table III*. The monozygotes were correlated but not the dizygotes. When albumin excretion calculated from total protein excretion and percentage of albumin obtained by paper electrophoresis was compared with albumin excretion determined immunochemically in 20 urines a correspondence was found, r = 0.85. The albumin values were 29 ± 20 mg and 19 ± 13 mg respectively. The biuret method used has earlier been shown to give too high values due to interference of protein-bound pigments, PISCATOR [1962].

Table III. Percentage albumin in urinary proteins after exercise

		n	Percentage
Mz	A	12	36 ± 9
Mz	B		36 ± 11
	r		0.67
Dz	A	19	39 ± 12
Dz	B		37 ± 13
	r		0.14

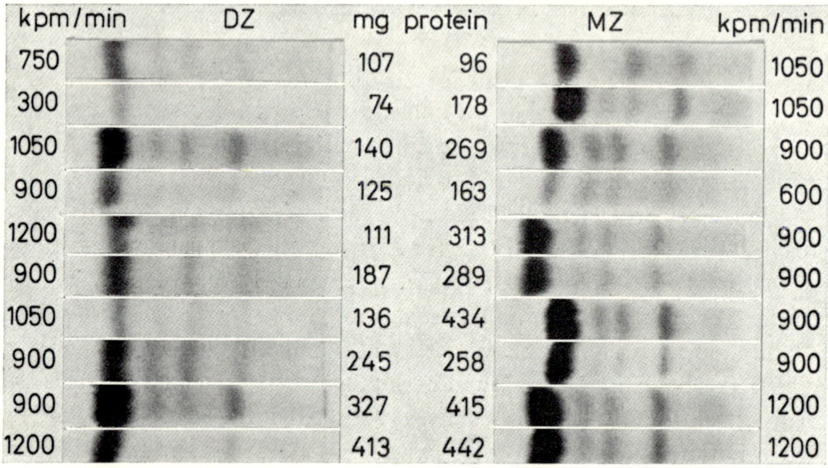

kpm/min	DZ	mg protein	MZ	kpm/min
750		107	96		1050
300		74	178		1050
1050		140	269		900
900		125	163		600
1200		111	313		900
900		187	289		900
1050		136	434		900
900		245	258		900
900		327	415		1200
1200		413	442		1200

Figure 1. Paper electrophoretic patterns for dizygotic and monozygotic pairs after exercise.

The paper electrophoretic examinations revealed as shown in *figure 1* that there were large similarities after exercise between the monozygotes, but many of the dizygotes A and B were also similar. *Figure 2* shows agarose patterns from all three periods in two pairs. In the pre-exercise period monozygote A has a tubular pattern, whereas the patterns seem to be identical after exercise. The dizygotes in the same figure differed considerably in the morning urine, but were similar in the following periods. *Figure 3* shows patterns for two dizygotic pairs, where in the one to the left A has a tubular pattern in all three periods, whereas B on the other hand has a glomerular pattern after exercise. In the pair to the right it can be seen

Exercise Proteinuria in Monozygotic and Dizygotic Twins

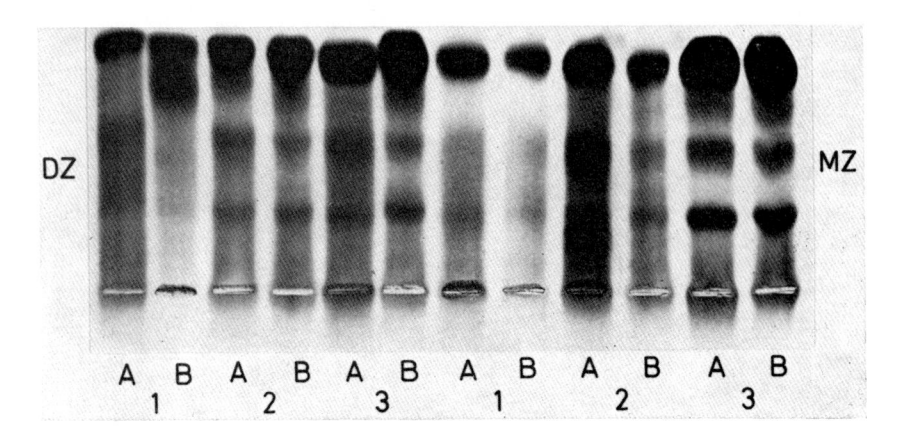

Figure 2. Agarose electrophoretic patterns from all three periods for a dizygotic pair and a monozygotic pair. 1. Morning; 2. Before exercise; 3. After exercise.

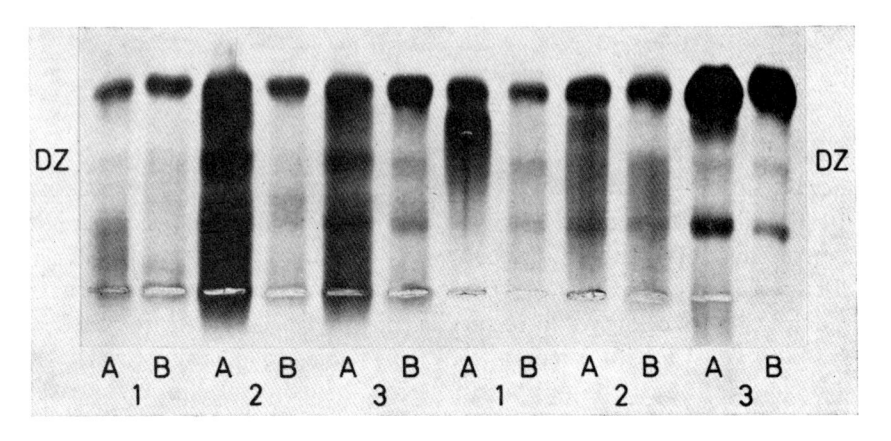

Figure 3. Agarose electrophoretic patterns from all three periods for two dizygotic pairs. 1. Morning; 2. Before exercise; 3. After exercise.

that both change to glomerular patterns after exercise. *Figure 4* shows paper electrophoretic patterns for one pair that was excluded from *table II*. This was a dizygotic pair where there were large differences in medical history and morning excretion of protein. In B there was a steady output of protein in all periods, whereas in A the increase between the morning and the post-exercise output was tenfold.

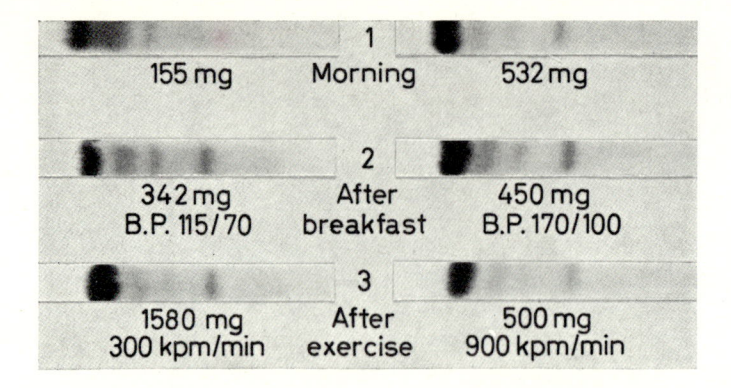

155 mg	1 Morning	532 mg
342 mg B.P. 115/70	2 After breakfast	450 mg B.P. 170/100
1580 mg 300 kpm/min	3 After exercise	500 mg 900 kpm/min

Figure 4. Paper electrophoretic patterns for a dizygotic pair.

Aorctic and mitral incompetence
Serum creatinine
1.2 mg/100 ml

Hypertension, nephrectomized
Aorctic incompetence?
Serum creatinine
0.8 mg/100 ml

Discussion

The present material consisted of men considerably older than those examined in earlier investigations by POORTMANS and VAN KERCHOVE [1962] and CASTENFORS [1967]. This was reflected in a high incidence of hypertension, especially in the monozygotic group. CASTENFORS [1967] has discussed the mechanisms for exercise proteinuria and both changes in glomerular permeability and renal vasoconstriction were held responsible. The individual protein excretion was usually related to intensity of work. He also indicated that a constitutional factor in the glomerular membrane was of greater importance in the development of exercise proteinuria than intensity of work.

The present study supports this theory as the monozygotic twins behaved similarly even when work loads were not the same, i.e. this constitutional factor must be determining the magnitude and type of proteinuria. This is supported by the fact that normotensive dizygotes also behaved similarly, whereas hypertension in the dizygotes influenced the response to exercise.

It is difficult to explain why in some cases protein excretion decreased after exercise. One possibility is that if there is no change at all in glomerular permeability, the decreased urine flow will result in better reabsorption.

It is also possible that precipitation of mucoproteins from the urinary tract results in decreased protein concentration. PATEL [1964] showed that these substances often lose their solubility in exercise urines due to increases in salt concentration.

Summary

Urinary protein excretion was measured in 19 monozygotic twin pairs and in 31 dizygotic twin pairs in the morning, before and after exercise. In the monozygotes total protein excretion was correlated both before and after exercise. In 12 pairs it could be shown that also albumin excretion was correlated. In the dizygotes no correlation at all was found. When only normotensive dizygotes were compared, correlations were found in total protein excretion before and after exercise. It is concluded that a constitutional factor plays an important role in the changes in glomerular permeability which are thought to cause exercise proteinuria. This factor appears to be more important than work intensity.

References

1. CASTENFORS, J.: Renal function during exercise. Acta physiol. scand. *70:* suppl. 293 (1967).
2. CASTENFORS, J.; MOSSFELDT, F. and PISCATOR, M.: Effect of prolonged heavy exercise on renal function and urinary protein excretion. Acta physiol. scand. *70:* 194–206 (1967).
3. CEDERLÖF, R.: The twin method in epidemiological research. Diss. Stockholm (1966).
4. GLASS, R. H.; RISINGER, C.; WIDE, L. and GEMZELL, C. A.: Quantitative determination of albumin in normal urine by an immunochemical method. Scand. J. clin. Lab. Invest. *15:* 266–272 (1963).
5. HARE, R. S.: Endogenous creatinine in serum and urine. Proc. Soc. exp. Biol. *74:* 148–151 (1950).
6. PATEL, R.: Urinary casts in exercise. Austr. Ann. Med. *13:* 170–173 (1964).
7. PISCATOR, M.: Proteinuria in chronic cadmium poisoning. 2. The applicability of quantitative and qualitative methods of protein determination for the demonstration of cadmium proteinuria. Arch. environm. Hlth *5:* 325–332 (1962).
8. POORTMANS, J. et VAN KERCHOVE, E.: La protéinurie d'effort. Clin. chim. Acta *7:* 229–242 (1962).

Author's address: Dr. MAGNUS PISCATOR, Institute of Hygiene, Karolinska Institutet *10401 Stockholm* (Sweden).

Etude qualitative de la protéinurie intermittente au repos et après effort modéré

M. Segers, J. R. Poortmans, J. s'Jongers et A. Segers

Laboratoire de l'Effort, Université Libre de Bruxelles

Nous nous sommes proposés de déterminer les pourcentages respectifs des protéines urinaires au repos et à l'effort chez quatre sujets offrant une protéinurie intermittente. Cette étude a été effectuée de façon à pouvoir être comparée avec les pourcentages relevés au repos et à l'effort chez les sujets normaux par l'un de nous [1]. Les sujets d'expérience ont été choisis dans le groupe de jeunes adolescents de 12 à 18 ans offrant une protéinurie intermittente et sélectionnés par l'un de nous [A. Segers, 1968].

Les dosages ont été effectués pour sept des protéines urinaires à savoir l'albumine, la transferrine, l'a_1-glycoprotéine acide, l'a_2HS-glycoprotéine, la Zna_2-glycoprotéine et les globulines γA et γG, selon la technique d'immunodiffusion radiaire [1]. Les valeurs quantitatives obtenues ont été exprimées en pourcentage de la protéinurie totale.

Pour chaque sujet les urines ont été prélevées d'une part avant l'effort et d'autre part après une épreuve sur cycle-ergomètre de 1,5 W/kg imposée pendant 15 min.

Les moyennes des résultats ainsi recueillis chez nos sujets d'expérience au repos et après cette épreuve d'effort modérée sont exprimées dans le tableau I.

Tableau I. Sujets atteints de protéinurie intermittente. Pourcentage relatif de 7 constituants protéiques exprimé par rapport à la protéinurie totale

	Repos	Effort
a_1-glycoprotéine acide	0,8	5,2
a_2HS-glycoprotéine	0,4	1,8
Zna_2-glycoprotéine	0,7	3,2
Albumine	41	40
Transferrine	1,5	1
γA-globuline	0,7	1
γG-globuline	4,9	10,1

Les chiffres correspondent aux moyennes recueillies chez 4 sujets immédiatement avant et après un effort modéré.

Tableau II. Pourcentage relatif de 7 constituants protéiques par rapport à la protéinurie totale
Sujets normaux d'après POORTMANS [2]

	Repos	Effort
a_1-glycoprotéine-acide	1,3	6,7
a_2HS-glycoprotéine	3,8	1,2
Zna_2-glycoprotéine	5,2	9,4
Albumine	40	59
Transferrine	0,5	1,9
γA-globuline	1,8	0,7
γG-globuline	8,9	11,2

Les chiffres correspondent aux moyennes recueillies d'une part au repos et d'autre part après effort.

Il est permis de comparer ces résultats avec ceux obtenus chez les sujets normaux par POORTMANS [2] et qui sont repris dans le tableau II.

Cette comparaison montre qu'au repos, entre les sujets de notre groupe expérimental et les cas normaux, les taux de 5 protéines ne diffèrent pas de plus de 2 à 3 fois. Toutefois pour les deux a_2-glycoprotéines le taux est de 8 à 9 fois moindre dans notre groupe expérimental.

Par contre en ce qui concerne les résultats obtenus après effort, l'écart entre les deux groupes de sujets est nettement plus faible. En effet, pour 6 des protéines examinées, les taux ne diffèrent que très peu, c'est-à-dire moins du simple au double. Seule la Zna_2-glycoprotéine offre un taux près de 3 fois plus faible chez les sujets atteints de protéinurie intermittente.

En conclusion, il existe entre la protéinurie normale et la protéinurie intermittente certaines différences de pourcentage relatifs des différents constituants protéiques. Cette différence est toutefois nettement moindre entre les urines d'effort qu'entre les urines de repos. En d'autres termes, dans notre groupe expérimental le comportement rénal à l'effort modéré paraît se rapprocher de celui observé chez les sujets normaux.

Remerciements

Nous remercions vivement Madame O. RUBIN pour son aimable aide technique, ainsi que la Direction de l'Ecole Ch. Janssens d'Ixelles qui nous a permis d'obtenir des sujets d'expérience.

Résumé

Entre la protéinurie normale et les cas de proténuries intermittentes il existe certaines différences dans les pourcentages relatifs des différents constituants protéiques. Cette différence diminue toutefois après effort.

Summary

In normal and in intermittent proteinuria the relative percentage of the protein components is not the same, but the difference is lower after exercise than at rest.

Bibliographie

1. Poortmans, J. R. and Jeanloz, R. W.: Quantitative immunological determination of 12 plasma proteins excreted in human urine collected before and after exercise. J. Clin. Invest. *47:* 386–393 (1968).
2. Poortmans, J.: Exercise proteinuria; in Jokl and Hebbelinck, M. (Ed.), International Research in Physical Education (Thomas, Springfield, in press).

Adresse des auteurs: Drs M. Segers, J. Poortmans, J. s'Jongers et A. Segers, Laboratoire de l'Effort, Université Libre de Bruxelles, *Bruxelles* (Belgique).

The Significance of Polarographic Pattern Changes in the Protein Double Waves of Sportsmen

J. Malomsoki

Research Laboratory, National Institute for Medicine of Physical Education and Sports, Budapest

Making polarographic analyses of a sulfosalicylic filtrate of serum, Brdicka et al. found a characteristic double wave pattern. In various disorders, so for example in cancer, the waves were higher than in normal sera. They attributed this elevation to a higher rate of protein decomposition, and thought it to be related to an increased serum level of cystine. Other investigators considered it as due to a rise of certain mucoproteids.

Polak and Nosek observed a decrease in the double wave along with an improvement of the physical condition of cancer patients who were treated by injections of a ferro-ascorbate complex. Other authors investigated sera of sportsmen by this method, but failed to find significant connexion between the height of the double wave and physical condition.

In his comprehensive survey, Cahn [1960] considered biological compounds having an -SH group to be essential both for carbohydrate and creatine metabolism, and for intracellular redox processes such as the H-ion transport of ascorbic acid. Since physical exertion is closely linked to these processes, some change in the double wave seemed to us rather probable to occur under the influence of sports activity.

8 male and 7 female cross-country runners volunteered as subjects. In order to determine their physical fitness, cardiorespiratory exercise function tests and electrophoretic fractionation of serum proteins were carried out. Previously [Malomsoki] we found that in well-trained sportsmen post-exercise shift of protein fractions was significantly slighter than in normal but untrained persons.

The studies took place in Budapest and during a training camp of 3 weeks in the country. In the camp the blood for polarography and paper electrophoresis was drawn immediately before and after the scheduled program of training in the middle of each week. Cardiorespiratory tests were performed the following day. After an alkaline hydrolysis of the serum samples polarographic analysis was done in an ammoniacal 10^{-3} mole stock solution of trivalent cobalt. Recording sensitivity was set to 3.10^{-7} A/mm.

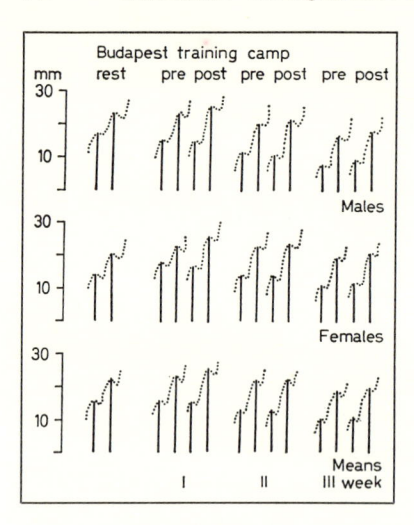

Figure 1. Polarography of serum. Curves obtained before and after exercise are plotted side by side. From left to right: Studies performed at rest in Budapest, first, second, and third week of camp, respectively.

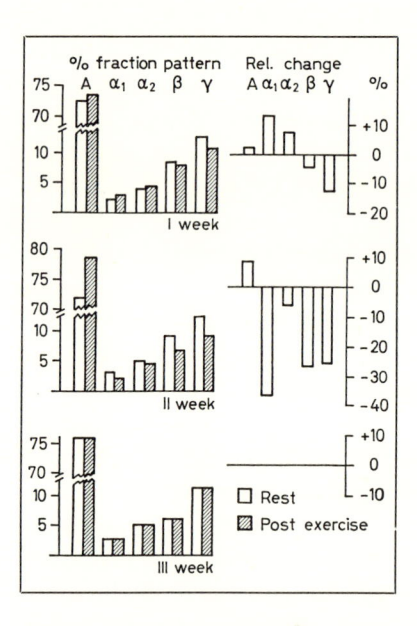

Figure 2. Serum electrophoresis. Relative change per cent refers to difference between respective pre- and post-exercise levels.

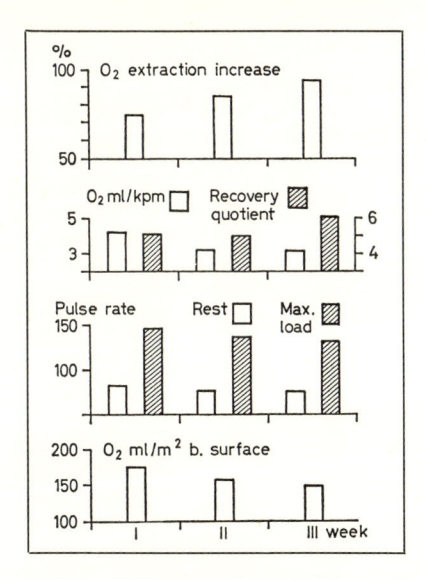

Figure 3. Cardiorespiratory function tests. Top row: Increase in the extracted oxygen fraction in expired air. Second row: Oxygen consumption per unit of work performed. Recovery quotient = Böhlaus Erholungsquotient: Excess oxygen uptake during exercise divided by excess uptake during recovery. Third row: Max. load designates highest pulse rate attained during identical exercise. Bottom row: Total excess oxygen consumption per unit of body surface.

Figure 1 illustrates the results as double waves that were constructed according to the mean heights of the respective curves. Regular training brought about a gradual diminution of the amplitudes so that those obtained from the last week samples were markedly smaller than the ones prior to the camp. Due to each training event the second wave was always higher after exercise, especially so during the first week. A difference between males and females could not be observed.

The electrophoretic patterns of the respective sera are shown in *figure 2*. The extent of relative changes is demonstrated on the right side of the diagram. While exertion of the 1st and 2nd weeks elicited marked shifts, training had practically no effect on the protein fractions in the 3rd week.

Figure 3 demonstrates some of the factors of the spiroergometric tests. The increase in the extracted oxygen fraction and in the recovery quotient [BÖHLAU, 1955] as well as the reduction of the other values unequivocally show the rise that occurred in the physical working capacity.

Summary

A reduction in the height of the Brdicka double wave could be observed in the sulfosalicylic filtrate of sera obtained from 15 cross-country runners who after three weeks of intensive training displayed objective spiroergometric signs of improved performance. A better physical fitness was substantiated also by the post-training stabilization of serum electrophoretic pattern. Single training events brought about an increase of the second wave. These polarographic results lead us to conclude that due to exertion cystine or an other substance having an identical polarographic activity accumulates in the serum, which in recovery tends to fall below pre-exercise levels. Although a definitive answer concerning its nature has not yet been reached, the reaction seems to be useful for the appraisal of fitness changes in sportsmen.

References

1. Böhlau, V.: Prüfung der körperlichen Leistungsfähigkeit. p. 49 (VEB Georg Thieme, Leipzig 1955).
2. Brezina, M. and Zuman, P.: Die Polarographie in der Medizin, Biochemie und Pharmazie, pp. 546, 570, 579 (Akademische Verlagsgesellschaft, Leipzig 1956).
3. Cahn, J. et Hérold, M.: Importance des groupes sulfhydryles en biologie. Agressologie *ii:* 157–168 (1960).
4. Malomsoki, J.: Die Dynamik der Veränderung von Serumeiweissfraktionen bei Sportlern. Medizin und Sport (in press).

Author's address: J. Malomsoki, Research Laboratory, National Institute for Medicine of Physical Education and Sports, *Budapest* (Hungary).

Rapports entre la variation de la tyrosinémie et certaines modifications de l'excitabilité neuromusculaire, déterminées par un effort dosé chez les sportifs

Fl. C. Ulmeanu, Al. Partheniu et G. Haralambie

Chaire de Physiologie, Laboratoire de Recherches de l'Institut de Culture Physique de Bucarest

La présente communication aborde l'un des aspects de l'étude chez le sportif des corrélations entre l'excitabilité et le métabolisme, dont nous avons discuté le principe dès 1957 [12] et qui est systématiquement poursuivie dans nos laboratoires [4, 10, 13, 14].

Les investigations ont été faites chez 16 sportifs, sans déviations pathologiques et sans manifestations des indices d'une suprasollicitation physique. On a déterminé la courbe Intensité/Durée de l'excitabilité neuromusculaire au niveau d'un muscle phasique, le vaste interne du quadriceps [11, 15], avant et dans les minutes 4 à 8 après l'effort (180 W pendant 10 min) au cycloergomètre. Avant et immédiatement après le travail on a pris des épreuves de sang de la veine cubitale, sans stase, sous anticoagulant (héparine). Dans le plasma, aussitôt séparé, on a dosé la tyrosine libre [2]. Le même dosage a été fait dans la sueur récoltée sur le front des sujets à la fin de l'effort et dans l'urine.

Un premier groupe expérimental (9 pentathlètes et 1 sprinteur) a fourni une première orientation qui a été vérifiée sur 6 autres sujets pratiquant l'haltérophilie, le tennis et le judo, sélectionnés au préalable d'après les éléments de l'excitabilité du vaste interne qui avaient un rapport avec les modifications de la tyrosinémie.

Résultats

Chez 23 sportifs, y compris nos sujets, la valeur moyenne de la tyrosinémie au repos était de $11,2 \pm 2,6$ µg/ml, en bonne concordance avec la littérature [7, 9, 16]. La tyrosinurie au repos était de $6,5 \pm 2,94$ mg/h; à noter que par ce procédé sont dosés aussi: le tyrosine-O-sulfate, la tyrosine des dipeptides et l'acide p-hydroxyphényl-pyruvique.

Tableau I. Valeurs individuelles de l'excitabilité neuromusculaire et des variations de la tyrosine

Sujet N°	Excitabilité en mA t = 0,1 ms repos	effort	t = 0,2 ms repos	effort	Trosine du plasma µg/ml repos	effort	Tyrosinurie µg/ml repos	effort	mg/heure repos	effort	Tyrosine dans la sueur µg/ml	Observations
1	12,2	14,6	8,5	10,1	10,25	8,7	75	68,5	–	7,2	9,7	
2	11,6	12,5	6,7	7,3	11,4	10,3	77,7	70,5	10,4	4,75	22,2	Groupe de contrôle
3	11,5	18	6,6	9,6	9,8	5,6	83	75	–	12,26	8,2	
4	10,4	12	6,4	7,5	10,1	9,6	109	104	3,19	1,43	20,7	Groupe de contrôle
5	10	15	7	7,5	12,3	11	87	97	10,2	8,1	14,0	
6	9,3	11,8	4,7	7,1	10,0	10,1	85	86,5	4,29	2,58	23	Groupe de contrôle
7	9,0	11,2	6,2	8,5	9,5	9,6	30	50	5,71	5,79	18	Groupe de contrôle
8	8,7	11,2	7,0	8,7	6,0	9,7	138	114	3	3,48	–	Groupe de contrôle
9	8,0	9,7	5,7	7,0	8,7	13,9	66,5	97	–	6,43	–	
10	7,6	13,7	5,7	9,8	9,5	13,8	64,8	85	–	6,8	38,6	
11	6,8	6,2	5,2	4,7	15,2	23,0	140	172	7,56	5,1	32,6	Groupe de contrôle
12	6,7	8,8	3,8	5,6	14,0	19,0	44,5	29	–	6,12	33,6	
13	6,2	11,1	5,3	9,6	15,5	22,5	78,7	92	–	5	30,5	
14	5,2	8,9	3,7	6,1	14,6	16,8	168	162	–	19,1	39	
15	4,2	9,6	2,7	7,6	11,3	12,5	89,5	83,8	7,78	9,72	17	
16	2,9	4,3	2,2	3,5	13,0	17,4				8,3	27,4	

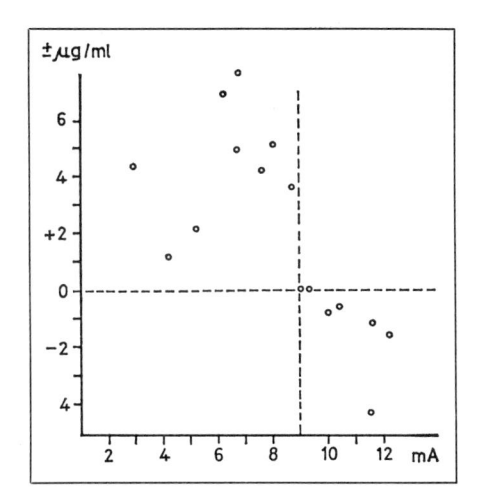

Figure 1. Valeur de repos de l'excitabilité du m. vaste interne du quadriceps pour 0,1 ms (abscisse) et modifications de la tyrosinémie après l'effort (ordonnée).

Le tableau présente les données obtenues, ordonnées d'après la valeur de l'excitabilité du vaste interne pour un stimulus de 0,1 milisec. Nous avons trouvé :

Une augmentation notable de la tyrosine du plasma chez tous les sujets pour lesquels la valeur de l'intensité du courant-seuil d'excitation pour 0,1 ms était *au repos*, inférieure à 9 mA;

une diminution de la tyrosinémie chez les sujets chez lesquels cette valeur dépassait nettement 9 mA;

chez 2 sujets, ayant la valeur de l'excitabilité de 9 et respectivement 9,3 mA, les modifications de la tyrosine étaient pratiquement nulles (figure 1).

On ne trouve pas de relation systématique de ces éléments avec la tyrosinurie. Une certaine relation directe peut être observée entre l'élimination sudorale de la tyrosine et sa concentration dans le plasma après l'effort, confirmant nos données antérieures [3] (figure 2).

Chez 15 des 16 sujets on trouve une diminution de l'excitabilité neuromusculaire (ENM) après l'effort (intensité-seuil pour 0,1 ms plus élevée de 0,9 à 6,5 mA). Il n'y a pas de corrélation systématique entre l'ampleur des variations de la tyrosinémie et celle de l'ENM. On peut seulement noter que le seul sujet dont l'ENM *augmente* après l'effort, présente la plus grande augmentation de la tyrosinémie, cependant que la plus nette diminution de l'ENM est rencontrée chez le sujet avec la plus importante chute de la tyrosine.

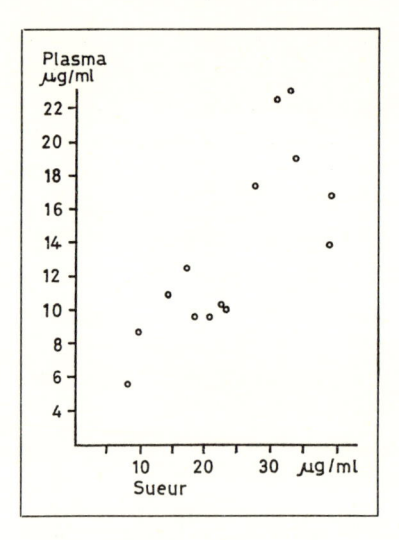

Figure 2. Elimination sudorale de la tyrosine en fonction de son niveau plasmatique après l'effort.

Discussion

Les modifications de la tyrosinémie après l'effort ne peuvent pas être simplement expliquées par l'hémoconcentration, ni par l'élimination urinaire ou sudorale. L'intervention de l'hémoconcentration ne rend d'ailleurs pas compte des relations entre la tyrosinémie d'effort et les valeurs *de repos* de l'excitabilité.

PARTHENIU [11] a montré, dans une étude portant sur plus de 400 sportifs que l'éxcitabilité moyenne du vaste interne, au repos, pour 0,1 ms est de 7,6 ± 1 mA. Les sujets avec hypérexcitabilité à ce niveau présentent, d'après cet auteur, des réactions de type hypersympathicotone, cependant que les sujets hypoexcitables ont diverses réactions d'hypervagotonie. On sait, par ailleurs, que la tyrosine est le principal précurseur métabolique de la synthèse des catécholamines dans divers tissus [6, 8, 9], ainsi que de la triiodothyronine; les deux types d'hormones sont directement intéressés dans l'adaptation ergotrope immédiate de l'organisme à l'effort.

Tenant compte de ces aspects on pourrait formuler une hypothèse de travail concernant la signification des faits trouvés. Lors de la sollicitation ergotrope déterminée par l'effort, accompagnée de l'augmentation de la formation d'hormones d'origine tyrosinique, le besoin accru en cet aminoacide déclenche peut-être sa mobilisation sous forme libre dans le sang; chez certains sujets, cette mobilisation serait, pour des considérents neuro-endocrins, moins efficace; ces sujets ont, au repos encore, une hyporéactivité du muscle phasique, «de vitesse»; chez eux, l'élimination de la tyrosine par la sueur, soit qu'elle reflète simplement le niveau sanguin, soit qu'il s'agit d'une réaction compensatrice à la perte sudorale, est basse.

La question d'une «consommation» exagérée de la tyrosine dans divers organes (foie, rein et peut-être muscle) peut encore se poser pour ces sujets. Ce serait aussi un aspect négatif, en relation avec le mauvais rendement sportif des sujets «hypoexcitables» pour l'instance étudiée.

Il ressort de certains travaux que les variations de la tyrosinémie pendant l'effort ne suivent pas nécessairement celles de l'azote aminé, ou des autres aminoacides [1, 5]. Cet aminoacide aurait ainsi un comportement propre, dépendant probablement de facteurs neuro-endocrins, non éllucidés.

Deux points résultant de nos observations doivent encore être soulignés:

La nécessité d'appliquer dans de telles recherches des méthodes de précision élevée, dépassant nettement celles qui sont couramment employées dans l'examen médico-sportif; il s'agit notamment ici des relations entre *microgrammes* de tyrosine et *microcoulombs* de courant pour le niveau de l'ENM;

la confirmation du comportement individuel – sur le plan des corrélations: excitabilité-métabolisme – des trois types de fibres musculaires squelettiques; il n'y a pas, en effet, de relation entre l'excitabilité des fibres «à temps longs» ou intermédiaires et les variations de la tyrosine; seules les fibres «rapides» du muscle phasique étudié sont intéressées.

Si l'on admet en principe qu'il y aurait un contrôle neuroendocrin de la libération de la tyrosine pour fournir le matériel de départ de la synthèse des hormones ergotropes, cet aspect est susceptible de développements ultérieurs utiles pour la physiologie de l'effort physique.

Bibliographie

1. CARLSTEN, A.; HALLGREN, B.; JAGENBURG, R.; SVANBORG, A. and WERKÖ, L.: Arterial concentrations of free fatty acids and free amino acids in healthy human individuals at rest and at different work loads. Scand. J. clin. Labor. Invest. *14:* 185 (1962).

2. CERIOTTI, S. et SPANDRIO, L.: Colorimetric determination of tyrosine. Biochem. J. *66:* 607 (1957).
3. HARALAMBIE, G.: L'élimination de la tyrosine pendant l'effort physique. Méd. éduc. phys. Sport *39:* 325 (1964).
4. HARALAMBIE, G.: Excitabilité neuro-musculaire et magnésiémie chez les sportifs. Int. Z. angew. Physiol. *25:* 181 (1968).
5. HARALAMBIE, G.; KEUL, J. and DOLL, E.: (to be published).
6. IYER, N. and MCGEER, P.: Conversion of tyrosine to catecholamines by rat brain slices. Canad. J. Biochem. *41:* 1565 (1963).
7. KEPPLER, D. and HOFFMANN, G.: Glucocorticoidwirkung auf freie Plasmaaminosäuren. Klin. Wschr. *46:* 106 (1968).
8. MATSUOKA, D. and ALCARAZ, A.: Biosynthesis of heart catecholamines. Arch. Int. Pharmacodyn. *159:* 144 (1966).
9. MEISTER, A.: Biochemistry of the Amino Acids, 2nd ed. vol. 2 (Academic Press, London/New York 1965).
10. PARTHENIU, AL.; HARALAMBIE, G. und CHIRIAC, D.: Beobachtungen über den biologischen Zustand der rumänischen Basketballspielerinnen vor Beginn der Europameisterschaften 1964. Sportarzt u. Sportmed. *18:* 161 (1967).
11. PARTHENIU, AL.: L'intervalle phasico-tonique de l'excitabilité neuro-musculaire. Observations chez les sportifs. Int. Z. angew. Physiol. *24:* 333 (1967).
12. ULMEANU, FL. C.; PARTHENIU, AL. et PETRESCU, N.: Etude sur la neurodynamique cérébrale, les caractéristiques de l'activité motrice, la dynamique circulatoire-respiratoire et le comportement sportif chez les gymnastes. Congr. Féd. Int. Gymnast.: p. 231, Zagreb (1957).
13. ULMEANU, FL. C.; PARTHENIU, AL.; HARALAMBIE, G. et MURESANU, I.: Influence de l'acide glutamique sur l'adaptation à l'effort 1er Congr. Européen Méd. Sport.: p. 491, Prague, 1963 (paru 1965).
14. ULMEANU, FL. C. et PARTHENIU, AL.: Actions de la tri-iodothyronine sur quelques effets aigus de l'effort physique chez les sportifs. XVI Weltkongress Sportmed. Hannover 1966: S. 478, Dtsch. Ärzte-Verlag, Köln-Berlin (1967).
15. ULMEANU, FL. C. et PARTHENIU, AL.: Asupra conditiilor de explorare a excitabilitatii neuromusculare in studiul adaptarii la efort. Fiziol. Norm. Patol. (Bucarest), *5:* 419 (1963).
16. ZIMMERMANN-TELSCHOW, H.; BETHGE, H.; HERLBERG, L. und ZIMMERMAN, H.: Untersuchungen am Menschen über die Veränderungen der Aminosäuren im Plasma im Verlauf des Insulin-Stress Testes. Klin. Wschr. *45:* 768 (1967).

Adresse des auteurs: Prof. Dr FL. C. ULMEANU, Dr AL. PARTHENIU and Dr G. HARALAMBIE, Laboratoire de Recherches de l'Institut de Culture Physique de Bucarest, Str. Maior Ene 12, *Bucarest* (Roumanie).

Influence of Increasing Activity on the Protein Level in Serum, Urine and Sweat

E. Delforge, B. Delforge and J. R. Poortmans

Laboratoire de l'Effort, Université Libre de Bruxelles, Bruxelles 5 (Director: Prof. M. Segers)

It is well known that strenuous exercise enhances the protein content in serum and urine (see p. 312), during and after activity. However, the importance of the registered modifications is different from one author to another. It was of some interest to appreciate the evolution of proteinemia and proteinuria for subsequent increase of local intensity in a same subject.

The present paper deals with the variation in the level of proteins in serum, urine and sweat, which occurs after exercise with increasing load.

Methods

Six male subjects (18–22 years) performed an exercise on a bicycle ergometer. After 15 min with a light load of 75 W per min, the intensity of the work was increased to 120 W per min and sustained during 15 min. On subsequent days, the same schedule was repeated, but with a rise in the last 15 min to 140 W, 160 W and 180 W per min, respectively.

Venous blood samples and urine collection were taken at rest, immediately after stopping the exercise and at the 30th min of the recuperation period. All subjects were dressed with a whole sweating suit and sweat was collected during the post-exercise period. Sweat was also obtained after a sauna bath.

Total proteins in serum was analysed by the biuret method [2], while the Amidoschwarz method [1] was used for the determination of proteins in urine and in sweat. The determination of lactic acid was performed with the UV test (Boehringer Test). Paper electrophoresis was performed on each serum and, after staining, the relative proportion of the protein fractions was recorded automatically.

Results

Table I shows that proteinemia and proteinuria are progressively increased as the work intensity is enhanced. This is well correlated with the

Table I. Variations in the level of proteins in serum, urine and sweat, before and after exercise. Relative percentage

	Rest	120 W per min Ex	120 W per min Rec	140 W per min Ex	140 W per min Rec	160 W per min Ex	160 W per min Rec	180 W per min Ex	180 W per min Rec
Lactic acid	100	200	67	340	81	410	98	1,000	148
Proteinemia	100	100	97	105	103	107	107	110	99
Proteinuria	100	156	204	185	81	261	206	547	385
Proteins in sweat	100	125		290		430		300	

Ex: samples collected immediately after stopping the exercise.
Rec: samples collected at the 30th min after stopping the exercise.

stepwise increase of lactic acid in blood. Moreover, the data also reveal that at 120 W of intensity, proteinemia is not modified, although proteinuria is already enhanced. At a heavy load (180 W) the relative variation of proteinemia amounts to 10%, while the excretion of proteins in urine has a 5-fold increase as compared to rest period. After the 30th min of recuperation, lactic acid in blood has returned to a level lower than that obtained at rest, except for the heavy load (180 W) for which the level of lactic acid remains higher than prior to exercise.

The elimination of proteins through the skin slowly rises according to the stepwise increase of work. However, the maximal data are recorded at 160 W, while protein secretion in sweat is reduced at 180 W as compared to the previous work intensity.

Paper electrophoresis of serum has not revealed any statistically valuable change in the protein distribution during and after exercise when related to rest conditions.

Discussion

The present investigation has shown that the changes of proteinemia and proteinuria observed on the same subject, after exercise, are intimately connected to work intensity. The increase of the level of proteins in serum is presumably to be related to the hemoconcentration phenomenon. However, one of us (see p. 312) has mentioned that the withdrawal of water from the plasma, during strenuous exercise, may not explain the whole concentration phenomenon in blood.

It is a common observation that strenuous exercise induces a heavy sweat secretion. This increased effectiveness of the sweating mechanism is generally associated with a decreased concentration of sodium and chloride in the sweat, which allows progressively better conservation of salt. Therefore, it is usually assumed that large quantities of sweat which are secreted by the sweat glands provide a rapid evaporative cooling of the body. Meanwhile, the present study emphazises that the protein concentration in sweat is not reduced by a dilution process of increasing water secretion. On the contrary, the level of total proteins in sweat expressed in terms of $\mu g/min$, is enhanced after exercise. Further investigations are to be undertaken to elucidate the precise mechanisms of this protein secretion through the skin.

Summary

The level of proteins in serum, urine and sweat has been analyzed on subjects who underwent four different exercises on bicycle ergometer with increasing load. The results have shown that there is a stepwise rise in the values of proteinemia, proteinuria and protein sweat secretion as the intensity of the exercise is increased.

References

1. HEREMANS, J. F.: La réaction de Donaggio. Ses fondements biochimiques et ses applications en pathologie. III. La réaction de Donaggio dans les urines. Rev. Belge Pathol. Méd. Expér. *26:* 264–311 (1958).
2. O'BRIEN, D. and IBBOTT, F. A.: Laboratory Manual of Pediatric. Micro- and Ultramicro-Biochemical Techniques; p. 260 (Harper and Row, Publ., 1962).

Author's address: E. DELFORGE, Laboratoire de l'Effort, Université Libre de Bruxelles, *Bruxelles 5* (Belgium).

The Proteins of Sweat[1]

J. Vanfraechem

Laboratoire de l'Effort, Université Libre de Bruxelles, Brussels

In a previous work [5] we have showed that sweat contains 17 plasmaproteins and non identified specific proteins.

These proteins are situated in 4 zones: albumin, a_2, β, γ and post-γ.

We intend to study the effect of calibrated efforts on an ergocycle, upon the separation of these zones.

Methods

Six subjects were submitted for 15 min to efforts of 120, 140, 160, 180 W/min. Sweat was collected in a sweating suit. The reference values were given by sweat obtained in sauna.

The content of total proteins was evaluated by the Hartmann-Fauvert method [2], and then after filtration, centrifugation and concentration by ultrafiltration under reduced pressure [1], the sweats were analysed by the high-voltage gel electrophoresis method of Wieme [6].

They were integrated on a vitatron, which gave us the relative percentage of each zone.

Each sweat was studied by immunoelectrophoresis with a A-WHS (Hyland goat). We evaluated then the level of the most important proteins (alb., Zna_2, β_{1s}, γG) by the radial immunodiffusion method [4]. We excluded from this study the important post-γ fraction for which we did not have the relevant anti-serums. The only one we had was an urinary anti-post-γ, which gave no positive identity reaction[1].

Results

1. The content of total proteins before concentration (table I), decreases at 120 W, when the sweat mechanism begins. From 140 W to

[1] The following abreviations have been used: alb. = albumin; Zna_2 = Zna_2-glycoproteins; β_{1s} = transferrin; γA = γA globulin; γG = γG globulin.

Table I. Total proteins of sweat in mg/min

Sujets	R	120 W	140 W	160 W	180 W
1	0.763	0.134	0.615	1.426	0.258
2	0.964	0.220	0.723	1.298	0.220
3	0.187	0.050	0.181	0.288	0.274
4	4.16	0.090	0.246	0.109	0.242
5	0.28	0.030	0.073	0.088	0.261
6	2.11	0.138	1.11	0.519	0.822

Table II. Mean concentrations of the electrophoretic fractions (mg/min)

	Prealb.	Alb.	a_2	β	γ	Post-γ
R	0.082	0.252	0.272	0.051	0.106	0.064
120 W	0.007	0.027	0.025	0.007	0.023	0.016
140 W	0.017	0.097	0.098	0.026	0.092	0.032
160 W	0.026	0.151	0.118	0.068	0.067	0.105
180 W	0.018	0.086	0.115	0.022	0.058	0.051

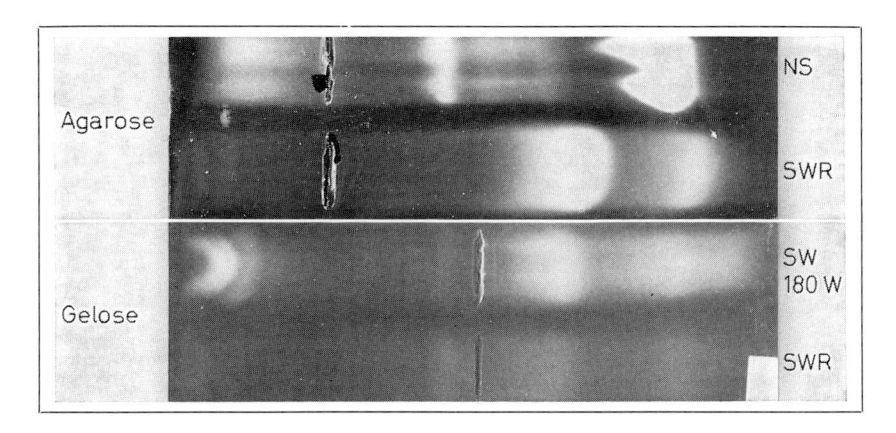

Figure 1. Electrophoreses on Agar Gel and on Agarose. NS = Normal serum; NSW R = Normal Sweat at Rest; SW 180 W = Normal Sweat at 180 W/min.

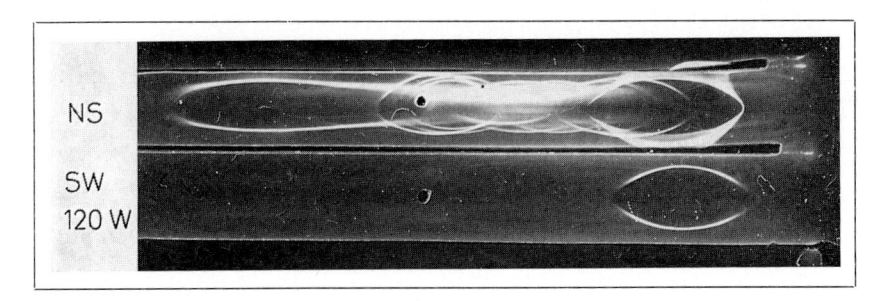

Figure 2. Immunoelectrophoresis. NS = normal serum; SW = Normal Sweat; A-WHS = Anti Whole Human Serum; 120 W = 120 W/min.

Table III. Individual proteins. Mean concentrations in mg/100 ml

	$Zn\alpha_2$	Alb.	γG	$\beta_1 S$
R	86.96	3.48	0.84	0.12
120	11.44	0.86	0.36	0.09
140	37.82	1.63	0.92	0.13
160	29.24	0.98	0.53	0.27
180	26.80	0.78	0.43	0.18

180 W/min we have individual variations, showing a different adaptation of the sweat mechanism at the different levels of effort.

2. Therefore we studied the variation of the electrophoretic zones at these efforts (fig. 1).

We can see that all the electrophoretic fractions decrease at 120 W/min and then increase until they reach a maximal value at 160 W/min, except for the γ-globulins, which reach their maximal value at 140 W/min (table II). The increase is particularly important for the post-γ and β levels which are higher than the reference values. At 180 W/min we have a decrease of all the fractions.

3. In the immunoelectrophoreses we do not see differences between the thermal and effort sweats, with regard to the plasma proteins (fig. 2).

4. We have also investigated the albumin and α_2 zones. In these zones, we only studied the plasma proteins which appeared distinctly in immunodiffusion. So the quantitative immunodiffusion is performed on the albumin, $Zn\alpha_2$, γG and β_{1s} (table III).

The concentration of $Zn\alpha_2$ is higher than the concentration of the other proteins we studied.

The concentrations of $Zn\alpha_2$ and Alb. are higher in the thermal sweats. They decrease at 120 W and reach higher values at 140 and 160 W/min like on the electrophoresis. γG and β_{1s} are present at very low concentration, and they vary little at the various efforts.

Discussion

For calibrated efforts on ergocycle: the level of total proteins is higher in the thermal sweats than in the effort sweats.

For a light effort (120 W/min) the level of total proteins as well as the level of each protein reaches low values.

These values increase at 140 and 160 W/min. At 180 W/min the 'fatigue sudorale' mechanism [3] seems to be responsible for a fast decrease of the protein excretion at strenuous efforts.

The electrophoreses show that the important zones are, the albumine, α_2 and post-γ zones.

In the albumine and α_2 fraction the most important plasma proteins are the albumin and $Zn\alpha_2$ proteins, γG and β_{1s} only appear in traces.

These proteins have a maximal concentration in the thermal sweats. The optimal value is reached at 140 and 160 W/min.

The level of $Zn\alpha_2$ in sweat is very high; this is confirmed by the result of the preparative electrophoresis which confirms that the α_2-zone is quite completely composed of $Zn\alpha_2$ protein.

Acknowledgements

We thank Dr. J. R. POORTMANS (Brussels) for his gift of specific antisera against albumin, Zn-α_2-glycoprotein, transferrin and γG-globulin, and Dr. C. LATERRE for his antiserum against urinary post-γ-globulin.

The author is endebted to B. and E. DELFORGE for their kind technical collaboration.

References

1. EVERALL, PH. and WRIGHT, GH.: Low pressure ultrafiltration of proteins containing fluids. J. Med. Lab. Technol. *15:* 209 (1958).
2. HARTMANN, L. et FAUVERT, P.: in Pasteur Valery Radot (Red.) – Les albuminuries, p. 41 (Masson, Paris 1954).

3. HOUDAS, Y.: Etude critique des méthodes de repérage de la contrainte thermique. Rev. des Corps de Santé *8, 6:* 854 (1967).
4. MANCINI, PH.; CARBONARA, O. A. and HEREMANS, J. F.: Immunochemical quantitation of antigens by single radial immunodiffusion, Immunochemistry *2:* 235 (1965).
5. VANFRAECHEM, J. et POORTMANS, J. R.: Protéines plasmatiques de la sueur humaine normale. Rev. franc. Et. clin. biol. *4, XIII:* 383 (1968).
6. WIEME, R. J.: Procédé simple d'identification des lignes de précipitation spécifiques dans l'immunoélectrophorèse. Bull. Soc. Chim. biol. *37:* 995 (1955).

Author's address: J. VANFRAECHEM, Laboratoire de l'Effort, Université Libre de Bruxelles, *Brussels* (Belgium).

Répercussions des activités physiques modérées sur le taux de la protéinurie intermittente des adolescents

A. Segers

Laboratoire de l'Effort, Université Libre de Bruxelles

Nous nous sommes proposés d'examiner les conséquences d'un effort modéré sur le taux de la protéinurie intermittente observée chez certains jeunes gens.

Nous avons notamment eu pour but de préciser les modifications quantitatives de cette protéinurie sous l'influence d'épreuves physiques imposées sur cycle-ergomètre ou bien encore lors d'activités de la vie courante telles que la natation, les séances de gymnastique scolaire, les cross-promenades et les après-midi sportives.

Notre groupe expérimental a été sélectionné de la façon suivante. Nous avons effectué, au cours de 3 après-midi différentes la recherche de la protéinurie au repos parmi les 250 jeunes gens de 12 à 18 ans d'une même école. Nous avons retenu 43 sujets qui au cours de ces 3 dépistages ont présenté au moins une fois un taux de protéinurie totale dépassant 0,1 g/l. Rappelons que Poortmans [1] et d'autres ont précisé que le taux moyen de la protéinurie des sujets normaux au repos est nettement plus bas, de l'ordre de 0,03 g/l: Le seuil au dessus duquel nous avons sélectionné nos sujets est certes arbitraire, mais il nous paraît difficile de procéder autrement tant que la protéinurie intermittente n'aura pas pu recevoir une meilleure définition.

Notre groupe correspond à 17% de la population totale de cette école, pourcentage nettement plus élevé que celui habituellement cité qui est de l'ordre de 5% des sujets [2].

Nous ne nous proposons pas de discuter ici les raisons de cette différence, mais soulignons toutefois que nous n'avons eu que 8 à 10% de cas positifs au cours de chaque série d'examens et que le taux de 17% est le résultat cumulatif de nos trois contrôles, 14 ont été positifs deux fois et 22 n'ont été positifs qu'une fois.

Nous avons tout d'abord examiné chez les sujets la fluctuation spontanée de leur taux de protéinurie au repos. En exprimant ce taux en g/l/min les valeurs mesurées se sont réparties de la façon suivante au cours de 106 contrôles effectués au repos (tableau I).

Tableau I. Taux de protéinurie (exprimé en g/l/min) l'après-midi au repos

Taux de protéinurie	% des cas
> 0,10	33%
de 0,01 à 0,10	54%
< 0,01	13%

Tableau II. Taux de protéinurie (exprimé en g/L/min) après effort modéré

Taux de protéinurie	% des cas
> 0,10	29%
de 0,01 à 0,10	54%
< 0,01	17%

Au cours de contrôles successifs effectués l'après-midi au repos, un même sujet passe au point de vue quantitatif d'une catégorie dans l'autre et la plupart se révèlent certains jours négatifs. C'est-à-dire que leur protéinurie se révèle fluctuante et intermittente.

Nous avons ensuite effectué les déterminations après séances de natation, de gymnastique scolaire, d'après-midi sportive ou après épreuve d'effort imposée sur cycle-ergomètre de 1,5 W/kg durant 15 min.

Après ces divers types d'effort modéré chez les sujets de ce groupe les taux de protéinurie totale se sont répartis de la façon suivante au cours de 35 contrôles (tableau II).

La comparaison des deux tableaux montre que l'effort modéré n'entraîne que des modifications peu importantes de la répartition des taux de protéinurie.

Nous avons examiné ces effets de l'effort modéré en les exprimant non plus de façon globale, mais en précisant pour chaque sujet dans quelle mesure sa protéinurie a présenté un taux différent avant et après l'effort. Nous avons classé nos résultats en considérant comme négligeables les modifications inférieures à 0,05 g/l/min. Dans ces conditions nous pouvons les exprimer par le tableau III.

Tableau III. Modification du taux de protéinurie après effort modéré par rapport à celui existant immédiatement avant, au repos

Modification	Nombre de cas
+	6
0	20
–	6

Ce tableau confirme que lorsqu'il existe une protéinurie intermittente au repos, son taux ne présente pas de modification systématique sous l'influence d'efforts modérés. Signalons cette particularité assez inattendue, à savoir que dans un cas l'activité physique a fait disparaître totalement une protéinurie de 0,05 g/l/min présente immédiatement avant l'effort.

Nous pouvons conclure de ces résultats que la protéinurie intermittente chez les jeunes gens ne subit dans l'ensemble pas d'aggravation par les activités physiques courantes. Nous pouvons même dire qu'il n'y a apparemment pas pour ces sujets de contre-indication à pratiquer les mêmes activités sportives que leurs camarades de classe.

Remerciements

Nous remercions vivement J. POORTMANS pour ses précieux conseils, Madame O. RUBIN pour son aimable aide technique, ainsi que la Direction de l'Ecole Ch. Janssens d'Ixelles qui nous a permis d'obtenir des sujets d'expérience.

Résumé

Le taux de la protéinurie intermittente observé chez les jeunes gens ne présente pas de modification appréciable sous l'influence d'une épreuve d'effort modérée. La pratique de la gymnastique et des activités sportives scolaires ne paraît donc pas contre-indiquée chez eux.

Summary

Intermittent proteinuria of young people does not present quantitative changes after moderate physical activity. The usual physical exercise does not seem to be avoided in such cases.

Bibliographie

1. POORTMANS, J.: La protéinurie physiologique au repos et à l'effort, Ann. Soc. roy. Sc. Méd. Nature, Bruxelles *17:* 89–188 (1964).
2. ROBINSON *et al.:* Orthostatic Proteinuria. Amer. J. Path. *39:* 11 (1961).

Adresse de l'auteur: Dr ANDRE SEGERS, Laboratoire de l'Effort, Université Libre de Bruxelles, *Bruxelles* (Belgique).

Protéinurie de fatigue: Détermination quantitative de certaines fractions protéiques[1]

G. DOMINICI, E. ROTTINI, U. MILIA et G. COZZOLINO

Istituto di semeiotica medica della Università di Perugia

Poursuivant les recherches sur la protéinurie due à la fatigue (les résultats préliminaires de ces recherches ont fait l'objet de publications récentes DOMINICI et al. [1, 2]), nous avons accompli une détermination immunologique quantitative de 6 plasmaprotéines sur les urines excrétées par 2 groupes d'athlètes avant et après une activité musculaire intense et prolongée, un match de football d'une durée de 90 min par exemple.

Les plasmaprotéines examinées sont les suivantes: albumine, céruloplasmine, transferrine, IgA, IgG et IgM. La méthode employée est l'immunodiffusion radial simple selon MANCINI, CARBONARA et HEREMANS [3]; la Behringwerke nous a fourni les relatifs Partigen.

Comme nous l'avons déjà signalé, nous avons considéré 2 groupes d'athlètes, le premier composé de 11 footballeurs amateurs de 16 à 18 ans, le second composé de 11 footballeurs professionnels âgés de 24 à 30 ans qui pratiquent ce sport sans interruption depuis au moins 8 ans.

On a recueilli aussi les urines des athlètes en conditions de repos durant les 24 h qui ont précédé le match de football.

Dans 10 des 22 échantillons ainsi obtenus, 5 appartenant au premier groupe (footballeurs amateurs) et 5 appartenant au second groupe (footballeurs professionnels), on a déterminé après concentration préalable le contenu dans les 6 plasmaprotéines dont les valeurs sont résumées dans le tableau I. En analysant ce tableau on peut émettre les considérations suivantes: la concentration en albumine, céruplasmine, transferrine, IgA et IgG ne présente pas de différences substancielles entre les échantillons du 1er groupe et ceux du 2e groupe; les différentes oscillations sont toutes comprises dans les limites de la norme, c'est-à-dire que les valeurs relevées pour chaque protéine s'accordent bien avec les valeurs normales données par la littérature; la concentration en IgM est inférieure à mg 0,02/1; l'albumine est la fraction protéique qui prévaut, vient ensuite la IgG.

---

[1] Travail publié avec la contribution de la Fédération Italienne de Médicine du Sport.

Tableau I. Concentration urinaire en albumine, céruloplasmine, transferrine, IgG, IgA, IgM (mg/l) en 10 athlètes en condition de repos

	Albumine	Cerulo plasmine	Trans-ferrine	IgG	IgA	IgM
1	10	0,02	0,14	3	0,06	– 0,02
2	18	0,09	0,20	4	0,10	– 0,02
3	12	0,05	0,16	4	0,08	– 0,02
4	9	0,03	0,10	2,4	0,05	– 0,02
5	9	0,08	0,20	5	0,06	– 0,02
6	7	0,04	0,10	2	0,05	– 0,02
7	13	0,06	0,18	3,4	0,10	– 0,02
8	9	0,04	0,15	3	0,04	– 0,02
9	20	0,1	0,24	2,2	0,12	– 0,02
10	12	0,06	0,16	3	0,08	– 0,02
Media	11,9	0,057	0,16	3,2	0,074	

La moyenne des concentrations urinaires (mg/l) permet de relever, pour les différentes plasmaprotéines examinées, les valeurs suivantes: albumine 11,9, céruloplasmine 0,057, transferrine 0,16, IgA 0,074 et IgG 3,2.

Nous avons ensuite recueilli les urines excrétées par 22 athlètes immédiatement après un match de football et selon la même méthode nous les avons examinées dans leur contenu dans les susdites 6 plasmaprotéines. Les concentrations des différentes fractions protéiques sont reportées dans les tableaux II et III.

Dans le tableau II on peut remarquer que les valeurs en albumine, céruloplasmine, transferrine, IgA et IgG des athlètes numéros 3 et 6 sont supérieures aux valeurs relevées chez les neuf autres athlètes de ce groupe. Il est bon de rappeler à ce propos que les deux athlètes avaient participé grippés au match (diagnostics à postérieurs).

Un premier examen, même approximatif, des tableaux II et III permet de formuler quelques considérations. Que ce soit dans son ensemble ou dans les différentes fractions protéiques examinées, la valeur de la protéinurie relevée dans les athlètes du premier groupe est sensiblement inférieure à celle des athlètes du second groupe; l'albumine demeure, même après effort, le composant le plus élevé de cette protéinurie, viennent ensuite la IgG et la transferrine; la concentration de la IgM est inférieure à mg 0,2/l chez tous les athlètes.

Dans le but de recueillir les informations les plus précises et significatives sur la marche et l'entité de la protéinurie on a élaboré en statis-

Tableau II. Escrétion urinaire de plasmaprotéines (mg/l) en des joueurs amateurs après un match de football de 90′. – Les athlètes ont l'âge de 16/18 ans. – Le n° 3 et 6 avaient de la fièvre (grippe)

	Albumine	Cerulo-plasmine	Trans-ferrine	IgA	IgG	IgM
1	126	0,4	16,6	0,18	20	– 0,2
2	182	0,6	12,5	0,20	25	– 0,2
3	336	1	22,7	0,34	48	– 0,2
4	140	0,6	15,6	0,16	22	– 0,2
5	164	0,5	14,2	0,20	24	– 0,2
6	362	1	25	0,32	50	– 0,2
7	175	0,6	12,8	0,20	24	– 0,2
8	190	0,5	14	0,18	20	– 0,2
9	124	0,3	12,6	0,15	19	– 0,2
10	148	0,3	13,5	0,16	21	– 0,2
11	138	0,4	12,8	0,14	20	– 0,2

Tableau III. Escrétion urinaire de plasmaprotéines (mg/l) en des joueurs professionnels après un match de football de 90′. – Les athlètes ont l'âge de 24/30 ans et pratiquent le sport depuis 8 années

	Albumine	Cerulo-plasmine	Trans-ferrine	IgA	IgG	IgM
1	260	0,9	18,6	0,30	42	– 0,2
2	234	0,8	18,2	0,28	36	– 0,2
3	252	0,9	20	0,30	38	– 0,2
4	210	0,7	16,4	0,26	34	– 0,2
5	196	0,6	16,2	0,24	32	– 0,2
6	224	0,8	17,8	0,28	34	– 0,2
7	240	0,8	18,2	0,30	36	– 0,2
8	274	0,9	21,4	0,32	42	– 0,2
9	312	1	22,6	0,38	46	– 0,2
10	238	0,8	19,4	0,30	36	– 0,2
11	360	1,1	26,8	0,38	46	– 0,2

tiques les données expérimentales acquises grâce à cette recherche et reportées dans les tableaux précédents.

Dans cette élaboration statistique on a mis surtout en évidence l'augmentation du contenu urinaire des plasmaprotéines examinées, con-

Tableau IV. Incrément moyen des plasmaprotéines urinaires (rapport entre la valeur moyenne après l'effort et la valeur moyenne normal)

	m/n Normal	m/n Amateurs	m/n Professionnels
Albumine	1	13,0 $\sigma_r = 0{,}05$	21,4 $\sigma_r = 0{,}06$
Ceruloplasmine	1	8,2 $\sigma_r = 0{,}08$	14,8 $\sigma_r = 0{,}05$
Transferrine	1	86,5 $\sigma_r = 0{,}03$	122,5 $\sigma_r = 0{,}05$
IgA	1	2,4 $\sigma_r = 0{,}04$	4,1 $\sigma_r = 0{,}04$
IgG	1	6,8 $\sigma_r = 0{,}03$	12,0 $\sigma_r = 0{,}04$

m = valeur moyenne après l'effort
n = valeur moyenne normal
σ_r = déviation standard relative

sidérant les différentes rapports (et par conséquent le rapport moyen) entre les valeurs des concentrations des diverses fractions protéiques dans chaque individu après l'effort et une valeur moyenne présumée «normale» obtenue en étudiant la concentration des protéines en question dans les urines excrétées par 10 athlètes à repos (5 amateurs et 5 professionnels). En outre, pour avoir un critérium de jugement sur la dispersion des mesures, on a préféré utiliser, plutôt que la déviation standard, la déviation standard relative, σ_r, rapport entre la déviation standard et sa valeur max théorique:

$$\sigma \max = \mu\sqrt{n-1}$$

et ceci parce que les différentes déviations standard simples sont très diverses les unes des autres et par conséquent (tout en restant un excellent indice de dispersion de l'échantillon) ne permettent pas d'établir des comparaisons entre un échantillon et un autre, lors que la déviation standard relative qui en un certain sens rapporte les déviations simples à la même unité de mesure les facilite.

Les résultats de l'évaluation statistique ainsi accompli sont illustrés dans le tableau IV et représentés dans la figure 1.

Le résultat le plus saillant après analyse du comportement des différentes fractions protéiques examinées est le suivant: l'augmentation

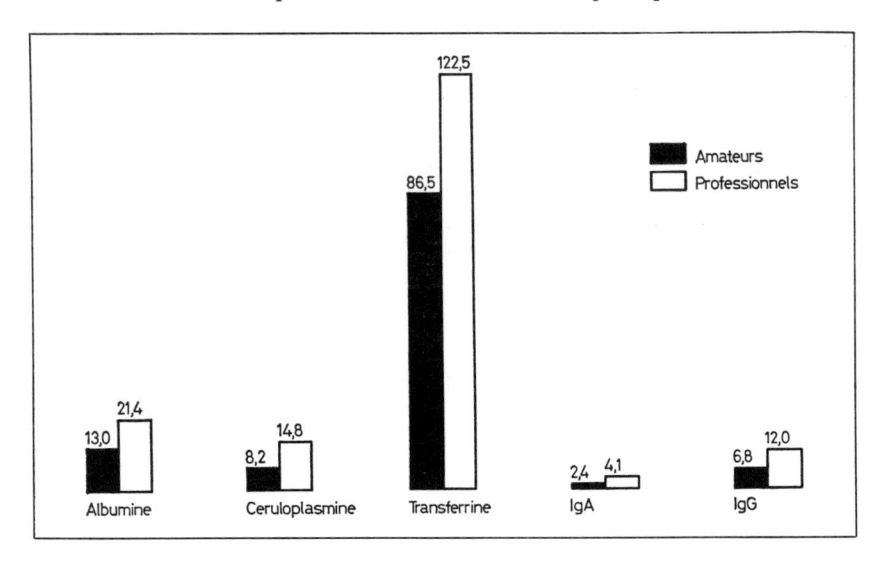

Figure 1. Rapport moyen de la concentration in plasma-proteinse urinaires après l'effort.

moyenne maximum, exprimée en tant que rapport entre la valeur moyenne après effort et la valeur moyenne normale est celui de la transferrine (86,5 chez les footballeurs amateurs et 122,5 chez les professionnels), viennent ensuite l'albumine (13 et 21,4), la céruloplasmine (8,2 et 14,8), la IgG (6,8 et 12) et enfin la IgA (2,4 et 4,1). Il n'a pas été possible d'analyser le comportement de la IgM ; en effet, la concentration urinaire de cette globuline n'a pas subi de modifications substancielles à la suite d'une activité sportive.

Sur la basc des résultats relevés dans cette expérience nous pouvons conclure que la concentration urinaire des plasma-protéines examinées ne varie pas proportionnellement à leur poids moléculaire.

En substance tout ceci est en accord avec ce que POORTMANS et JEANLOZ [4] ont relevé dans une intéressante étude à ce propos, en accord aussi avec ce que nous avons postulé dans une étude précédente.

Il semble qu'on puisse rapporter le déterminisme de la protéinurie due à la fatigue à une augmentation de la perméabilité glomérulaire et à une réabsorption tubulaire sélective.

Bibliographie

1. DOMINICI, G.; ROTTINI, E. e LATINI, P.: Presenza di albumina, transferrina e gamma G-globulina nelle urine di atleti affaticati. Boll. Soc. ital. Biol. sper. *XLIII:* 982–984 (1967).

2. Dominici, G.; Rottini, E.; Latini, P. e Pistolesi, S.: Rilievi sperimentali sulla proteinuria da fatica. Recenti Progr. Med. *XLIV:* 1–12 (1968).
3. Mancini, G.; Carbonara, A. O. and Heremans, J. F.: Immunochemical quantitation of antigens by single radial immunodiffusion. Immunochemistry *2:* 235 (1965).
4. Poortmans, J. and Jeanloz, R. W.: Quantitative immunological determination of 12 plasma proteins excreted in human urine collected before and after exercise. J. clin. Invest. *47:* 386 (1968).

Adresse des auteurs: Dr G. Dominici, Dr E. Rottini, Dr U. Milia et Dr G. Cozzolino, Istituto di Semeiotica Medica dell'Università di Perugia, *Perugia* (Italie).

Etude expérimentale sur le comportement des mucoprotéines dans les conditions de l'effort physique

C. Rotaru

Laboratoire de Physiologie, Institut de Médecine et de Pharmacie, Iassy

L'intérêt soulevé par les recherches sur les mucoprotéines est multilatéral. Quoique non spécifiques elles sont intéressées dans les phénomènes humoraux et artériosclérotiques; dans le domaine de l'effort physique et de la fatigue leur étude acquiert un intérêt tout particulier.

Les modifications dans la composition du sang et de l'urine comme répercution de la fatigue physique sont exposées par Tayeau [7] dans le tableau du syndrome humoral de la fatigue, et les investigations effectuées par Poortmans [1] élucident le mécanisme fonctionnel de la protéinurie au cours de l'effort musculaire.

Nos recherches antérieures nous ont démontré que dans les conditions de l'effort physique et dans l'état de fatigue il se produit une augmentation de la concentration sérique des mucoprotéines [4] à laquelle correspond une augmentation importante et constante de leur concentration dans le liquide cephalo-rachidien [3 b] ainsi que l'intensification de l'excrétion par l'urine [5, 3 a].

En tenant compte de nos résultats expérimentaux nous nous sommes proposé d'analyser certaines corrélations qui peuvent être établies entre l'évolution des composants protéiques séro-sanguins et urinaires au cours de l'effort physique comparativement à leur fond de repos, dans le but de discerner certains aspects qui pourraient élucider les considérations actuelles sur l'origine et l'évolution des mucoprotéines dans le cadre du syndrome humoral de la fatigue.

Méthode de recherches

Nos recherches ont été effectuées sur des lots de chiens, soumis à l'effort de la course sur bande roulante jusqu'à l'apparition de la fatigue.
Les déterminations faites au repos de même qu'à la cessation de l'effort ont eu en vue: le sang (récolté par ponction veineuse) dans lequel on a apprécié la protéinémie – microdosage par précipitation à l'amidoschwartz 10 B [J. Badin et B. Herve, 1965];

[1] Mme Rosca Valeria, chimiste, a collaboré pour les analyses.

Tableau I. La moyenne, la dispersion, la déviation standard, le coefficient de variation et l'intervalle de sûreté statistique des composants du sérum sanguin et de l'urine au repos et dans la fatigue

Serum sanguin

	Protéine totale g⁰/₀₀ repos	fatigue	Protéine préc. percl. g⁰/₀₀ repos	fatigue	Mucoprotéine g⁰/₀₀ repos	fatigue	Mucoprotéine/ protéine totale % repos	fatigue	Mucoprot. active Donaggio UD/ml repos	fatigue
$\overline{X}$	63,77	67,43	63,20	66,77	0,57	0,66	0,90	0,99	7,45	11,78
σ^2	18,07	34,28	8,00	34,21	0,0079	0,0079	0,0211	0,0239	2,57	6,04
σ	4,25	5,85	4,24	5,85	0,088	0,088	0,15	0,15	1,60	2,16
$\dfrac{\sigma \times 100}{\overline{X}}$	6,7%	8,7%	6,7%	8,8%	15,4%	13,3%	16,7%	15,2%	21,5%	18,3%
$\overline{X} \pm 2\sigma$	55,3–72,3	55,7–79,1	54,7–71,7	55,1–78,5	0,4–0,8	0,5–0,8	0,6–1,2	0,7–1,3	4,2–10,6	7,5–16,1
	F** r = 0,63		F** r = 0,63		F** r = 0,72		F**		F** r = 0,65	

la mucoprotéinémie (mucoprotéines totales) – précipitation à l'acide phosphoungstitque [A. Varay et M. Masson, 1960]; les mucoprotéines actives dans la réaction d'obstacle – dosage au bleu de méthylène B. Extra [J. Heremans, 1957]; fractionnement électrophorétique des protéines – sur papier filtre; l'urine (récolté par des fistules vésicales chroniques) dans laquelle on a apprécié la protéinurie – dosage à l'amidoschwartz 10 B (J.Heremans, 1958); les mucoprotéines actives Donaggio – responsables du phénomène d'obstacle – dosage au bleu de méthylène B. Extra [J. Heremans, 1958].

Les résultats analysés du point de vue statistique-mathématique sont présentés dans le tableau I.

On relève une augmentation en proportions variées de la valeur des protéines et des mucoprotéines dans la fatigue par rapport au repos, avec des différences fortement significatives tant dans le sang que dans les urines.

Discussions

Dans les conditions de l'effort physique nous constatons une augmentation de la concentration sérique des mucoprotéines totales et de celles actives (dans la réaction d'obstacle) qui est constante et avec des différences fortement significatives par rapport aux valeurs au repos; entre ces valeurs il existe une corrélation nette.

Ces aspects du comportement des mucoprotéines suggèrent l'idée d'une relation d'origine avec une substance fondamentale du tissu conjonctif. Dans ce sens nous remarquons que malgré une certaine correspondance avec l'augmentation des protéines (totales et de celles précipitées par l'amidoschwartz), le poids spécifique des mucoprotéines relevé par le rapport mucoprotéines/protéines totales %, bien qu'augmenté dans l'effort physique n'est pas significatif.

Donc: les mucoprotéines du sérum sanguin, dans l'effort physique, peuvent être considérées de manière indépendante comme une expression du rapport avec le métabolisme de la substance fondamentale et de la correlation avec les influences endocrino-humorales, présentes dans le syndrome humoral de la fatigue.

L'analyse des électrophorégrammes relève, à la cessation de l'effort physique, des modifications, tant des valeurs pour-cent que de celles absolues des fractions électrophorétiques, de manière constante – dans le sens d'une augmentation – des concentrations pour le groupe de globulines alfa.

Concomitamment aux concentrations élevées des mucoprotéines actives dans la réaction d'obstacle elles évoluent dans le même sens et ce mode de comportement met en évidence une corrélation étroite.

Des équations et des lignes de régression qui expriment la loi de l'augmentation des mucoprotéines par rapport au niveau des globulines

Urine

	Protéine Conc. mg/ml repos	fatigue	Excr. mg/min repos	fatigue	Excr. mg/24 h repos	fatigue
$\overline{x}$	0,038	1,88	0,011	0,516	16,1	746,4
σ^2	0,000089	0,5328	0,000016	0,0626	34,6	131,846
σ	0,009	0,73	0,004	0,25	5,88	363
$\dfrac{\sigma \times 100}{\overline{x}}$	23,7%	38,8%	30,4%	48,4%	36,4%	48,6%
$\overline{x} \pm 2\sigma$	0,02–0,06	0,42–2,34	0,003–0,019	0,016–1,016	4,38–27,90	401–1127
	F**		F** r = 0,82		F**	

alfa se détache la constatation que le niveau de leur augmentation dans les conditions de repos est plus accentué par rapport aux globulines alfa 2, tandis qu'après l'effort il est plus accentué par rapport aux globulines alfa 1.

La relation constatée se base aussi sur les faits suivants, dans les conditions du même mode expérimental:

Par des saignements abondants et répété chez le lapin, TAYEAU [7] réalise une augmentation de l'élimination de mucoprotéines actives dans la réaction d'obstacle comme résultat de l'augmentation de leur concentration dans le sang. RASCANU et al. [2], en étudiant les variations des constantes physico-chimiques du sang pendant le collapsus hémoragique et la réanimation chez le chien, constate une augmentation marquée du pourcentage d'alfa globulines après le saignement, en particulier des alfa 2 globulines.

La corrélation étroite dans l'évolution des deux composants sanguins étudiés dans les conditions d'un organisme soumis à l'effort physique poursuivi jusqu'à la fatigue peut faire supposer ou bien que cette double évolution est l'expression du même phénomène complexe – la fatigue physique – ou que l'évolution de chaque composant sanguin exprime un aspect séparé du phénomène (intensité de l'effort musculaire, et degré de la fatigue).

Par des explorations fonctionnelles effectuées antérieurement [6] chez des sportifs soumis à l'effort physique dosé au cycloergomètre nous avons relevé l'existence d'une forte corrélation entre l'intensité de la dépense énergétique et de la consommation d'oxygène d'une part, et l'évolution des alfa globulines d'autre part, ces dernières apparaissant comme un indicateur de l'intensité de l'effort déposé, tandis que la majorité des auteurs considèrent la mucoprotéinurie comme l'expression de l'installation du phénomène de fatigue.

dans les conditions de l'effort physique

Mucoprotéine active Donaggio						Diurèse	
Conc. UD/ml		Excr. UD/min		Excr. UD/24 h		ml/min	
repos	fatigue	repos	fatigue	repos	fatigue	repos	fatigue
1,48	6,93	0,45	1,88	6,38	2748	0,293	0,266
0,12	2,96	0,0284	0,47	4,9694	9818,734	0,003844	0,002777
0,34	1,72	0,17	0,69	223	1044	0,062	0,053
23,0%	24,8%	37,8%	36,7%	35,0%	38,0%	21,2%	20,0%
0,80–2,16	3,49–10,87	0,11–0,79	0,50–3,26	192–1084	660–4836	0,17–0,42	0,16–0,37
F**		F**		F**		F**	
		r = 0,86					

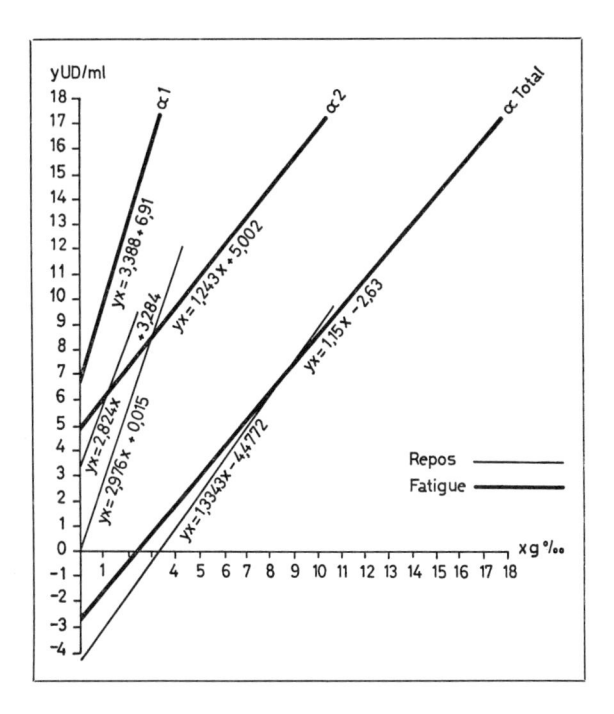

Figure 1. Les lignes et les equations de régression des valeurs des mucoprotéines actives dans la réaction d'obstacle en fonction des valeurs des alfa globulines.

En considérant parallèlement les composants étudiés, d'une part dans le sang et d'autre part dans les urines, il résulte qu'il n'est permis de mettre en évidence aucune corrélation, tant dans l'état de repos que dans l'effort physique, de même qu'on ne peut établir une corrélation entre les différences d'augmentation du repos à l'effort.

L'explication du mécanisme d'une intensification de la concentration en mucoprotéines dans les urines est discutable. On peut considérer que les mucoprotéines, présentes en quantité habituelle dans le sang, peuvent passer en abondance dans les urines par suite d'une perméabilité rénale augmentée, ou bien par suite d'une concentration excessive dans le sang.

En analysant nos résultats on peut remarquer une forte corrélation entre les valeurs, au repos ou à la fatigue, des protéines et des mucoprotéines, ainsi que l'existence d'une parallélisme avec leur évolution dans les urines quand on prend en considération l'excrétion/min. On constate en même temps qu'entre les différences du repos à la fatigue des protéines et des mucoprotéines il existe une très forte corrélation.

Ces constatations viennent étayer la supposition que la perméabilité rénale intervient de manière efficace au cours de la fatigue pour établir le niveau de la concentration de ces substances dans les urines, ce qui est important car cette perméabilité peut intervenir de manière isolée ou en association avec l'augmentation de la concentration de protéines et de mucoprotéines sanguines.

Résumé

Les déterminations ont été effectuées sur des lots de chiens. Dans la fatigue on a constaté une augmentation de la concentration sérique des mucoprotéines qui évolue dans le même sens que les fractions globuliniques du groupe alfa. Le poids spécifique des mucoprotéines dans les protéines totales, bien qu'augmenté, n'est pas significatif, ce qui fait que la mucoprotéinémie peut être considérée de manière indépendente, comme l'expression du rapport avec le métabolisme de la substance fondamentale. Dans les urines l'augmentation de mucoprotéines suit une évolution parallèle dans le cadre de la protéinurie. L'analyse comparative des composants sanguins et urinaires ne met en évidence aucune corrélation, ce qui justifie la participation des phénomènes rénaux dans l'intensification de la mucoprotéinurie dans la fatigue.

Bibliographie

1. POORTMANS, J.: La protéinurie physiologique au repos et à l'effort. Ann. Soc. Roy. Sci. Méd. Nat. *17:* 89–188 (1964).

2. Rascanu, V.; Dorogan, D.; Rotaru, C.; Stefan, I. et Dragan, P.: Variations des constantes physico-chimiques du sang au cours du collaps hemorragique experimental. Stud. Cercet. St. Med. Iassy *2:* 265–272 (1962).
3. Rotaru, C.: L'étude de l'origine de la mucoprotéinurie au cours de la fatigue. Rev. méd. chir., Iassy *1:* 173–179 (1968a) – L'évolution des mucoprotéines dans liquide cephalo-rachidien au cours de la fatigue. *2:* 540–552 (1968b).
4. Rotaru, C.; Pruteanu, P. et Rosca, V.: Le rapport entre les protéines et les mucoprotéines du sérum sanguin dans la fatigue. Rev. méd. chir. Iassy *4:* 1007–1013 (1966).
5. Rotaru, C. et Rosca, V.: La relation entre la protéinurie et la mucoprotéinurie dans la fatigue. Rev. méd. chir. Iassy *1:* 163–170 (1967).
6. Rotaru, C. et Stefan, I.: L'étude électrophorétique dans la fatigue. Rev. méd. chir. Iassy *1:* 91–98 (1959).
7. Tayeau, F.: Le syndrome humoral de la fatigue. Exp. Ann. Bioch. Méd. *16:* 215–250 (1954).

Adresse de l'auteur: Dr Constantin Rotaru, Strada 23 August nr. 40, Bloc B2 ap. 38, *Iasi* (România).

Subject Index

Acid-Base, balance, 15, 52
–, equilibrium, 47
–, imbalance, 2
a_1-acid-glycoprotein, serum, 312
–, urine, 319
– –, intermittent proteinuria, 340
Adrenalin, urinary excretion, 170, 202
– –, hypoxia, 190
Adenosine triphosphate, activity in muscle, 249
–, production, 42
β-adrenolytic drug, effect on swimming, 163
Adrenosympathic activation, non esterified fatty acid metabolism, 209
Aerobic work capacity, 2
–, urinary excretion of catecholamines, 202
Agar gel electrophoresis, urine, 320
–, sweat, 322, 356
Agarose gel electrophoresis, urine, 333
–, sweat, 356
Albumin, serum, 78, 314, 329
–, sweat, 356
–, thyroxine-binding, serum, 182
–, urine, 319, 365
– –, intermittent proteinuria, 340
– –, twins, 333
Aldolase, 225
–, diminished atmospheric pressure, 268
–, muscle, 249
–, serum, 280
Alveolar-arterial PO_2 difference, 4
Alveolar carbon dioxide, 47
Alveolar oxygen pressure, 7
Amino acids, serum, 316
Ammonia, biological fluids, 284
–, serum, 316
Amylase, serum, 274
Anaerobic capacity, urinary excretion of catecholamines, 202

Anterior pituitary hormones, effect on knee ligaments, 192
Antidiuretic hormone, serum, 323
a_1-antitrypsin, serum, 314
–, urine, 319
Arterial-coronarvenous difference, O_2, 36
Arterial-femoralvenous difference, β-hydroxybutyrate, 41
–, free fatty acids, 41
–, glucose, 41
–, lactate, 41
Arterial free fatty acids, 132
Arterial glucose, 132
Arterial hematocrit, 81
Arterial lactate, 3, 15, 81, 132
Arterial PCO_2, 53, 71, 81
Arterial pH, 81
Arterial PO_2, 2, 81
Arterial pyruvate, 15, 81, 132
Arterial-venous difference, O_2, 4, 68
–, pH, 70

Base excess, blood, 55, 71, 78
Bicarbonate, plasma, 55, 71, 90
Blood, cholesterol, 96, 148
–, coagulation, 316
–, coronarvenous, PCO_2, 35
– –, pH, 35
– –, PO_2, 35
–, eosinophils, 73
–, femoralvenous, PCO_2, 35
– –, pH, 35
– –, PO_2, 35
–, gas tensions, 66
–, glucose, 144, 274
–, hematocrit, 152, 274, 314
–, lactate, 62, 78, 89, 96, 152
–, non esterified fatty acids, 96, 274
–, PCO_2, 78
–, pH, 78, 90
–, pyruvate, 78, 90, 96

Subject Index

Body water, 159
Brachial artery, pH, lactate, 66
Brachial vein, pH, 66

Calcium, biological fluids, 284
–, serum, 301
Cardiac output, maximal exercise, 66
Catecholamines, urinary excretion, 170, 202
Ceruloplasmin, urine, 319, 366
Chloride, biological fluids, 284
Cholesterol, muscle, 116
–, plasma, 96, 102, 148
– –, children, 152
Chylomicrons, plasma, 102
Citrulline, sweat, 294
Competition, turnover of sympathicoadrenal hormones, 205
Coronarvenous blood, PCO_2, pH, PO_2, 35
Creatine phosphokinase, 217, 249, 259, 280
Cytochrome C oxidase, 217
Diet, effect on performance, 297
Diminished atmospheric pressure, enzymes, 268
2,4-dinitrophenol, effect on oxidation of free fatty acids, 128
Donaggio substances, 299, 323, 372
Dopamine, urinary excretion, 202

Electrolytes, biological fluids, 284
–, serum, 73, 284, 301
–, sweat, 284, 294
Enzymes, heart, 254
–, liver, 245, 254
–, muscle, 245, 254, 268
–, plasma, 216, 254, 259, 268, 274, 280, 301
Eosinophils, 73
Epinephrine, see adrenalin
Excess lactate, 30
Exercise training, metabolism of glucose 122
–, metabolism of free fatty acids, 122

Fat content, heart, 137
–, skeletal muscle, 137
Femoral vein, blood gas tensions, pH, 66
Femoral venous blood, PCO_2, pH, PO_2, 35

Free fatty acids, arterial-femoralvenous difference, 41
–, metabolism, 100, 122
–, oxidation by skeletal muscle, 128
–, plasma, 96, 100, 274

Gas exchange, 2
Gel filtration, urine, 319
Glucose, arterial, 132
–, arterial-femoralvenous difference, 41
–, regulation, 114
–, serum, 96
–, skeletal muscle, 122
–, synovial fluid, 156
–, urine, 299
Glucose-6-phosphatase, muscle and liver, 245
Glucose-6-phosphate, muscle and liver, 245
Glucose-6-phosphate dehydrogenase, muscle and liver, 245
–, serum, 280
Globulin, thyroxine-binding, serum, 182
a_2-Gc-globulin, urine, 319
γA-globulin, serum, 314
–, urine, 312, 365
– –, intermittent proteinuria, 340
γD-globulin, urine, 319
γG-globulin, serum, 314
–, sweat, 356
–, urine, 317, 365
– –, intermittent proteinuria, 340
$3S\gamma_1$-globulin, urine, 319
γM-globulin, serum, 314
–, urine, 319
post-γ-globulin, sweat, 322, 356
Glutamate dehydrogenase, 221
Glutamate oxaloacetate transaminase, serum, 225, 249, 259, 268, 301
Glutamate pyruvate transaminase, serum, 226, 249, 259, 268
Glyceraldehyde phosphate dehydrogenase, 220
Glycogen, diaphragm and heart, 163
–, metabolism, 245
–, skeletal muscle, 107, 122, 159
Glycoprotein, serum, 312, 328, 343, 371
–, urine, 371
Glycoprotein, a_1-acid, serum, 314
– –, urine, 319
– – –, intermittent proteinuria, 340

Subject Index

a_2HS-glycoprotein, urine, 319
--, intermittent proteinuria, 340
Zn-a_2-glycoprotein, sweat, 356
--, urine, 319
--, intermittent proteinuria, 340
β_2-glycoprotein I, urine, 319

Haptoglobin, urine, 319
Heart, enzyme level, 268
--, fat content, 137
--, lactic dehydrogenase, 254
--, lipoproteinase activity, 137
--, oxidative metabolism, 41
--, necrosis, muscular activity, 137
--, triglycerides, 109
Hematocrit, 274, 314
--, arterial blood, 81
Hemoglobin, 328
Hemopexin, urine, 319
Hexokinase, muscle and liver, 245
Hexosamines, urine, 299
Homovanillic acid, urine, 202
β-hydroxybutyrate, arterial-femoralvenous difference, 41
Hydroxymethoxymandelic acid, serum, 189, 205
Hyperoxia, 9
Hypoxia, 9, 52
--, heart, 41
--, PCO_2, pH, PO_2, 35
--, skeletal muscle, 41
--, sympathoadrenal response, 188

Immunoelectrophoresis, quantitative, 318
--, sweat, 356
--, urine, 317
Immunoglobulins, serum, 314
--, sweat, 356
--, urine, 319, 340, 365
Insulin, secretion, 199
--, clearance, 115
Intermittent proteinuria, 340, 361
Interstitial cell-stimulating hormone, 192
Iron, biological fluids, 284

Kallikrein, effect on proteinuria, 324
17-OH-Ketosteroids, 73
Knee joint, glucose, 156
Knee ligaments, influence of anterior pituitary hormones, 192

Lactate, arterial, 15, 55, 62, 71, 81, 89, 132

--, arterio-femoralvenous difference, 41
--, skeletal muscle, 62, 122
--, venous, 73, 96, 153, 353
Lactic dehydrogenases, 225, 280
--, isoenzymes, serum, 254, 259
--, tissues, 254
--, muscle, 249
Lean body mass, 140, 153
Lipids, metabolism, 100
--, serum, 329
--, skeletal muscle, 116
Lipoproteinase activity, heart and skeletal muscle, 137
Lipoproteins, plasma, 101
Liver, enzyme level, 268
--, lactic dehydrogenases 254
Low oxygen tension, acid-base balance, 52

Magnesium, biological fluids, 284
Malic dehydrogenase, 225, 280
Metabolism, lipids, 100
--, oxidative, heart, 41
--, muscle, free fatty acids, 103, 122, 128
--, glucose, 15, 122
--, lipids, 100, 116
3-methoxy-4-hydroxy-mandelic acid, urine, 190, 205
Muscle, enzyme activity, 249
--, diminished atmospheric pressure, 268
--, fat content, 137
--, free fatty acids, 103, 122, 128
--, glucose, 122
--, glycogen, 159, 245
--, lactate, 62, 122
--, lactic dehydrogenase isoenzymes, 254
--, lipoproteinase activity, 137
--, mitochondria, 239
--, oxidation of free fatty acids, 128
--, pyruvate, 122
--, subcellular fraction, lipids, 119
--, triglycerides, 103
Mucoproteins, serum, 371
--, urine, 299, 371

Nicotinamide adenine dinucleotide, dehydrogenase, 224
--, cytochrome C reductase, 224
Non esterified fatty acids, see free fatty acids
Noradrenalin, urine, 170, 188, 202

Subject Index

Norepinephrine, see noradrenalin
Normoxia, acid-base balance, 2, 54
–, adrenalin and noradrenalin, 188

Oxidative metabolism, heart, 41
Oxygen, consumption, 2
–, debt, 62
–, supply, heart and skeletal muscle, 36

H^3 palmitic acid, skeletal muscle, 122
Paper electrophoresis, serum, 314, 343
–, urine, 333
PCO_2, arterial, 55, 81
–, coronarvenous and femoralvenous blood, 35
–, venous, 78
Pentoses, urine, 299
pH, arterial, 81, 90
–, coronarvenous and femoralvenous blood, 35
–, venous, 78
Phosphate, biological fluids, 284
Phosphatidyl choline, muscle, 116
Phosphofructokinase, 222
Phosphoglucomutase, 246
Phosphohexoisomerase, 268
Phospholipid, muscle, 116
Phosphorylase, 222
–, muscle and liver, 246
Pilocarpine, effect on sweat secretion, 294
Plasma volume, 159
PO_2, arterial, 81
–, coronarvenous and femoralvenous blood, 35
Potassium, biological fluids, 284
–, effect on performance, 297
–, serum, 301
Prealbumin, thyroxine-binding, serum, 182
–, tryptophan-rich, urine, 319
Prediction of performance, hematological indicators, 73
Proteins, biological fluids, 312
–, perchlorosoluble, 314, 372
–, plasma, renal clearance, 321
–, polarographic pattern, 343
–, serum, 78, 314, 328, 353, 372
–, sulfosalicylic-soluble, 343
–, sweat, 322, 353, 356
–, thermosoluble, 314, 372
–, urine, 316, 340, 353, 362, 365, 372

––, monozygotic and dizygotic twins, 333
Pulmonary diffusion capacity, 4
Pyruvate, arterial, 15, 81, 90, 132
–, venous, 78, 96
–, skeletal muscle, 122

Renal clearance, plasma proteins, 321
Renin, effect on proteinuria, 324

Seromucoids, serum, 328
Serum, carbohydrates, 96, 114, 328
–, electrolytes, 73, 284, 301
–, electrophoretic patterns, 314, 343
–, enzymes, 226, 249, 254, 259, 268, 274, 280
–, hormones, 114, 323
–, immunoelectrophoretic patterns, 314
–, lipids, 96, 100, 148, 329
–, proteins, 78, 182, 312, 328, 343, 353, 371
–, tyrosine, 347
Sialic acid, serum, 328
Sodium, biological fluids, 284
–, serum, 301
Stress indicators, 73
Succinate oxidase, 224
Sweat, electrolytes, urea and citrulline, 294
–, electrophoretic patterns, 322, 356
–, immunoelectrophoretic patterns, 322
–, protein content, 322, 353, 356
–, tyrosine, 347
Swimming, muscle glycogen, 163
–, test in rats, 297
Sympatho-adrenal activity, 170
–, normoxia and hypoxia, 188
–, turnover in sportsmen, 205
Synovial fluid, glucose, 156

Testosterone, effect on knee ligaments, 192
Thyroid-stimulating hormone, effect on knee ligaments, 192
Thyroxine, free, serum, 182
Thyroxine-binding albumin, serum, 182
Thyroxine-binding globulin, serum, 182
Thyroxine-binding prealbumin, serum, 182
Training, blood cholesterol, 148
–, enzyme level, 349

–, muscle lipids, 116
–, turnover of sympathico-adrenal hormones, 205
Transferrin, serum, 314
–, sweat, 356
–, urine, 319, 365
– –, intermittent proteinuria, 340
Triglycerides, plasma, 101
–, tissues, 103, 116
Tryptophan-rich prealbumin, urine, 319
Twins, proteinuria, 333
Tyrosine, biological fluids, 347

Urea, serum, 316, 328
–, sweat, 294

Uridine diphosphoglucose, glycogen synthethase, 246
–, pyrophosphorylase, 246
Urine, carbohydrates, 299
–, catecholamines, 170, 189, 202
–, electrolytes, 284
–, electrophoretic patterns, 320, 333
–, immunoelectrophoretic patterns, 317
–, protein excretion, 299, 316, 333, 340, 353, 362, 365, 371
–, tyrosine, 347

Vanilmandelic acid, urine, 202

Zn-α_2-glycoprotein, sweat, 356
–, urine, 319, 340

Author Index

AGNEVIK, G. 62
ALESSANDRO, G. D' 96, 280
BABIN, J.P. 284
BADJOU, R. 259
BANISTER, E.W. 52
BECKER, E.J. 188
BLOCK, P. 259
BÖHMER, D. 249
BRUNNENGRABER, H. 14
BULA, B. 268, 271
CIAMPOLINI, E. 274
COBB, L.A. 116, 122
CONARD, V. 114
COZZOLINO, G. 365
CURETON, T. 73
DE COSTER, A. 15
DEGRÉ, S. 15
DELFORGE, B. 353
DELFORGE, E. 353
DE NAYER, PH. 182
DENOLIN, H. 15
DE SCHAEPDRIJVER, A. 114, 202
DE VISSCHER, M. 182
DIAMANT, B. 62
DOLEŽEL, J. 148, 152
DOLL, E. 35, 41, 132
DOMINICI, G. 365
DRINGOLI, R. 209, 274
EULER, U.S. v. 170
FRANCKSON, J.R.M. 114
FRÖBERG, S.O. 100
GEROLA, A. 209
GOLLNICK, P.D. 239
HARALAMBIE, G. 328, 347
HARTLEY, L.H. 62
HEBBELINCK, M. 202
HOLLMANN, W. 81
JEFLEA, G. 328
JIRKA, Z. 152
JONGERS, J. S' 340
KARLSSON, J. 62

KASTNER, K. 81
KEPPLER, D. 132
KERSTING, U. 144
KEUL, J. 35, 41, 132
KING, D.W. 239
KLAUS, E.J. 144
KOPECKÁ, J. 294
KOSIEK, J.-P. 144
KRÁL, J.A. 294
KREUZER, F. 188
KÜSTERS, F. 144
LEONE, D. 297
LILJEFORS, I. 333
LUKASIK, S. 268, 271
MALAISSE, W.J. 199
MALOMSOKI, J. 343
MARMO, E. 163
MATERA, A. 163
MERGNER, W. 192
MESSIN, R. 15
METIVIER, G. 301
MILIA, U. 365
MITOLO, M. 297
MOERMANS, E. 114
MORGAN, T.E. 116, 122
MOSKWA, J. 156
NOVOSADOVÁ, J. 254
NOWACKI, P. 205
OLSSON, K.E. 159
ORSUCCI, P.L. 209, 274
OSTIJN, M. 182
PAŘIZKOVÁ, J. 137
PARTHENIU, AL. 347
PIOVANO, G. 96
PISCATOR, M. 333
POORTMANS, J.R. 312, 340, 353
RAVAIOLI, P. 209, 274
RISINGER, C. 333
ROTARU, C. 371
ROTTINI, E. 365
ROUGIER, G. 284

Author Index

Saltin, B. 62, 66, 159
Sandage, D.S. 192
Scherrer, M. 2
Schmid, E. 205
Schmidt, E. 216
Schmidt, F.W. 216
Segers, A. 340, 361
Segers, M. 340
Shephard, R.J. 47
Short, F.A. 116, 122
Spitzer, J.J. 128
Tipton, C.M. 192

Topi, G.C. 96, 280
Ulmeanu, Fl. 347
Vandermoten, P. 15
Vanfraechem, J. 356
Van Melsem, A.Y. 259
Van Eijmenant, M. 259
Vanroux, R. 89, 114
Vogeleer, R. 259
Weist, F. 205
Wright, P.H. 199
Yakovlev, N.N. 245
Ženíšek, A. 294

Medicine and Sport, Vol. 4 (in preparation)

Physical Activity and Aging

With Special Reference to the Effect of Exercise and Training on the Natural History of Arteriosclerotic Heart Disease
Edited by D. BRUNNER, Jaffa, and E. JOKL, Lexington, Ky.
Ca. 200 p., 88 fig., 69 tab., 1969

Contents

I. Physiology of Exercise
II. Physiology of Aging
III. Biochemical Studies
IV. Functional Analyses of Cardiovascular Performance of Coronary Patients
V. Electrocardiography
VI. Experimental and Descriptive Pathology
VII. Epidemiology
VIII. Miscellaneous

This volume contains the proceedings of the First International Symposium on 'Physical Activity and Aging', held at the College of Medicine, University of Tel Aviv, Israel, under the auspices of the International Council of Sport and Physical Education of Unesco. The symposium in which many of the world's leading authorities on applied physiology of exercise, clinical cardiology, epidemiology, and pathology participated led to a clarification of the implications of the aging process in respect of the decline of form, the decline of function, and the decline of health, traditionally assumed to be characteristic of aging. Among the few known modifiers of all three of the above mentioned categories of aging, exercise occupies a place of special relevance. The evidence presented at the Tel Aviv seminar leaves no doubt that the decline of form, the decline of function, as well as at least certain facets of the decline of health, can be slowed down and at times even inhibited. More particularly, the natural history of the ischemic heart diseases is significantly influenced by sustained physical activity.

S. Karger Basel (Switzerland) New York

RC1200
I54
1968